WORKSHOP ON

DISABILITY IN AMERICA

A NEW LOOK

Summary and Background Papers

Based on a Workshop of the Committee on Disability in America:
A New Look

Board on Health Sciences Policy

Marilyn J. Field, Alan M. Jette, and Linda Martin, editors

INSTITUTE OF MEDICINE
OF THE NATIONAL ACADEMIES

THE NATIONAL ACADEMIES PRESS
Washington, D.C.
www.nap.edu

THE NATIONAL ACADEMIES PRESS • 500 FIFTH STREET, N.W. • Washington, DC 20001

NOTICE: The project that is the subject of this report was approved by the Governing Board of the National Research Council, whose members are drawn from the councils of the National Academy of Sciences, the National Academy of Engineering, and the Institute of Medicine. The members of the committee responsible for the report were chosen for their special competences and with regard for appropriate balance.

This study was supported by Contract No. 200-2000-00629, TO #32 between the National Academy of Sciences and the Centers for Disease Control and Prevention. Any opinions, findings, conclusions, or recommendations expressed in this publication are those of the author(s) and do not necessarily reflect the view of the organizations or agencies that provided support for the project.

Library of Congress Cataloging-in-Publication Data

Workshop on Disability in America, a New Look (2005 : Washington, D.C.)
    Workshop on Disability in America, a New Look : summary and papers : based on a workshop of the Committee on Disability in America: a New Look, Board on Health Sciences Policy / Marilyn J. Field, Alan M. Jette, and Linda Martin, editors.
        p. ; cm.
    Includes bibliographical references and index.
    ISBN 0-309-10090-9 (pbk.)
    1. People with disabilities—United States—Congresses. 2. People with disabilities—Health and hygiene—United States—Congresses. 3. Disabilities—Age factors—United States—Congresses. 4. Health promotion—United States—Congresses.
    [DNLM: 1. Disabled Persons—United States—Congresses. 2. Age Factors—United States—Congresses. 3. Chronic Disease—epidemiology—United States—Congresses. 4. Comorbidity—United States—Congresses. 5. Disabled Persons—classification—United States—Congresses.] I. Field, Marilyn J. (Marilyn Jane) II. Jette, Alan M. III. Martin, Linda G., 1947- IV. Institute of Medicine (U.S.). Committee on Disability in America: a New Look. V. Title.
    HV1553.W67 2005
    362.40973—dc22
                                        2005036811

Additional copies of this report are available from the National Academies Press, 500 Fifth Street, N.W., Lockbox 285, Washington, DC 20055; (800) 624-6242 or (202) 334-3313 (in the Washington metropolitan area); Internet, http://www.nap.edu.

For more information about the Institute of Medicine, visit the IOM home page at: **www.iom.edu.**

"Knowing is not enough; we must apply.
Willing is not enough; we must do."
—Goethe

INSTITUTE OF MEDICINE
OF THE NATIONAL ACADEMIES

Advising the Nation. Improving Health.

THE NATIONAL ACADEMIES
Advisers to the Nation on Science, Engineering, and Medicine

The **National Academy of Sciences** is a private, nonprofit, self-perpetuating society of distinguished scholars engaged in scientific and engineering research, dedicated to the furtherance of science and technology and to their use for the general welfare. Upon the authority of the charter granted to it by the Congress in 1863, the Academy has a mandate that requires it to advise the federal government on scientific and technical matters. Dr. Ralph J. Cicerone is president of the National Academy of Sciences.

The **National Academy of Engineering** was established in 1964, under the charter of the National Academy of Sciences, as a parallel organization of outstanding engineers. It is autonomous in its administration and in the selection of its members, sharing with the National Academy of Sciences the responsibility for advising the federal government. The National Academy of Engineering also sponsors engineering programs aimed at meeting national needs, encourages education and research, and recognizes the superior achievements of engineers. Dr. Wm. A. Wulf is president of the National Academy of Engineering.

The **Institute of Medicine** was established in 1970 by the National Academy of Sciences to secure the services of eminent members of appropriate professions in the examination of policy matters pertaining to the health of the public. The Institute acts under the responsibility given to the National Academy of Sciences by its congressional charter to be an adviser to the federal government and, upon its own initiative, to identify issues of medical care, research, and education. Dr. Harvey V. Fineberg is president of the Institute of Medicine.

The **National Research Council** was organized by the National Academy of Sciences in 1916 to associate the broad community of science and technology with the Academy's purposes of furthering knowledge and advising the federal government. Functioning in accordance with general policies determined by the Academy, the Council has become the principal operating agency of both the National Academy of Sciences and the National Academy of Engineering in providing services to the government, the public, and the scientific and engineering communities. The Council is administered jointly by both Academies and the Institute of Medicine. Dr. Ralph J. Cicerone and Dr. Wm. A. Wulf are chair and vice chair, respectively, of the National Research Council.

www.national-academies.org

WORKSHOP COMMITTEE ON DISABILITY IN AMERICA: A NEW LOOK

ALAN M. JETTE (*Chair*), Director, Health & Disability Research Institute, Boston University

ELENA ANDRESEN, Professor and Chief, Epidemiology Division, Department of Health Services Research, Management, and Policy, University of Florida Health Sciences Center

DUDLEY S. CHILDRESS, Professor of Biomedical Engineering and Physical Medicine and Rehabilitation, McCormick School of Engineering and Feinberg School of Medicine, Northwestern University

VICKI A. FREEDMAN, Professor, Department of Health Systems and Policy, School of Public Health, University of Medicine and Dentistry of New Jersey

PATRICIA HICKS, Associate Professor of Pediatrics and Director, Continuity of Care Clinic, University of Texas Southwestern Medical School, University of Texas Southwestern Medical Center at Dallas

LISA I. IEZZONI, Professor of Medicine, Harvard University and Beth Israel Deaconess Medical Center

JUNE ISAACSON KAILES, Associate Director, Center for Disability Issues and the Health Professions, Western University of Health Sciences

LAURA MOSQUEDA, Director of Geriatrics, College of Medicine, University of California, Irvine

P. HUNTER PECKHAM, Donnell Professor of Biomedical Engineering and Orthopaedics, Case Western Reserve University

JAMES MARC PERRIN, Professor of Pediatrics, Harvard Medical School and Massachusetts General Hospital

---

Following the workshop and with the initiation of the second phase of the disability study, additional members were appointed to the committee: Michael Chernew, Ph.D., professor of health management and policy, School of Public Health, University of Michigan; Margaret A. Turk, M.D., professor of physical medicine & rehabilitation, State University of New York Upstate Medical University at Syracuse; Gregg Vanderheiden, Ph.D., professor of industrial and biomedical engineering and director, Trace Research and Development Center, University of Wisconsin at Madison; and John Whyte, M.D., Ph.D., director, Moss Rehabilitation Research Institute, Philadelphia.

Study Staff

MARILYN J. FIELD, Study Director
AFRAH ALI, Senior Project Assistant
FRANKLIN BRANCH, Research Assistant
LINDA MARTIN, Institute of Medicine Scholar in Residence

Board on Health Sciences Policy Staff

ANDREW POPE, Director, Board on Health Sciences Policy
AMY HAAS, Administrative Assistant

Contents

Boxes, Figures, and Tables

BOXES

FIGURES

ix

TABLES

Reviewers

This workshop summary has been reviewed in draft form by individuals chosen for their diverse perspectives and technical expertise, in accordance with procedures approved by the National Research Council's Report Review Committee. The purpose of this independent review is to provide candid and critical comments that will assist the institution in making its published reports as sound as possible and to ensure that the report meets institutional standards for objectivity, evidence, and responsiveness to the study charge. The review comments and draft manuscript remain confidential to protect the integrity of the deliberative process. We wish to thank the following individuals for their review of this report:

Diane L Damiano, Ph.D., P.T., Research Associate Professor, Department of Neurology, Washington University, Saint Louis

John Ditunno, M.D., Professor of Rehabilitation Medicine, Jefferson Medical College, Thomas Jefferson University

Corinne Kirchner, Ph.D., Director, Policy Research and Program Evaluation, American Foundation for the Blind

John Melvin, M.D., Chair, Department of Rehabilitation Medicine, Jefferson Medical College, Thomas Jefferson University

Kenneth J. Ottenbacher, Ph.D., Associate Director, Sealy Center on Aging, University of Texas Medical Branch, Galveston

Susan Palsbo, Ph.D., Principal Research Associate, Center for Health Research, Policy, and Ethics, George Mason University

Although the reviewers listed above have provided many constructive comments and suggestions, they were not asked to endorse the report nor did they see the final draft before its release. The review of this report was overseen by **Mel Worth, M.D.,** Scholar in Residence at the Institute of Medicine. Appointed by the National Research Council and the Institute of Medicine, he was responsible for making certain that an independent examination of this report was carried out in accordance with the institutional procedures and that all review comments were carefully considered. Responsibility for the final content of this report rests entirely with the authors and the institution.

WORKSHOP ON
DISABILITY IN AMERICA

A NEW LOOK

Introduction

"Disability is an issue that affects every individual, community, neighborhood, and family in the United States" (IOM, 1991, p. 1). The Institute of Medicine's (IOM's) 1991 report *Disability in America: Toward a National Agenda for Prevention* began with these words. They are as true today as they were 15 years ago.

In fact, a demographic imperative—the aging of the baby boom generation—will soon substantially increase the proportion and numbers of Americans in the older age groups that are most at risk of physical and mental impairments, limitations, and disabilities (U.S. Census Bureau, 2004). At the same time, certain trends in other age groups—for example, the increased rates of survival of extremely premature infants and increases in the prevalence of obesity in younger populations—are putting more children and younger adults at risk of disabling conditions. Thus, the promotion of good health, independence, and social integration for people with disabilities and the prevention of disabling injuries, diseases, and disorders are more important objectives than ever.

In the years since the publication of the 1991 report, the country has seen positive changes in the understanding of disability and a growing recognition that health promotion is as an important a goal for people with disabilities as it is for other members of the community. Increasingly, disability is understood not as an intrinsic characteristic of an individual but rather as "a gap between a person's capabilities and the demands of the environment" (IOM, 1991, p. 1). *Healthy People 2010*, which is a statement of national health objectives, cited inattention to environmental fac-

1

tors as a contributor to the neglect of health promotion opportunities for people with disabling conditions (USDHHS, 2000). The World Health Organization's *International Classification of Functioning, Disability and Health* (a revision of the 1980 *International Classification of Impairments, Disabilities and Handicaps* [WHO, 1980]) likewise stresses the critical role of environmental factors in enabling the participation in society of people with physical or mental impairments and activity limitations (WHO, 2001).

The 1991 IOM report and a subsequent report, *Enabling America* (IOM, 1997), emphasized that much disability is preventable. Prevention extends beyond primary prevention (e.g., improving automobile safety) to include the prevention of progressive or secondary health problems (e.g., pressure sores related to spinal cord injury), the development of more effective rehabilitation strategies, the use of appropriate assistive technologies, and the elimination or mitigation of environmental barriers that restrict the participation in society of individuals with disabling conditions.

Beginning in late 2004, the IOM began a project to take a new look at disability in America. It will review developments and progress since the publication of the 1991 and 1997 Institute reports. For technical contracting reasons, the new project was split into two phases. During the limited first phase, a committee appointed by IOM planned and convened a 1-day workshop to examine a subset of topics as background for the second phase of project. As was agreed upon with the sponsor of the workshop, the Centers for Disease Control and Prevention (CDC), the topics were

- methodological and policy issues related to the conceptualization, definition, measurement, and monitoring of disability and health over time;
- trends in the amount, types, and causes of disability;
- disability across the age spectrum and in the context of normal aging; and
- secondary health conditions.

The phase-one workshop was held in Washington, D.C. on August 1, 2005. Its participants included researchers, clinicians, social service professionals, policy experts, and consumer representatives and advocates. The meeting agenda and list of participants are included in Appendix A.

This report summarizes the workshop presentations and discussions. The background papers prepared for the workshop are included in Appendixes B through O. Some papers were submitted and circulated in advance of the meeting, whereas others were first presented at the meeting. The analyses, definitions, and views presented in the papers are those of the paper authors and are not necessarily those of the IOM committee. Likewise, the discussion summary is limited to the views of the workshop participants. Although the discussion was wide ranging, it did not offer a comprehensive review of the topics considered. Consistent with the policies of the National Research Council for workshop summary reports, this report includes no committee conclusions or recommendations.

The workshop summary and the background papers will serve as resources for the second phase of the committee's work. This phase, which began in fall 2005, expands the focus to cover additional topics, including the roles of assistive technologies and universal design, financing issues, and directions for public policy and research. For this work, the National Institute for Disability and Rehabilitation Research and the National Center for Medical Rehabilitation Research have joined the CDC as sponsors. Reflecting the expansion of activity in the project's second phase, new members have been added to the study committee (see note in Appendix P). Unlike this workshop summary, the committee's consensus report, which should be released in early 2007, will include recommendations.

REFERENCES

IOM (Institute of Medicine). 1991. *Disability in America: Toward a National Agenda for Prevention*. Washington, DC: National Academy Press.

IOM. 1997. *Enabling America: Assessing the Role of Rehabilitation Science and Engineering*. Washington, DC: National Academy Press.

U.S. Census Bureau. 2004. U.S. Interim Projections by Age, Sex, Race, and Hispanic Origin. Available online at: http://www.census.gov/ipc/www/usinterimproj/natprojtab02a.pdf. (Last accessed November 22, 2005.)

USDHHS (U.S. Department of Health and Human Services). *Healthy People 2010: Understanding and Improving Health*. 2nd ed. Washington, DC: U.S. Government Printing Office, November 2000. Available online at: http://www.healthypeople.gov/Document/tableofcontents.htm#volume1. (Last accessed November 22, 2005.)

WHO (World Health Organization). 1980. *International Classification of Impairments, Disabilities and Handicaps: a Manual of Classification Relating to the Consequences of Disease*. Geneva, Switzerland: WHO.

WHO. 2001. *International Classification of Functioning, Disability and Health*. Geneva, Switzerland: WHO.

Summary of Workshop Presentations and Discussions

A lan Jette, chair of the Institute of Medicine (IOM) committee that planned the workshop, began by welcoming the participants. He noted that the workshop was the first step in a broader IOM project that would revisit the 1991 IOM report *Disability in America* and the 1997 report *Enabling America*. Dr. Jose Cordero (Centers for Disease Control and Prevention), Mr. Steven Tingus (National Institute on Disability and Rehabilitation Research), and Dr. Michael Weinrich (National Center on Medical Rehabilitation Research) provided additional welcomes. They also offered brief comments on the relevance of the workshop and the broader IOM project to the priorities and agendas of their organizations.

The morning session of the workshop was organized around two panels, the first of which focused on models and concepts of disability. The second panel provided overviews of disability trends in childhood, midlife, and late life. The first of the afternoon panels considered disability issues over the human life span, specifically, risk factors for disability late in life and transitions or transfers in care for adolescents and young adults. The other two afternoon panels provided perspectives on the nature and the prevention of secondary health conditions.

As noted in the introduction, this summary is based on the presentations and discussion during the workshop and does not necessarily reflect the views of the IOM committee that organized the meeting. The committee is preparing a comprehensive report that will cover a range of issues, including the topics discussed in the workshop. That report, which will include recommendations, should be released in early 2007.

MODELS AND CONCEPTS OF DISABILITY

Presentations

Dr. Gale Whiteneck began with a brief history of models of disability. (The paper prepared by Dr. Whiteneck appears in Appendix B.) He noted in particular the seminal contribution of Saad Nagi in differentiating disability-related outcomes at three levels, namely, the organ, the person, and society. Dr. Whiteneck then focused on an assessment of the transition from the *International Classification of Impairments, Disabilities and Handicaps* (ICIDH) to the *International Classification of Functioning, Disability and Health* (ICF), which were published by the World Health Organization (WHO) in 1980 and 2001, respectively (WHO, 1980, 2001). ICF and its associated description offered one major conceptual step forward but also one step backward. Drawing on his experience with the classification revision process, Dr. Whiteneck proposed that several additional steps are needed to revise and apply the model.

The major step forward with ICF was the inclusion of physical, social, and other environmental factors that interact with an individual's health conditions and other characteristics to produce outcomes, including activity (defined as the execution of a task or action by an individual) and participation (defined as an individual's involvement in a life situation). This step was consistent with the recommendations of the IOM committees in 1991 and 1997 (IOM, 1991, 1997) and also with the provisions of the Americans with Disabilities Act (ADA; P.L. 101-336), which became law in 1990.

Other improvements in the classification involved the incorporation of neutral as well as negative ways of describing an individual's status. For example, the ICF model uses the neutral phrase "body function and structure" as well as the term "impairment" and includes the term "activity" as well as "activity limitation." The revised model also emphasized the complexity of possible interactions among its components (e.g., as shown by the two-way arrows rather than one-way "causal" arrows in the model's graphic representation).

The step backward with ICF was the blurring of the conceptual distinctions between activity and participation (and between activity limitations and participation restrictions). Rather than identifying certain difficulties as activity limitations and other difficulties as participation restrictions, ICF grouped them together in a single list. Among the many differences between the two concepts, the foremost is that activity (e.g., walking) operates primarily at the person level, whereas participation (e.g., working) operates at the social and societal level. Activities are generally simpler than participation, and participation is more dependent on environmental factors than activity. Participation also appears to be more relevant to the individual's quality of life.

Dr. Whiteneck proposed that a first step in future revisions of ICF should be to distinguish between the elements of activity and the elements of participation. Such distinctions would be particularly useful in helping to understand and respond to environmental barriers to participation. Dr. Whiteneck emphasized the complexity of linkages between environmental factors and participation. For example, those who have higher levels of social participation may report higher levels of environmental barriers because they encounter and perceive more such barriers than those who participate less.

In addition to distinguishing between difficulties with activities and difficulties with participation, Dr. Whiteneck offered six additional steps to complete the ICF. These steps were to

- add quality of life (an individual's subjective assessment of his or her overall well-being) to the ICF model as recommended by the 1997 IOM report;
- provide more theoretical and empirical specificity about the nature and complexity of environmental factors as they affect participation;
- identify and assess personal factors, including psychological and behavioral characteristics, that affect activity and participation;
- refine the graphic representation of the model so it would better help people to understand and use the model's concepts and relationships;
- develop a research strategy, including better measures and data resources, to test the model and its complex set of interrelations; and
- design and test interventions that are consistent with the model to assess whether they improve the lives of people with disabilities.

In the second presentation, Dr. Rune Simeonsson noted his agreement with Gale Whiteneck's discussion of ICF and his conclusions. He then highlighted current issues in defining and classifying disability among children and youth. (The paper prepared by Dr. Simeonsson appears in Appendix C.) He emphasized the need to move beyond classifications designed solely for health care to those applicable to educational and other service systems. Dr. Simeonsson also argued that we can learn from history, specifically, the evolution of models and concepts of disability across different disciplines.

Dr. Simeonsson reviewed historical models of child disability, emphasizing the transactional model of Sameroff and Chandler (1975). The premise of the transactional model is that outcomes for children with disabilities result not only from an initial cause—for example, having genetic syndrome—but also result from ongoing "transactions" in the child's life, including medical and educational interventions intended to improve outcomes. Both nature and nurture contribute.

Among the top current issues or challenges in conceptualizing, modeling, and measuring childhood disability are the changes in functional capacities that occur as children develop and the scientific complexity of differentiating developmental delay from impairment. Children are "moving targets." What defines normal development in a two-year old is very different from that in a four-year old or a 14-year old. For very young children, their developmentally limited verbal and behavioral repertoires complicate assessments. The interviews and self-report tools that are frequently used with adults are not appropriate.

Dr. Simeonsson noted that additional challenges are presented by the inconsistency and arbitrariness of language used to describe disabilities and the lack of uniformity in how government agencies and service systems identify and categorize children with disabilities. He noted that some programs work more from a medical model and focus on diagnostic categories, whereas others—consistent with a social model of disability—focus on functional abilities and limitations, which is consistent with the ICF model.

Dr. Simeonsson suggested a number of priorities for researchers and policymakers. These include

- adoption of the version of the ICF for children and youth (ICF-CY), when it is completed; and
- development of measures of human functioning that operationalize all the components of the ICF for adults and children.
- implementation of uniform concepts of child functioning and disability for health, education, and related services nationally and internationally; and
- identification and refinement of developmentally relevant measures risk indicators for disability among children.

In her presentation, Dr. Julie Keysor tackled the question raised by both earlier speakers: how does the environment influence social participation and disability? In the absence of data on participation and participation restrictions, she focused on conceptual work and research related to mobility limitations and the environment. (The paper prepared by Dr. Keysor appears in Appendix D.)

Dr. Keysor reviewed several conceptual frameworks, beginning with ICF. The ICF explicitly mentions three general environmental domains: the physical, the social, and the political (WHO, 2001). It also identifies specific aspects of the environment that should be considered in research, policy, and other work: (1) products and technology; (2) natural and human-made changes; (3) social support and relationships; (4) attitudes of other people; and (5) services, systems, and policies.

Dr. Keysor noted that the Quebec Group (Fougeyrollas and colleagues) has identified generally similar environmental factors ranging from the political-economic (e.g., public policies) to the socio-cultural (e.g., attitudes and norms) to the physical (e.g., natural or built features of the environment) (see, e.g., Fougeyrollas, 1995 and Fougeyrollas et al., 1997). Shumway-Cook, Patla and colleagues (2002) have elaborated specifically on aspects of the physical environment that influence mobility. They have identified eight dimensions related to distance, terrain, time (e.g., time to cross a street), physical load (e.g., carrying objects), need for postural transitions (e.g., change of direction), crowding or density, attentional demands (e.g., familiarity of surroundings), and weather and light levels.

Dr. Keysor also observed that she and her colleagues, including Alan Jette, have proposed a different way of classifying physical domains (Keysor et al., 2005). Their classification identifies home mobility barriers, community mobility barriers, mobility technology facilitators, communication technology facilitators, and transportation facilitators.

Related to these frameworks and others are several measurement instruments that can be used for epidemiological and observational studies. The research challenges are to assess which domains of the environment have the greatest influence on participation or disability and also to identify which elements act as participation barriers and which as facilitators.

Dr. Keysor described the Craig Hospital Inventory of Environmental Factors, which was developed by Gale Whiteneck and his colleagues (Whiteneck et al., 2004). This is a self-report instrument that asks people how often in the past 12 months an environmental barrier has been a problem and for an identified problem whether has it been a big problem or a little problem. Other self-report instruments, for example, the Measure of the Quality of the Environment developed by Fougeyrollas and the Quebec group, add a focus on environmental facilitators as well as barriers.

Based on her search of the research literature from 1991 to 2005 related to rehabilitation, stroke, spinal-cord injury, and arthritis, Dr. Keysor reviewed the handful of studies relating mobility limitations to environmental factors. In general, these studies found that people with mobility limitations do report facilitators and barriers in their environments and that they try to avoid the barriers. The research findings are, however, not that consistent or strong, and they raise many questions. For example, it is not clear from the research how long environmental effects or perceptions endure. Perhaps people adapt to the barriers they encounter, for example, by finding technologies, social supports, or other means to cope with the barriers, or perhaps they change their perceptions of their environment.

Although the growing number of measurement instruments is a plus, the lack of consensus on domains of environment presents challenges. The paucity of studies argues for further investigations, especially ones that are prospective and experimental. In addition, researchers need to focus more on how people interact with their environments at work, school, and elsewhere. Finally, Dr. Keysor seconded Dr. Whiteneck's call for more emphasis on assessing quality of life and life satisfaction.

Discussion

One participant noted the lack of use of ICF in framing surveillance and research activities and asked if it is necessary to modify the conceptual framework or just move forward with the research. Dr. Simeonsson responded that one reason for this lack of use is that thus far most of the research relies on preexisting instruments and data sets, although new resources have been developed since the publication of ICF. Drs. Whiteneck and Keysor supported the need for feedback from research use of the models to refine or elaborate on the conceptual and classification model, but they said that it is not necessary to wait for the perfect model. ICF can be used now. In a similar vein, another participant wondered—given the different meanings of words to different people—whether or not the limits of communication have been reached and whether it should just be recognized that there is noise and uncertainty in the use of these concepts.

One participant probed further the proposal that models of disability incorporate quality of life. Dr. Whiteneck suggested that the best approach would be to keep quality of life in a separate domain and not try to integrate it into all domains of ICF. He argued that the essential aspect is a person's subjective, overall assessment of well being rather than only health-related quality of life, which tends to dominate now. Dr. Simeonsson noted that quality of life is not isomorphic or perfectly correlated with activity or participation. That is, people with similar limitations in those areas may have very different assessments of their quality of life.

The remaining discussion focused on the relation to ICF of particular concepts that have been highlighted in the disability literature. One question involved the implications of all the two-way arrows in the ICF graphic model, including the implications for a life-course perspective and the malleability of health. Dr. Simeonsson responded that the concept of early intervention certainly existed before ICF.

Another participant asked where the family fits into ICF. All the panelists agreed that families are a critical part of the environment. Dr. Whiteneck added that involvment in family life is an important dimension of participation but that family structure or behavior can also be an environmental barrier or facilitator of participation. For example, people with traumatic brain injury have cited family attitudes as an important barrier. A final question was whether ICF includes the concept of psychological accommodation, in which, over time, people with disabilities change their perspectives about the adequacy of their own functioning and develop a subjective sense of well being that may be quite different from what an outside observer might expect. Dr. Simeonsson responded that he was not sure where it fits into ICF, but there is ample evidence that individuals' conceptions of what is important in life change as they live with disability.

TRENDS IN DISABILITY

Presentations

Dr. Vicki Freedman, whose task was to discuss trends in late-life disability, reviewed perspectives on the implications of increased life expectancy for morbidity and disability in late life. (Dr. Freedman's paper appears in Appendix E.) Life expectancy was 68 in 1950 and reached over 77 in 2002. This increase has raised the question: are these extra years of life associated with longer periods of morbidity and disability? Some have predicted increases in late-life morbidity and disability, some have predicted decreases, and others have hypothesized an increase in chronic conditions but a decrease in their progression to disability in late life.

Dr. Freedman stressed that disability in late life is a socially-defined concept that reflects the intersection of an older person's capabilities, their environment, and the nature of the tasks that they wish to accomplish. In practice, most studies of trends in disability among the older population focus on self-reports of difficulty or assistance with activities of daily living (ADLs; e.g., bathing, dressing, and eating) and instrumental activities of daily living (IADLs; e.g., preparing meals and managing money). Ideally, measures and studies would focus not just on activities but also on participation in society (as conceptualized in the ICF) and the environmental factors that limit or assist participation. Dr. Freedman observed that no published epidemiologic studies, at this time, have consistently focused on these other dimensions of disability.

The earliest trend analyses for the 1960s and 1970s showed no increase in the levels of disability in old age, but for the 1980s and early 1990s, Manton and colleagues found declines in disability (Manton et al., 1993, 1997). Others, using different data sets, have found conflicting results (Crimmins et al., 1997). A review and evaluation of eight unique surveys that allow trend analysis reported that studies rated fair or good in their methods showed that IADL disability had declined substantially among older Americans (Freedman et al., 2002). Declines have been concentrated in activities central to living independently, for example, shopping, managing money and doing laundry. A technical working group found that there were also declines in the number of older Americans who had difficulty with ADLs and who received help with ADLs, but these changes were relatively small. The group found that inconsistencies across previously published survey analyses of ADL trends could be attributed to differences in the wording of the questions, the period of analysis used, age standardization, and the inclusion of the institutional population.

Less evidence exists regarding demographic and socioeconomic disparities in trends in late-life disability, and at times the evidence has conflicted. One recent analysis of data from the National Health Interview Survey (NHIS) from 1982 to 2002 shows that racial and ethnic gaps in the need for help with ADLs and IADLs have persisted, and disparities related to education and income gaps appear to be growing (Schoeni et al., 2005). For example, ADL disability has been declining more rapidly for those with higher levels of education and income.

Also limited is the research on the causes of the trends in late-life disability. Given the strong negative relation between disability and education in the cross-sectional analyses, the dramatic increase in the educational attainment of the older population can explain some, but by no means all, of the change in rates of disability. One can hypothesize many ways in which education may influence functioning and disability, for example, by influencing the work-related risk of disease, injury, or impairment; the use of the healthcare system; the use of assistive technologies; adherence to medical regimens; and risk-taking behaviors.

Disability declines do not appear to be the result of declines in chronic disease. To the contrary, based on self-reports, the prevalence of many chronic diseases has increased, even as their disabling effects have declined. This pattern could reflect improved medical diagnosis and treatments, but studies thus far have yielded little insight. There has been a decline in physical functional limitations (such as the ability to stoop or climb, which are precursors to disability in the simplified linear models of the disablement process), but evidence about trends in cognitive and sensory functioning is mixed. Finally, recent data suggest that the increased use of assistive technology (e.g., for mobility and bathing) has contributed to the decline in people needing help with ADLS. But the role of other modern conveniences not specifically designed for people with disabilities (e.g., direct deposit banking and microwaves) is unclear.

Dr. Jay Bhattacharya discussed trends in disability among the U.S. working-age population. (The paper by Dr. Bhattacharya, coauthored by Kavita Choudhry and Darius Lakdawalla, appears in Appendix F.) Will the decreases in rates of disability in old age described by Vicki Freedman in the preceding presentation continue? The answer will depend on trends among the current working-age group, who are the elderly of the future. Dr. Bhattacharya discussed reasons for concern related to the recent worrying increases in the rates of obesity, diabetes, and asthma among the working-age population. He also noted that a continuation of recent declines in disability in late life would have positive implications for Medicare's solvency.

Dr. Bhattacharya observed that a challenge in measuring disability among those of working age is that reports of work disability (e.g., difficulty working because of a health problem) may be influenced by public policies, for example, changes in the generosity of disability insurance programs and in the application of the Americans with Disabilities Act. ADL- and IADL-based measures avoid this problem (although they have conceptual and other limitations as measures of disability).

The analysis that Dr. Bhattacharya presented used NHIS reports of the need for help with ADLs for 1984 to 1996 and 1997 to 2000. The division of the analysis into two parts reflects changes in the NHIS questions on disability after 1996. For the period from 1984 to 1996, disability rates for the working-age groups increased, but the rates were basically flat in the period from 1997 to 2000.

The next step in Dr. Bhattacharya's analysis was to decompose or separate the trend in disability (i.e., needing assistance with ADLs) from 1984 to 1996 into three components: the change in the prevalence of chronic disease, the change in the probability of being disabled given that a chronic disease is reported, and the change in the probability of being disabled given no chronic disease. To illustrate the results, Dr. Bhattacharya presented data for three ages: 30, 45, and 60 years. (These data were developed using a "data smoothing" technique [described in Appendix F] that adjusts data on people not in these specific age groups, e.g., those one year older or younger, to provide more robust estimates.)

For all three age groups, there was a decline in disability among those without chronic diseases. For the 30- and 45-year-old age groups, the data showed an increase in the prevalence of chronic diseases and of disability due to chronic diseases. For these groups, the largest source of disability due to chronic disease was obesity. Those in the 60-year-old age group showed reductions in disability because a substantial decrease in the prevalence of disability among those with chronic illnesses offset a smaller increase in the prevalence of such illnesses. Although 60-year-olds with chronic disease showed decreased disability overall, the increase in obesity was a major countervailing influence in this group.

Beyond the increased prevalence of obesity in the two younger age groups, other highlights were as follows:

- for 30-year-olds, increased disability related to heart disease and the combination of heart disease and obesity;
- for 45-year-olds, increased disability among those with hyperten-

sion, chronic obstructive pulmonary disease (COPD), and obesity combined with diabetes; and

• for 60-year-olds, an increased prevalence of asthma combined with COPD, heart disease combined with stroke, and obesity combined with diabetes (despite a decrease in obesity alone) and decreases in disability related to many chronic conditions but increased disability because of COPD and stroke combined with hypertension.

In concluding, Dr. Bhattacharya stressed the increase in obesity among the working-age population and the increase in disability rates among the younger segments of this population. Noting that he was speculating, Dr. Bhattacharya concluded by observing that the data suggest that the United States may not see a continuing decline in disability among those over age 65 as the current working-age population enters old age.

In the final presentation of the morning, Dr. Ruth Stein discussed trends in disability in early life. She began by reviewing demographic trends, including the growth and increasing racial and ethnic diversity of the child population in the United States. She also highlighted the strong association between poverty and poor health among children. (Dr. Stein's paper appears in Appendix G.)

Dr. Stein argued that the two traditional measures of disability used for adults, namely, work disability and ADLs-IADLs, do not apply well to developing children, and to young children, in particular, for whom independence in activities is not expected. Instead of these measures, limitations in other activities, such as school and play, have been assessed, although very few children are not able to play.

Dr. Stein presented data on activity limitations among children from a variety of sources that have used different questions about disability or activity limitations. As reported by Newacheck and colleagues (1986), the prevalence of activity limitations among children under 18 years old rose from less than 2.0 percent in 1960 to about 3.5 percent in 1980. More recent data from NHIS show increases to greater than 6.0 percent in 2000 (Child Trends Data Bank, 2005). Most of this activity limitation is related to participation in special education, which is more common among boys than girls.

Supplemental Security Income enrollment for children, which primarily involves those in poverty, has increased. This increase reflects the addition of the mental health conditions list to the program's eligibility categories and a 1990 Supreme Court decision (*Sullivan v. Zebley*) that broadened the eligibility criteria.

For childhood disability, major measurement challenges include the lack of an appropriate baseline measure of normal function against which functional deficits can be assessed. Across different parts of society, wide variations exist in what is viewed as "normal" childhood physical and mental development. Another complexity is presented by the increasing recognition that the core tasks of childhood are development and maturation rather than playing or going to school per se. Dr. Stein cited a recent IOM report (joint with the National Research Council) on children's health that stressed this point (NRC/IOM, 2004). She argued that it is important to investigate chronic conditions in early life that lead to disability in both childhood and adult life. It is likewise important to understand better the consequences of those conditions, such as a dependence on compensatory mechanisms or the use of services above the usual levels for the age group.

Dr. Stein reviewed the tools that have been developed to operationalize concepts of child health and disability. Based on one of those tools, the 1994–1995 NHIS Disability Supplement, 14.8 to 18.0 percent of children were identified as having special health care needs and about 50 percent of that group had functional limitations. The proportions of children affected increased with increases in age and poverty.

Dr. Stein also noted indirect evidence of overall trends determined from measures of particular child health problems. On the positive side, the rate of lead poisoning has declined substantially during the last 25 years, and the use of folic acid antenatally has been associated with declines in the numbers of children born with spina bifida and anencephaly since 1996–1997. On the negative side are increases in asthma rates and rates of the low birth weight and preterm births since the 1980s. Racial and ethnic disparities in infant mortality rates continue. Also troubling is the increase in the proportion of children ages 6 to 19 years who are obese from less than 5 percent in the mid-1960s to almost 15 percent in 1999–2000. Minority children are especially affected.

Dr. Stein closed by suggesting that if the goal is to minimize lifetime disability, then there is need for a conceptualization of disability for the young that is broader than the most severe degree of limitation. She pointed out that the genomic revolution is allowing the much earlier identification of children who are at biologic risk of later disability. It is, thus, providing an opportunity for early intervention to limit the progression or consequences of genetic conditions before they cause observable problems. If we enlarge the focus of disability policies beyond children and adults who are already severely disabled, the growing number of effective preventive strategies can be better applied.

Discussion

Several questions during the discussion focused on data and methodology issues. One question was whether there were data sets that would allow investigation of disability trajectories for those with child-onset conditions versus the trajectories for those with adult-onset conditions. Dr. Stein responded that such data were not available for the United States but might be for the United Kingdom. Another question was whether it would be possible to use current data sets to operationalize the two-way arrows that specify feedback from activity and participation to disease in the ICF graphic model. Dr. Bhattacharya indicated that it is not possible to capture such interactions in cross-sectional data sets and that useful longitudinal data are scarce.

One suggestion was that to predict future trends analysts need to understand the differences in environments and the rates of environmental change that different birth cohorts have experienced. Dr. Freedman responded that disentangling the large age, time period, and cohort effects is mathematically challenging. She argued that it would be helpful to focus somewhat less on describing what has happened in the past and somewhat more on using data to help guide society in acting to prevent disability in the future.

Responding to a question about the influence of the creation of Medicare on old-age disability trends, Dr. Freedman said that it was difficult to measure the influence of this key policy change. In general, studies that have focused on the influence of medical treatment on disability have suffered from serious data limitations. In addition, she suggested it would be useful to see more investigations about the impact of public policies in addition to Medicare.

When he was asked about any prevention messages that would follow from the morning's presentations, Dr. Bhattacharya emphasized that successful steps to reduce the rates of obesity would have a very large effect on future disability rates and that reducing the prevalence of chronic diseases would also diminish disability. Dr. Stein agreed strongly. She added that the lack of universal health care for children in the United States particularly affects the uninsured working poor whose children have the worst health status.

Dr. Stein also mentioned a body weight and cohort concern related to the increasing survival of extremely low birth weight infants. Recent data suggest that almost half of such infants are experiencing health problems or functional limitations eight to ten years later.

Another participant pointed to the recent controversy about the relation between weight and mortality and wondered if there were statistical pitfalls that should be taken into account when emphasizing obesity reduction as means of preventing future disability. Dr. Bhattacharya noted that part of the difficulty in the relationship between weight and mortality is that overweight (rather than obese) people have mortality rates similar to those of normal-weight people. So far, his research has focused on obesity and not on overweight. For those who are obese, the link to disability is very persuasive.

One participant expressed concern that focusing more on children with less severe disabilities would leave behind those with the greatest disability because there are so many more children in the first group. Dr. Stein responded that there could indeed be a slippery slope, but from the perspective of the nation's future, it is important to develop a more comprehensive understanding of disability in the population and its sources. We must continue to be concerned about children and others with the most severe problems, but we will miss opportunities if we focus too narrowly on this group.

DISABILITY ACROSS THE AGE SPECTRUM

Presentations

Dr. Jack Guralnik began the afternoon panels with a review of research on risk factors for disability in old age. (Dr. Guralnik's paper appears in Appendix H.) He credited the Nagi model of disability and its further articulation in the IOM reports for helping guide epidemiologic research and hoped that the new IOM study would produce equally valuable direction. Dr. Guralnik also cited the value of the more recent ICF model and the work of Verbrugge and Jette (1994). He encouraged the current IOM committee to continue with an approach or model that is practical and that can be operationalized in a valid and reliable way for population-based and other studies.

Dr. Guralnik explained that many of the data that he reviewed came from work performed at the National Institute on Aging that employed a set of population-based studies called the Established Populations for Epidemiologic Studies of the Elderly (Guralnik et al., 1993). By monitoring populations over time, it was possible to assess the developing incidence of mobility limitations and other problems and to identify chronic health conditions as risk factors for these problems. For purposes of their work, mobility problems were defined as the inability to walk a quarter mile and the inability to climb a set of stairs. By way of overview, the research group found that the odds ratio for the loss of mobility was in the range of about 1.2 to 1.5 for people who had baseline reports of heart attack, stroke, diabetes, dyspnea, or exertional leg pain. Other analyses have focused behavioral risk factors such as smoking, drinking, and physical inactivity.

Dr. Guralnik noted differences between chronic conditions as risk factors for women and men. He presented data showing that women reported arthritis as the main cause of problems for walking one-half mile, doing heavy housework, and bathing. The pattern for men differed. Men also reported arthritis as the top cause of difficulty walking one-half mile. However, for disability in doing heavy housework, the top cause was heart disease, and for bathing disability, stroke led by a small margin.

It is important to examine both the difficulty in performing an activity and the inability to perform the activity at all. For example, Leveille and colleagues (1999) have found that although pain has a significant impact on difficulty with climbing, lifting, and ADLs, it is not significantly related to whether people can or cannot perform these activities at all.

In identifying health risk factors for disability, it is also important to consider comorbid conditions. As the number of comorbid conditions increases, the risk of developing a new disability increases rather dramatically. Individuals with four or more conditions at the baseline were almost three times as likely as those with no conditions to have lost mobility at follow up. He noted that this kind of epidemiologic study is very difficult to do, even with datasets as large as the one he and his colleagues were using.

Dr. Guralnik discussed research that attempts to explain the mechanism underlying the association between diabetes and problems with lower-extremity function. When he and his colleagues examined specific diabetes-related conditions and impairments (e.g., peripheral neuropathy and visual impairment), they found that entering each condition into the group's statistical model reduced the initial statistical association between diabetes and the measures of lower-extremity function. Collectively, the diabetes-related conditions explained about 80 percent of the statistical association between diabetes and (especially) mobility outcomes (Volpato et al., 2002).

Although most of his work has focused on health conditions as risk factors for disability, Dr. Guralnik reported that his group has examined some socioeconomic and demographic factors. He presented data for white and black women that showed more years of disability-free life expectancy for those with higher levels of education (Guralnik et al., 1993).

In closing, Dr. Guralnik reviewed data on the level of disability among people over age 65 in the years before death. For people in their 90s, disability rates are very high. Thus, although age-adjusted or age-specific rates of disability are declining in the United States, the overall number of people affected and the impact on society will grow because so many more people will be entering the very old age groups. Identification of the causes of late-life disability and interventions that can mitigate these causes or their effects will be increasingly important.

The presentation by Dr. John Reiss shifted the focus from the oldest segment of the U.S. population to the youngest and from risk factors for disability to certain difficulties that children with disabilities or special needs may experience as they move from adolescence into adulthood and from pediatric to adult health care providers. (Dr. Reiss's paper, which is coauthored by Robert Gibson, is presented in Appendix I.) He distinguished between the narrow concept of an individual's transfer from pediatric to adult health care services (an event) and the broad concept of transition, which refers to a planned process that should support the development of the knowledge and the skills needed to support a young person's full participation and decision making in the adult world.

Any discussion of disability among children needs to recognize the centrality of children's physical and mental development, a process that begins with the normal dependency of infancy and that is, for most children, marked by increasing independence and by an emphasis on actions and policies to "enable" children's greatest development. Dr. Reiss discussed a conceptual framework—represented graphically as a sort of kaleidoscope—that was proposed in a 2004 report, *Children's Health, the Nation's Wealth: Assessing and Improving Child Health*, from the National Research Council and the Institute of Medicine (NRC/IOM, 2004). That framework depicts the complex and dynamic nature of child health and the social and policy factors that affect a child's physical and social environment and that interact with a child's biological and other characteristics to affect the child's health.

Dr. Reiss noted the support by the Maternal and Child Health Bureau for studies of health care transitions for children with special health care needs and for work to identify the policies and services that can help these children live more independently as adults. He also cited the consensus statement by the American Academy of Pediatrics, the American Academy of Family Physicians, and the American College of Physicians (2002) endorsing the provision of uninterrupted, high-quality, developmentally appropriate health care services to maximize individual functioning and support the transition of young people from pediatric to adult health care.

The reality appears to fall short of this goal. Results from the 2000 National Survey of Children with Special Health Care Needs found that only about half of the parents with children between the ages of 14 and 17 years said that their child's pediatrician or family physician discussed how the child's needs might change as he or she moved toward adulthood (Lotstein et al., 2005). Only 30 percent reported that they had a plan for addressing those changing needs, and just 20 percent had a plan for transferring their child to adult health care providers. These findings, combined with other information and experience, point to significant problems, including unplanned, abrupt transfers from pediatric to adult health care services. Data on what happens after unplanned transfers are, however, limited.

Dr. Reiss observed that transfers from pediatric to adult health care are typically based on age rather than the individual readiness of a young person. Policies for Medicaid and other health insurance and social service programs play a role, since many supportive services for children end at age 18.

Dr. Reiss suggested that internists and other physicians for adults tend to be less comfortable with a significant role for parents. Even young people without special needs often are still developing the decision-making and other capacities and knowledge needed to navigate the adult health care system. An associated need for some degree of parental involvement and support may continue for many years after an individual reaches age 18.

Dr. Reiss proposed that more research is needed on what happens to individuals, especially those with special needs, after transfer to the adult health care system. Are there consequences for the utilization of resources, health outcomes, the development of secondary conditions, and the quality of life? Research should also focus on understanding what is expected of young adults in the adult health care system. What are the key competencies that youth need to move into the adult health care system, and what adjustments in that system may be necessary to provide developmentally appropriate services for young people with special needs?

Dr. Reiss concluded by suggesting that pediatric health care has changed over time to become much more child and family centered and that this change stems in part from successful advocacy by families and advocacy organizations. He argued that we need youth leaders to advocate for an adult health care system that is more responsive to youth and young adults with special health care needs.

Discussion

The first question in the discussion focused on what the IOM committee should consider in terms of analysis and recommendations about making the transition to adult health care services work for children with disabilities or special health care needs. Dr. Reiss repeated his view that young adults are still developing their capacities, including their ability to assert themselves in encounters with health care professionals. Physicians and others need to recognize this. Particularly when they see young people with special health care needs, physicians need to become more accepting of a role for parents. He also suggested that the board requirements for internal medicine be revised to cover the transition needs of young adults.

Another participant questioned such broad requirements, arguing that few internists see enough young adults with conditions such as cerebral palsy to become experts in their management. Specialized requirements will go for naught if the actual practice volume is not high enough to reinforce and build on the internist's initial training.

One of the next questions dealt with priorities for research to advance understanding of the epidemiology of disability in late life. Dr. Guralnik responded that researchers have investigated pieces of the pathway to disability for particular health conditions or limitations but that the overall picture is still very partial. The epidemiologic monitoring of people over the life course and the development of better and less burdensome instruments for assessing disability would help.

In response to another question, Dr. Guralnik added that it is particularly important to illuminate aspects of the pathway to disability that are amenable to interventions—for example, certain kinds of exercise—that will prevent or reduce disability. Suggestive observational data are available, but much still remains to be learned. For example, some data suggest that if a person has good balance, that person needs less strength to maintain mobility, so that might point to more of a focus on balance but also on the identification of the basic strength levels needed to maintain functional independence. The collection of some important data will require controlled trials of exercise and other interventions.

Dr. Reiss added the observation that young people who have had functional limitations from a very young age, for example, children who had needed a wheelchair for years, may find disability a foreign concept because they have developed special skills or have found assistive technologies or other means to do what they need to do. What they want and how they want to interact with health care providers and others may differ from the desires of someone who develops limitations as a result of an injury or a medical condition in later life. The perceptions of these young people may also differ from those of health care providers accustomed to working with older adults. Dr. Reiss also endorsed the focus on "enabling America" (as in the 1997 IOM report) as particularly appropriate for young people with special needs.

Dr. Guralnik observed that it is a challenge for those who do research on disability in old age to talk to people interested in childhood disability. Discussions can have an almost "apples and oranges" aspect. Among those doing research on aging, disability is viewed as a kind of final common pathway of many chronic diseases, and measures of disability are useful in summarizing health status. Young people, however, tend to be uncomfortable with and even insulted by data on how disability, for example, predicts institutionalization. Working and learning together are important but not easy.

SECONDARY HEALTH CONDITIONS: PART I

Presentations

Dr. Margaret Turk led off the panel with an overview of secondary conditions. (Dr. Turk's paper appears as Appendix J.) She proposed definitions of several concepts, suggesting that it would be helpful for researchers, analysts, and clinicians to be consistent and use the same terms or labels to refer to related but distinct health circumstances. Use of the same words to mean different things can impede communication.

Interest in secondary conditions seems to have been stimulated in the 1980s, when Dr. Michael Marge began to use the label "secondary condition" in his work with the National Council on Disability (Marge, 1988).

Use of the term in two IOM reports in 1991 and 1997 further focused attention on secondary conditions as subjects for study and intervention. Secondary conditions are important because they can create or intensify activity limitations, make participation in society more difficult, and decrease the quality of life.

Dr. Turk proposed several definitions and clarifications to distinguish secondary conditions from other conditions. A secondary condition is directly related to a primary disabling condition; the primary condition is a risk factor for the secondary condition. An example for people with cerebral palsy is contractures. Depending on the primary condition, other examples include pain, renal insufficiency, pressure ulcers, osteoporosis, and chronic edema in the lower limbs.

Dr. Turk argued for limiting the term "secondary condition" to health states (physical or mental) and not extending it to cover the social correlates or the potential societal consequences of having a primary disabling condition. Examples of such correlates include reduced access to employment or companionship. Such outcomes are important to our understanding of disability and quality of life, but lumping them together with secondary health conditions is not helpful. Doing so dilutes the concept and understanding of secondary health conditions. More important, perhaps, such a broad definition of secondary conditions blurs the focus on key elements in current models of disability, specifically, restrictions on participation in society and performance of social roles and the environmental and personal contributors to such restrictions.

The relationship between particular primary conditions and particular secondary conditions—including the likelihood and ways that an individual with a primary condition will experience a secondary condition—may be quite variable. Several general factors will influence the expression, prevention, or modification of a given secondary condition. These factors include (1) the state of scientific knowledge about the primary condition and its consequences, (2) the existence of proven clinical interventions or assistive technologies, (3) social and physical environments and public policies (including health insurance coverage for services and equipment), and (4) family and personal factors (including an individual's age or stage of development and personality traits).

Dr. Turk said that it is important to recognize that a primary condition will have a number of features that are aspects of the basic pathology or nature of the condition, what we may call associated conditions. With cerebral palsy, for example, seizures, mental retardation, and spasticity are considered features—albeit variable features—of the primary condition. They are not secondary conditions that result from the primary condition. She recognized that there may sometimes be a fine line between the basic pathology of a primary disabling condition and its secondary health consequences, and the new research can change perspectives.

A "comorbid condition" is one that is neither part of nor the result of a primary condition. For example, an individual who experiences a spinal cord injury may have skin cancer at the time that the injury occurs or may develop the disease later. Skin cancer is a comorbid condition in either case. Sometimes, increased scientific knowledge leads to an understanding that what was thought to be an unrelated comorbidity is actually a related secondary condition. For example, spinal cord injury is now recognized as a risk factor for insulin-resistant diabetes.

Dr. Turk also considered the relevance of aging to secondary health conditions. Aging is a normal developmental process. It is variable and modifiable to some degree across individuals, but manifestations of aging are an expected part of human life. People with disabling conditions, however, may have a smaller reserve capacity for performance and function as they age. In addition, some conditions associated with aging may be accelerated. For example, depending on a person's primary condition, she might be at risk for pain from degenerative joint disease as part of normal aging or at risk for the early onset of symptoms.

If one thinks in terms of health and wellness of people with disabling conditions, then maintaining or improving health requires attention to the etiology, prevention, and management or modification of secondary conditions for which people are at risk because of their primary condition. Again, depending on the condition, a secondary condition can have serious consequences for a person's survival, quality of life, and capacity to take advantage of participation-enhancing equipment or environments. Despite confusion and differences in the use of the term "secondary conditions," the discussion overall has helped direct attention of physicians and others to issues and problems that are central to the lifelong health and well-being of many people with disabling conditions.

In the next presentation, June Kailes spoke primarily from a consumer perspective, describing herself as a "living aging-with-disability laboratory." (Ms. Kailes's paper appears as Appendix K.) As someone in midlife who has lived with cerebral palsy since birth, she observed that disability-specific health care programs treat many people with lifelong disabilities as if they disappear when they turn 21. People with disabilities between the ages of 21 and 65 find a dearth of experienced professionals and comprehensive services. Instead, they encounter access barriers, illogical bureaucracies, and professionals with little preparation to serve midlife adults with disabilities. They encounter a system focused on acute care rather than continuing and coordinated care and assistance for those living long term with disability and chronic conditions. Choices may be limited, if one is lucky, to a pediatric-focused health care professionals with teddy bears on their business cards or geriatrics-focused health care providers.

Navigating the current health care system requires great energy, good "health literacy," and strong skills in advocating for oneself. Not everyone can be expected to have these personal navigational resources.

Ms. Kailes noted that aging with disability is a particular concern. As they provide routine health care, medical professionals may not anticipate the early aging experienced by many people with disabling conditions such as cerebral palsy. Margaret Turk talked earlier about secondary conditions related to aging and living with disability. Progress in identifying these conditions has not yet translated into effective interventions.

Ms. Kailes reiterated that disability is not something one has or does not have. Instead, a continuum of activity limitations exists and affects most people to various degrees at some point in their lives, if not lifelong. Furthermore, for policy, service, and research purposes, disability should be defined on a functional basis and in a unified and comprehensive way rather than in fragmented and narrow categories. It is not helpful to have many different definitions of disability across government departments and programs.

With respect to research, a greater focus on functional limitations that are common across a number of disabling conditions makes sense, given the complexity and diversity of these conditions and the low prevalence of many discrete diagnoses. The science also needs to be coordinated across relevant federal agencies to infuse attention to disability content throughout the broad range of health research. Although people with disabilities have a wealth of experience to inform policy, they are just advocates with opinions if they do not have the support of sound research and data.

In addition, Ms. Kailes stressed that planning for services and research should be undertaken *with* people with disabilities rather than *for* but *without* them. People with disabilities bring important knowledge and perspectives to the planning process and also to implementation. They can contribute as managers, investigators, and collaborators. As an additional point, people with disabilities should not be routinely excluded from pharmaceutical and other clinical trials that are not related to their disabling condition.

Ms. Kailes contended that services that are initially denied because of antiquated and shortsighted policies, inaccessible medical facilities and equipment, and similar problems can lead to the subsequent downstream use of more health care and social services and increased costs. One specific problem is restrictive definitions of medical necessity in health insurance programs. Such definitions often exclude services and technologies, including durable medical equipment, that will prevent deterioration, injuries, and decline in people with disabilities and thus avert the subsequent use of additional acute health care services and social services. Wheeled mobility is not a "convenience" item, as it has been described by one insurer. A motorized scooter is not a fashion statement.

Medicare specifically should change its policy that restricts coverage of mobility devices to those that are reasonable and necessary for use inside a person's home. Many people with mobility limitations can get around the home by "wall walking" and "furniture surfing." Outside the home, these methods are unsafe and unacceptable. The current Medicare policy reflects an outdated mind set that places minimal value on participation in society by people with disabling conditions.

Another problem identified by Ms. Kailes is that the implementation of ADA in health care settings lags far behind its implementation in many other areas. The implementation of ADA requires more attention to physical access to facilities and equipment (e.g., scales and examination tables) and also to accessible communications and other program features. Ms. Kailes closed by emphasizing that the work of the current IOM committee on disability is serious business for those who need better services and tools to live productive and fulfilling rather than unnecessarily confined lives.

Dr. James Rimmer began his presentation by endorsing the participatory model of disability research described by June Kailes. (Dr. Rimmer's paper, coauthored by Swati Shenoy, appears as Appendix L.) With respect to the panel topic, he cited the impact of a conference held several years ago that focused on secondary conditions in individuals with spina bifida and cerebral palsy. The conference and publication of the conference proceedings were sponsored by the Spina Bifida Association and United Cerebral Palsy in conjunction with several federal agencies including the Centers for Disease Control and Prevention (Lollar, 1994).

Dr. Rimmer suggested that continued research on secondary conditions and their prevention and management is important because secondary conditions are a major contributor to health disparities among people with disabilities. In the literature on secondary conditions, exercise-related research is quite prominent. Most of this research is, however, descriptive, with few experimental studies that test exercise interventions to reduce secondary conditions.

Dr. Rimmer noted recent studies reporting that people with a limited exercise capacity were at higher risk of death than others in the population. As is often the case, this research excluded people with disabilities.

The literature reviewed by Dr. Rimmer and his colleagues covered the period from 1990 to 2005. For the literature search, key words included "exercise," "physical activity," "secondary conditions," and "disability," in addition to terms for specific disabling conditions, such as "multiple sclerosis" and "spinal cord injury." The search yielded 167 abstracts, of which 42 were exercise training studies.

Dr. Rimmer's presentation focused on the literature examining the effects of exercise on fatigue, pain, and deconditioning. The review yielded few controlled trials. Several nonrandomized controlled studies reported that long-term aerobic and resistance exercise increased both physical and psychological well-being. Some additional studies reported that after the end of the exercise intervention, participants reported increased stress and a decreased quality of life without exercise.

A number of design limitations characterize this research. One limitation is small sample sizes, which is not surprising, because the recruitment of large numbers of research participants for studies of conditions with a low prevalence in the population is difficult. In addition, various exclusion criteria eliminated a large fraction of the target population. Dropout rates can be high, often because of transportation problems or the emergence of some kind of health complication. The implications of dropout rates for study validity must be assessed. Another limitation is that most interventions lasted 12 weeks or less and did not provide long-term follow-up. A different problem is that studies often include such a large number of outcome measures that some outcomes are likely to be found to be present at a statistically significant rate just by chance.

Among the important directions for research, one priority should be more efforts to conduct randomized controlled trials and longitudinal studies on exercise interventions for people with disabling conditions. Such studies will generate a stronger evidence base for guidelines and recommendations on exercise interventions for people with different disabling conditions.

Notwithstanding the value of randomized controlled trials, Dr. Rimmer observed that prospective and cross-sectional observational studies have a role to play. A larger study population can often be included in such studies, thereby providing more opportunity to control for demographic and other variables. Observational studies may allow assessments of exercise dose-response relationships that are expensive to assess in clinical trials.

New assessment technologies have real potential to reduce some of the burdens of research participation and make enrollment and study continuation easier. Examples include the use of web-based reporting by research participants, the use of more time-efficient assessment tools, and the use of global positioning systems to track certain aspects of physical activity.

Dr. Rimmer noted the existence of a large number of outcome assessment instruments that complicate comparisons across different studies. He suggested that a better understanding of the strengths and limitations of different assessment instruments would help researchers make better decisions about which instruments they should use and would also allow them to weed out some of the instruments with low reliability and validity.

In addition to research on interventions and measurement tools, more basic work is also needed to identify the biological mechanisms associated with changes in conditions such as stress and fatigue. Such work can guide future interventions. Likewise, a better understanding of the effects of different elements of health promotion efforts that involve multiple components (e.g., exercise and peer support) would be helpful.

Discussion

One participant observed that the discussion of secondary conditions needed to distinguish different disabling situations. One situation is a catastrophic disability in an otherwise young and healthy person; that individual has a primary condition—a medical diagnosis—that is a risk factor for specific secondary conditions or diagnoses. In contrast is the situation in much geriatric care, in which the problem is general frailty rather than a clear, primary disabling condition and in which frailty-associated activity limitations are risk factors for further deterioration. There needs to be a common framework for these contrasting situations that map onto the same longitudinal, enabling-disabling model of disability.

Dr. Turk agreed that the secondary conditions concept had been primarily applied to people who had lifelong primary disabling conditions such as cerebral palsy or people who experienced disabling injuries or illnesses in adolescence or midlife. How the concept should be applied to frail elderly people and also to people with chronic conditions such as obesity or hypertension needs more attention.

Another commenter returned to the issue raised by Dr. Reiss in the previous panel, specifically, the lack of professional education and research that focuses on people with disabilities who are too old for pediatric care and not old enough for geriatric care. The relative lack of service models approximating the pediatric and geriatric models is why families and adolescents feel that they drop into an abyss when a young person reaches age 18 or 20 or so. What programs exist are mostly diagnosis specific (e.g., for people with AIDS) and even then are generally not available to all people with the diagnosis. Dr. Turk pointed out that some model programs help adolescents with the transition from pediatric to adult services, providers, and programs. Widely available federal support may be needed for such programs to become more widely established.

Another issue for adolescents with disabilities is the high level of secondary mental health morbidity. This kind of secondary morbidity is not only a problem in itself but is also a behavioral risk factor for further problems (including those resulting from risky or self-destructive behaviors). This point prompted mention of the Surgeon General's new "call to action" on the health and wellness of persons with disabilities (Surgeon General of the United States, 2005). The document covers a broad range of topics, including some discussed in the workshop papers and presentations and other topics that need further consideration, for example, mental health problems.

In a comment about issues related to conducting research on exercise interventions to prevent or reduce disability, one participant cited Dr. Rimmer's observation about high dropout rates in exercise studies. That participant observed that people in certain target populations see themselves as having a fixed budget of energy that requires them to make trade-offs each day, for example, between using energy to participate in an exercise study versus using energy to do laundry. In this context, might not effectiveness research be just as important as efficacy research? That is, researchers should look at people's daily lives to determine whether something works in the real world, not just in a controlled trial situation. This participant asked whether researchers considered and investigated how people actually implement exercise in their daily lives and how they make trade-offs in spending their limited store of energy?

Dr. Rimmer responded that researchers bring people into laboratories. Although they may compare the characteristics of people who drop out versus the characteristics of those who continue with the research, they usually do not learn much about the actual reasons that people drop out of studies. Also, the studies he reviewed generally did not do "intention-to-treat" analyses and this limits the validity of the results because those who complete the exercise intervention may differ from those who drop out in ways that confound comparisons. How researchers can adapt their studies to accommodate people's real-life problems with transportation, energy limitations, and other barriers to research participation and the long-term effectiveness of an intervention is an important issue.

Another question arose about the contribution of pain to disability (defined as a limitation in performing socially expected roles, such as work). Dr. Turk noted that data sets vary in the amount of information available for the assessment of how pain may limit activities or participation. She agreed that it is important to consider the role of pain, whether it is an inadequately treated aspect of a primary condition or an aspect of a related secondary condition.

A participant then returned the discussion to the issue of exercise as an effective intervention in people's actual lives. It is important to understand dose-response relationships and to identify the critical thresholds (e.g., 20 versus 30 minutes of exercise) to achieve positive results for different kinds of interventions. Studies of this kind will help people with disabilities judge how they should invest their limited energy in exercise. The identification of interventions for which underlying biological mechanisms of effect have been identified should also help people make decisions about intervention options.

More generally, bringing together what is known in the basic sciences with what is known in applied or clinical sciences and epidemiological sciences is important, and real opportunity exists in this area. One example involves research on the biology of muscle contractures among people with limited mobility, a secondary condition that is a major focus of clinical prevention and management efforts. If scientists could identify the molecular switch that causes fibrous ingrowth into muscle, then ways to control that switch and prevent contractures from forming in the first place might be found.

A further research area with considerable promise involves the interaction between exercise-patterned activity and pharmacological options. For example, investigators studying rats have found that amphetamine does nothing by itself to rehabilitate a rat and that exercise has some effect, but amphetamine in combination with exercise potentiates the effect of exercise dramatically. Although it is difficult to do these types of studies with humans, the potential of such pharmacological strategies to improve the outcomes of exercise interventions is significant.

One participant noted the importance of both social and personal responsibility for improving the health and well-being of people with disabilities. There is a social responsibility—which has been greatly inadequate in practice—to provide individuals with access to services and technology that allow them to function better and participate in the community. In addition, people with and without disabilities have a personal responsibility to lead the healthiest lives possible, for example, by looking after their diet, exercise, and similar elements important to health. Persuading people to adopt health-promoting practices and supporting them in that effort are, unfortunately, difficult tasks, whether the focus is on people with disabilities or not.

Another concern with health promotion is access by children with disabilities to school physical education activities. These activities provide opportunities for learning good health behaviors and improving physical fitness that can have both short-term and long-term benefits. Education and health personnel need to coordinate their attention to the benefits of school physical education, the barriers encountered by children with disabilities, and the options for overcoming these barriers.

The discussion for this panel ended with an expression of concern about an impending crisis with Medicare, Medicaid, and private insurance programs. The result could be potentially dangerous reductions in financial access to services and equipment for people with disabilities. Monitoring the allocation of health care dollars will be important.

SECONDARY HEALTH CONDITIONS: PART II

Presentations

Dr. William Bauman discussed secondary conditions in the context of spinal cord injury. (Dr. Bauman's paper appears as Appendix M.) His presentation covered pulmonary, cardiac, metabolic, gastrointestinal, and dermatologic secondary conditions. Dr. Bauman recalled that when he made his first presentation on this topic at a conference in 1990, the audience did not at that time appreciate the importance of understanding secondary conditions as problems. Now the topic is firmly established in the field of spinal cord medicine.

As in the broader population, heart disease and lung disease are common causes of mortality and morbidity for people with spinal cord injuries. Individuals with spinal cord injuries have restrictive ventilatory dysfunction, and those with higher cord lesions also show evidence of airflow obstruction. The higher the spinal cord lesion, the greater the effect on respiratory muscles and the more difficulty people have breathing and coughing effectively. The tubes in the lung can become blocked, causing infection. Research has helped identify the level of impaired expiratory function that begins to cause problems. Whatever the technique—mechanical, pharmacological, electrical, or other—used to help people breathe better, it is important to mitigate this important contributor to mortality and morbidity.

Initially, some of the secondary complications for people with chronic spinal cord injury were not recognized because patients often did not survive long term. With improvements in long-term survival has come recognition of excess heart disease deaths in this group.

One contributor to these excess deaths is the predisposition of individuals with spinal cord injuries to the metabolic syndrome. People tend to develop insulin resistance, become obese, and develop carbohydrate and lipid abnormalities—in particular, low levels of high-density lipoprotein (HDL) or "good" cholesterol. Those with lower cord lesions also tend to have elevations in blood pressure. Data from the Framingham (Massachusetts) Heart Study demonstrate the health risks of low levels of HDL. For every 1-milligram-per-deciliter rise in the HDL cholesterol level, the risk of a cardiac event decreases by about 2 or, possibly, 3 percent (Castelli et al., 1986). For those with spinal cord injuries, the role of low-density lipoprotein (LDL), or "bad" cholesterol, is more complex, but evidence suggests that these individuals have smaller, denser, more atherogenic LDL particles, which is a risk factor beyond the actual LDL level itself.

Another risk factor related to the metabolic syndrome involves changes in body composition and insulin resistance. In people with spinal cord injuries, such changes occur both immediately and chronically. In general, the less active that a person is and the greater their level of body fat, the greater their extent of insulin resistance is. The mechanisms for these changes appear complex, possibly including (in addition to paralysis and immobilization) a reduction in anabolic forces and an elevation of catabolic hormones. In addition, those with the greatest neurologic impairment have the lowest frequency of normal glucose tolerance.

Management options for prevention of the development of diabetes and heart problems include increased activity, dietary changes, smoking cessation, and drug therapies. Some evidence suggests that even a small increase in the amount of exercise performed may be beneficial. Given the difficulty, cited earlier, in engaging people in exercise, this is encouraging.

Dr. Bauman went on to describe other secondary problems associated with spinal cord injury, one of which is difficulty with evacuation related to their injury. Bowel care is time-consuming, and shortfalls in such care increase morbidity. Cholinergic agents are effective but have adverse effects on the heart and on the lung. One promising area is combination drug therapy that selectively blocks these adverse effects.

Osteoporosis is another serious secondary problem. Losses in bone density occur very rapidly after injury and continue for years. It is particularly crucial to prevent bone loss immediately after the injury to avoid a compromised bone architecture that cannot be restored. Preventive strategies include drug and mechanical interventions. Vitamin D deficiency is also important in individuals with spinal cord injuries. More remains to be learned about vitamin supplementation strategies to prevent or limit osteoporosis in this group. Overall, more effective therapies to prevent or treat bone loss would improve employment prospects and other kinds of social participation.

Pressure ulcers are a tremendous source of morbidity in those with spinal cord injury and in the general population—probably costing about $8 billion to $10 billion a year nationwide for all care provided for this condition. Again, much remains to be learned about the development of pressure ulcers; rates of ulcer healing; and the roles of nutrition, inflammatory, and endocrine factors. Dr. Bauman noted that the Veterans Administration had funded a cooperative study to compare treatment with an oral anabolic agent against a placebo (each in combination with optimal clinical care) and assess the effects on the percentage of complete healing for pelvic region pressure ulcers. We will also learn more about the effects on healing rates of nutrition, inflammatory factors, and endocrine factors.

Dr. Bauman observed that most individuals with spinal cord injuries have learned to adapt to being paralyzed. In many respects, the secondary complications of the injury may have a greater impact on a person's quality of life than the loss of ambulation itself. The knowledge gained from studying the secondary consequences of spinal cord injuries can probably be transferred in large measure to other immobilizing conditions. Prevention and early intervention are important both to people's quality of life and to the costs of health care.

For the next presentation, Dr. Bryan Kemp spoke about depression in adults with disabilities. (Dr. Kemp's paper appears as Appendix N.) Whether depression should be categorized as a secondary condition or something else, it has important consequences for health and well-being. It is also a common and expensive problem for the population generally and affects every aspect of life: physical health, behavior, functioning, participation, interpersonal relations, and more.

Data indicate that depression is more common in people with disabilities and, in some respects, is more serious in this group. Compared with the rates of depression among people with no disability, the rates of depression among those with post-polio syndrome, rheumatoid arthritis, cerebral palsy, spinal cord injury, or stroke have been reported to be higher. Perhaps 1 person in 10 or 12 overall has a depressive disorder that warrants treatment. Among people with disabilities, the number is more like 1 person in 3 or 4.

Depression affects health and well-being both directly and indirectly because it reduces important brain transmitters as well as compliance with exercise and other health promotion activities and diminishes participation and social connections. One study of people with stroke reported that the 10-year survival rate was about 65 percent for those without depression but only about 30 percent for people with depression (Morris et al. (1993). Studies of change in functioning over time for people with disabilities report that depressed individuals show greater rates of decline than individuals without depression.

Dr. Kemp explained that the effects of aging present additional concerns for those with certain kinds of disabilities and increase the risk of depression. About 25 years after the onset of a disability (in a younger person) or at about 45 years of age (seemingly, whichever comes first), people begin to develop an inordinate number of new medical and function-related problems as well as pain, fatigue, and weakness. These changes are associated with higher rates of depression.

The literature supports some general statements about the causes of depression in people with disabilities. It does not appear to be directly related to the severity of the impairment; for example, more severe spinal cord injuries are not associated with higher rates of depression. Depression also does not appear to be related to the duration of impairment.

Dr. Kemp suggested that depression is most likely related to a person's ability to cope with the changes and losses that are associated with a disabling condition rather than to the existence of the condition per se. Studies also suggest that depression in people with disabilities is related to their financial status, level of social support, and other resources. For example, a study by Dickens and Creed (2001) reported a substantial increase in depression among people with disabilities who reported the loss of valued social or family activities.

Several factors seem to account for the inadequate treatment of depression in people in the community who have a disability. Lack of access to care is an important factor. In addition, symptoms of depression (such as fatigue) often overlap with symptoms of other health problems or disability effects. Some symptoms, such as apathy or irritability, may be missed by health care professionals who focus on feelings of sadness. Further, if professionals believe that depression is normal for people with disabilities, they will tend to undertreat it.

Dr. Kemp noted that long-term studies of treatment for depression among individuals living in the community are limited and that relatively few controlled treatment studies have been conducted. He reported that his group's quasiexperimental studies of combined pharmacotherapy and psychotherapy suggest that treatment for depression can be effective in several respects (Kemp et al., 2004). The group found that treatment reduced the level of depression and increased community participation; subsequently, people reported increased life satisfaction.

Many important areas for research remain. Some involve the better measurement of depression and outcomes in people with disabilities. Others relate to the short-term and long-term effectiveness of different treatment strategies, for example, comparison of early and late interventions and of different durations of therapies.

Dr. Tom Seekins made the final presentation, which covered secondary conditions among people with intellectual or developmental disabilities. This group numbers about 2 million to 4 million people in the United States. Estimates indicate that more than 350,000 adults with such disabilities live in more than 110,000 supported arrangements around the country. (The paper of Dr. Seekins and his colleagues, which appears as Appendix O, includes an updated estimate that over 420,000 adults with developmental disabilities live in over 148,000 such arrangements nationwide.)

Dr. Seekins described a community-based intervention strategy—a wellness club—that was designed for the target population and community. The strategy employed a surveillance model and instrument to support the planning and assessment of wellness services within the larger context of community-based services for people with developmental disabilities. First steps were the initiation of annual surveillance of health status at the community level and the evaluation of surveillance results at the state level, which provided the basis for setting priorities and mobilizing resources for changes at the local level. The surveillance instrument asked people to rate 45 secondary conditions. Using the responses, the investigators created a problem index based on the reported prevalence and the average reported severity. Data were also collected on 36 behavioral risk and protective factors and medical service utilization.

In the survey, the top three problems measured by the problem index were communication difficulties, physical conditioning problems, and weight problems. For those people reporting a problem, however, mobility problems had the highest average severity level. Among the risk factors for problems were stressful life changes, living arrangements, and turnover of personal assistance. Behavioral risk factors included inadequate physical activity and poor dietary habits.

Dr. Seekins also discussed the design of individual service plans for adults with developmental or intellectual disabilities who are living in supported arrangements in the community. Individual service plans, which are required by law, guide the provision of services for consumers and provide the blueprint for organizing the treatment environment. Dr. Seekins noted some positive preliminary findings that suggest that individual service plans that took a secondary condition into account were associated with more declines in problems than plans that did not, but no well-designed controlled studies have been conducted.

The individual service plan directs the activities of personal assistants, who are critical environmental elements. Again, preliminary findings suggest that turnover and change involving assistants are risk factors for secondary conditions. Also, the worse that the condition is initially, the larger the effect is.

Dr. Seekins' group is also looking at the impact of nutrition with a study in group homes that analyzed the home's menus and pantry contents for consistency with the formal nutrition plans for residents. They did not find a good match. An analysis of oral health arrangements in the homes showed a better match between these arrangements and the individual service plans.

Such analyses provide only snapshots of a person's overall situation. As described by Dr. Seekins, the "wellness club" approach is designed to be comprehensive by integrating wellness goals into the individual planning process on an ongoing, annual basis. The approach covers healthy home environments, the individual's health and lifestyle, assessment procedures for identification of the individual's needs and priorities, staff instruction, and methods for program and progress evaluation. The club strategy is also designed to provide participants a sense of belonging to something that is fun. The approach is being pilot tested in Montana and Kansas. The formal evaluation process is just beginning.

Discussion

The discussion began with a question about depression as a primary condition that can be disabling and that may also give rise to secondary conditions. Dr. Kemp agreed that depression can certainly be a primary condition as well as a secondary condition and that it may be complex to sort this out for an individual patient. The identification of coexisting or primary depression and the assessment of prevention and management needs in this context are important.

Another question arose about the risk factors for depression as a secondary condition. Part of Dr. Kemp's response emphasized the importance of positive social relationships and, conversely, the potential for negative relationships to increase secondary depression. Also important are personal attitudes and appraisals; for example, self-blame for a disabling injury is associated with the development of depression.

One participant stressed the importance of considering behavioral health issues, noting that the primary disabling condition for 60 percent of Medicaid recipients is some kind of severe and persistent mental health problem. Also, for children and families, learning disabilities can be described as hidden disabilities because they may not be obvious. It may be difficult to convince people that a cognitive processing deficit or other learning condition exists, that it may not be susceptible to medical treatment, and that it will persist into adulthood with all sorts of possible negative consequences, including incarceration.

These observations prompted further discussion of the attitudes and expectations of health care professionals, for example, whether they consider depression to be a normal consequence of disability and then, to some extent, discount it or overlook it as a preventable and treatable source of distress and suffering that can complicate many aspects of care management. Dr. Kemp suggested that professionals who routinely care for people with disabilities are sensitive to depression as a potential problem and may evaluate an individual for depression when functional or other problems seem to be occurring or persisting to an extent that is not anticipated, given other aspects of the individual's medical, treatment, and personal circumstances.

The chair asked if there were any general comments. One participant noted the changing profile of the American population and the increasing significance of immigrants. This development has implications and presents challenges for the provision of services to people with disabilities. Another concern is emerging disabilities or the transformation of diseases such as AIDS into chronic conditions for which people require rehabilitation or other assistance. The role of cognitive limitations was raised again with the observation that such limitations were far more common in connection with traumatic brain injury and other conditions than many of the problems discussed in the workshop. A related question was what to do about disabling conditions that "come out of left field," with autism offered as an example.

One participant stated that the evidence base for understanding, preventing, and mitigating disabling conditions is getting stronger. She also cited a series of meetings that are being sponsored by the Agency for Healthcare Research and Quality and the Robert Wood Johnson Foundation to discuss alternative study designs to strengthen and promote research on these and other conditions. Given the practical and ethical challenges of conducting randomized, double-blind clinical trials, it is important to consider observational and other studies at the same time that efforts are made to improve the methods and tools for such studies. The capacity to undertake rehabilitation research is also relevant. Adequate funding for the support of such research is part of the picture, but more fundamental aspects of the research capacity or infrastructure may need attention.

A different research issue relates to the data used to describe and assess the delivery of rehabilitative services. The data in this area are much poorer than the data for emergency room services or physician office visits.

With respect to longitudinal data, one participant encouraged the committee to look at the National Children's Study (sponsored by the National Institute on Child Health and Human Development and the Centers for Disease Control and Prevention, among other agencies).[1] It may eventually generate long-term data relevant to secondary conditions and other problems discussed at the workshop.

Questions were raised about the extent to which an IOM study would examine problems that are not related primarily to health care, such as access to employment. Certainly, participation as a concept is itself not primarily medical. Likewise, the creation or modification of the built environment is not primarily a health care function, but that environment is very important not only to the participation of people in society but also to the maintenance of mobility and the prevention of mobility decline in people with chronic conditions. Schooling is another important arena that offers opportunities for prevention and health promotion.

The vulnerability of people with disabilities to physical or mental abuse by caregivers (which may range from the withholding of prostheses to sexual violence) is a further cross-cutting environmental issue. For example, inadequacies in adult protective services, inappropriate placements of people with certain kinds of disabilities, and a lack of treatment or protection in settings such as jails create conditions for abuse.

---

[1]Information of this study can be found online at http://www.nationalchildrensstudy.gov/about/mission/index.cfm.

One participant cautioned against getting too preoccupied with theoretical or conceptual models to the extent that attention is diverted from significant practical and policy issues. The experiences of the two earlier IOM committees and those involved with WHO and ICF suggests that such a preoccupation is a likely—and difficult to avoid—hazard. In a final observation, another participant urged the IOM committee not to forget the personal dimension, the direct experiences of people living with disabilities.

REFERENCES

American Academy of Pediatrics, American Academy of Family Physicians, and American College of Physicians-American Society of Internal Medicine. 2002. A consensus statement on health care transition for young adults with special health care needs. *Pediatrics* 110:1304–1306.

Castelli WP, Garrison RJ, Wilson PWF, Abbott RD, Kalousdian S, Kannel WB. 1986. Incidence of coronary heart disease and lipoprotein cholesterol levels: the Framingham Study. *Journal of the American Medical Association* 256:2835–2838.

Child Trends Data Bank. Available online at www.childtrendsdatabank.org. (Last accessed November 21, 2005.)

Crimmins EM, Saito Y, Reynolds SL. 1997. Further evidence on recent trends in the prevalence and incidence of disability among older Americans from two sources: the LSOA and the NHIS. *Journals of Gerontology* 52(2):S59–S71.

Dickens, C, Creed, F. 2001. The burden of depression in patients with rheumatoid arthritis. *Rheumatology* 40:1327–1330.

Fougeyrollas P. 1995. Documenting environmental factors for preventing the handicap creation process: Quebec contributions relating to ICIDH and social participation of people with functional differences. *Disability and Rehabilitation* 17(3-4):145-53.

Fougeyrollas P, Noreau L, St Michel G. 1997. Measure of the quality of the environment. *ICIDH and Environmental Factors International Network* 9(1):32-39.

Freedman VA, Martin LG, Schoeni RF. 2002. Recent trends in disability and functioning among older adults in the United States: a systematic review. *Journal of the American Medical Association* 288(24):3137–3146.

Guralnik JM, LaCroix AZ, Abbott RD, et al. 1993. Maintaining mobility in late life. I. Demographic characteristics and chronic conditions. *American Journal of Epidemiology* 137:845–857.

IOM (Institute of Medicine). 1991. *Disability in America: Toward a National Agenda for Prevention.* Washington, DC: National Press Academy.

IOM. 1997. *Enabling America: Assessing the Role of Rehabilitation Science and Engineering.* Washington, DC: National Academy Press.

Kemp BJ, Kahan JK, Krause JS, Adkins RH, Nava G. 2004. Treatment of major depression in individuals with spinal cord injury. *Journal of Spinal Cord Medicine* 27:22–28.

Keysor J, Jette A, et al. 2005. Development of the home and community environment (HACE) instrument. *Journal of Rehabilitation Medicine* 37(1):37–44.

Leveille SG, Guralnik JM, Hochberg M, Hirsch R, Ferrucci L, Langlois J, Rantanen T, Ling S. 1999. Low back pain and disability in older women: independent association with difficulty but not inability to perform daily activities. *The Journals of Gerontology. Series A, Biological Sciences and Medical Sciences* 54(10):M487–M493.

Lollar DJ. 1994 (February 17-19). *Preventing Secondary Conditions Associated with Spina Bifida or Cerebral Palsy: Proceedings and Recommendations of a Symposium,* Crystal

City, Virginia. Washington, DC: Spina Bifida Association of America. Available online at http://www.cdc.gov/ncbddd/dh/Publications/Conferences/1994aSB_CP/1994aTableof Contents.htm. (Last accessed September 26, 2005.)

Lotstein D, McPherson M, Strickland B, Newacheck P. 2005. Transition planning for youth with special health care needs: results from the National Survey of Children with Special Health Care Needs. *Pediatrics* 115:1562–1568.

Manton KG, Corder LS, Stallard E. 1993. Estimates of change in chronic disability and institutional incidence and prevalence rates in the U.S. elderly population from the 1982, 1984, and 1989 National Long Term Care Survey. *Journals of Gerontology* 48(4):S153–166.

Manton KG, Corder L, Stallard E. 1997. Chronic disability trends in elderly United States populations: 1982–1994. *Proceedings of the National Academy of Sciences* 94(6):2593–2598.

Marge, M. 1988. Health promotion for persons with disabilities moving beyond rehabilitation. *American Journal of Health Promotion* 2(4):29–35.

Morris PLP, Robinson RG, Andrzejewski MS, Samuels J, Price TR. 1993. Association of depression with 10-year post-stroke mortality. *American Journal of Psychiatry* 150:124–129.

Newacheck PW, Budetti PP, Halfon N. 1986. Trends in activity-limiting chronic conditions among children. *American Journal of Public Health* 76:178–184.

NRC/IOM (National Research Council and Institute of Medicine). 2004. *Children's Health, the Nation's Wealth: Assessing and Improving Child Health*. Washington, DC: The National Academies Press.

Sameroff AJ and Chandler MJ. 1975. Reproductive risk and the continuum of caretaking casualty. In Horowitz FD, Hetherington M, Scarr-Salapatek S, and Siegel G, eds. *Review of Child Development Research*, Vol 4, pp. 187–244. Chicago: University of Chicago Press.

Schoeni R, Martin L, Andreski P, Freedman V. 2005. Growing disparities in trends in old-age disability 1982–2001. *American Journal of Public Health* 95(11):2065-2070.

Shumway-Cook A, Patla AE, Stewart A, Ferrucci L, Ciol MA, Guralnik JM. 2002. Environmental demands associated with community mobility in older adults with and without mobility disabilities. *Physical Therapy* 82(7):670-81.

Surgeon General of the United States. 2005. *The Surgeon General's Call to Action to Improve the Health and Wellness of Persons with Disabilities*. Washington, DC: U.S. Department of Health and Human Services. Available online at http://www.surgeongeneral.gov/library/disabilities/calltoaction/calltoaction.pdf. (Last accessed September 26, 2005.)

Verbrugge LM, Jette AM. 1994. The disablement process. *Social Science Medicine* 38(1):1–14.

Volpato S, Blaum C, Resnick H, Ferrucci L, Fried LP, Guralnik JM. 2002. Women's Health and Aging Study. Comorbidities and impairments explaining the association between diabetes and lower extremity disability: The Women's Health and Aging Study. *Diabetes Care* 25(4):678–683.

Whiteneck G, Gerhart KA, et al. 2004. Identifying environmental factors that influence the outcomes of people with traumatic brain injury. *Journal of Head Trauma Rehabilitation* 19(3):191–204.

WHO (World Health Organization). 1980. *International Classification of Impairments, Disabilities and Handicaps: a Manual of Classification Relating to the Consequences of Disease*. Geneva, Switzerland: World Health Organization.

WHO. 2001. *International Classification of Functioning, Disability and Health*. Geneva, Switzerland: World Health Organization.

A

Workshop Agenda and Participants

INSTITUTE OF MEDICINE
WORKSHOP ON DISABILITY IN AMERICA
August 1, 2005
AGENDA

8:30   **Welcomes and Introductions**

Alan Jette, Ph.D., Chair
Institute of Medicine Committee on Disability in America

Jose Cordero, M.D.
Director, National Center on Birth Defects and Development
Centers for Disease Control and Prevention

Steven Tingus, M.S.
Director, National Institute for Disability and Rehabilitation
Research

Michael Weinrich, M.D.
National Center for Medical Rehabilitation Research

39

8:45   **Disability Concepts, Models, and Measures**

Issues and Questions Involving Adults
Gale Whiteneck, Ph.D.
Director of Research
Craig Hospital

Issues and Questions Involving Children and Adolescents
Rune Simeonsson, Ph.D.
Professor of Education
University of North Carolina

Research on Environmental Factors
Julie Keysor, Ph.D.
Assistant Professor of Physical Therapy
Boston University Sargent College of Health and
    Rehabilitation Sciences

Discussion

10:20   Break

10:45   **Trends in Disability**

Trends in Disability in Late Life
Vicki Freedman, Ph.D.
Professor of Health Systems and Policy
School of Public Health
University of Medicine and Dentistry of New Jersey

Trends in Disability in Midlife
Jay Bhattacharya, Ph.D.
Assistant Professor of Medicine
Center for Primary Care and Outcomes Research
Stanford University

Trends in Disability in Early Life
Ruth E.K. Stein, M.D.
Professor of Pediatrics
Albert Einstein College of Medicine/Children's Hospital at
    Montefiore

Discussion

Noon   Lunch

1:00   **Aspects of Disability Across the Life Span**

Risk Factors for Disability in Late Life
Jack Guralnik, M.D., Ph.D.
Chief, Epidemiology and Demography Section
National Institute on Aging

Transitions for Adolescents with Disabilities
John G. Reiss, Ph.D.
Chief, Division of Policy and Program Affairs
Institute for Child Health Policy
University of Florida College of Medicine

Discussion

2:00   **Secondary Health Conditions: Concepts, Data, and Examples
(Part I)**

Overview
Margaret A. Turk, M.D.
Professor of Physical Medicine and Rehabilitation
State University of New York Upstate Medical University

Secondary Health Conditions and Aging with Disability:
Consumer Perspective
June Kailes, M.S.W.
Disability Policy Consultant

Effects of Exercise on Specific Secondary Conditions
James H. Rimmer, Ph.D., Professor
Director, Center on Health Promotion Research for Persons
with Disabilities
University of Illinois at Chicago

Discussion

3:30   Break

3:50   **Secondary Health Conditions (Part II)**

Secondary Conditions with Spinal Cord Injury

William A. Bauman, M.D.
Professor of Medicine and Rehabilitation Medicine
Mount Sinai School of Medicine

Depression as a Secondary Condition in Adults with Disability
Bryan Kemp, Ph.D.
Professor of Medicine and Psychology
University of California, Irvine

Preventing the Progression of Secondary Conditions with
Developmental Disabilities
Tom Seekins, Ph.D.
Director
University of Montana Rural Institute

Discussion

Adjourn

WORKSHOP PARTICIPANTS

Registrants

Gerald Adler
Office of Research
Centers for Medicare and Medicaid
  Services
U.S. Department of Health and
  Human Services

Noreen M. Aziz
Senior Program Director
Division of Cancer Control &
  Population Sciences
National Cancer Institute
National Institutes of Health

M. Nell Bailey
Rehabilitation Engineering and
Assistive Technology Society of
  North America

Laura Beckwith
Executive Director
Helen Keller Foundation

Helena Berger
Chief Operating Officer
American Association of People
  with Disabilities

Janis Berman
March of Dimes

Edward Brann
Director
Division of Human Development
  and Disability
Centers for Disease Control and
  Prevention

Ruth Brannon
Associate Director
Division of Research Sciences
National Institute on Disability and
  Rehabilitation Research

Hazel Breland
Occupational Therapist
University of Pittsburgh

Ethel Briggs
Executive Director
National Council on Disability

Tricia Brooks
Director of Government Relations
Christopher Reeve Foundation

Mary Cerreto
Associate Professor of Family
  Medicine
Boston University

Daofen Chen
Program Director of Systems and
  Cognitive Neuroscience
National Institute of Neurological
  Disorders and Stroke

Barney Cohen
Director, Committee on Population
National Academies

Jose Cordero
Director
National Center on Birth Defects
  and Developmental Disabilities

Deborah Cotter
Senior Legislative Assistant
Public Policy Office
American Psychological
  Association

David Coulter
Associate Professor, Neurology
Harvard Medical School

John Crews
Lead Scientist, Disability and
  Health
Centers for Disease Control and
  Prevention

M. Doreen Croser
Executive Director
American Association on Mental
  Retardation

Diane Damiano
Research Associate Professor of
  Neurology
Washington University
Representative, American Academy
  for Cerebral Palsy and
  Developmental Medicine

Gerben DeJong
Senior Fellow
National Rehabilitation Hospital

Robert Demichelis II
Legislative Liaison
Brain Injury Association of
  America

Brian Denger
Director of Education
Parent Project Muscular Dystrophy

Ketki Desai
Graduate student researcher of
occupational therapy
University of Pittsburgh

John Ditunno
Project Director
Rehabilitation Medicine
Regional Spinal Cord Injury Center
  of the Delaware Valley
Thomas Jefferson University

Sheila Fitzgerald
President
American Association of
  Occupational Health Nurses

Karen Flippo
Executive Director
National Association of Councils
  on Developmental Disabilities

Bruce M. Gans
Kessler Rehabilitation Corporation

Turner Goins
Associate Professor
West Virginia University

Suzanne Goldberg
National Heart, Lung, and Blood
  Institute
National Institutes of Health

Martin Gould
Director of Research and
  Technology
National Council on Disability

Andrew Guccione
Senior Vice President
Division of Practice and Research
American Physical Therapy
  Association

Kenneth Harwood
Director
American Physical Therapy Association

Ann A. Hohmann
Chief
Methods & Disablement Program
National Institute of Mental
  Health

Ann Huston
Executive Director
American Therapeutic Recreation
  Association

George Jesien
Executive Director
Association of University Centers
  on Disabilities

Maureen Kameda
Association of Occupational
  Health Professionals
Chapter Member, Virginia

Anne M. Kennedy
Muscular Dystrophy Association

Anju Khubchandani
Disability Issues Officer
Public Interest Directorate
American Psychological
  Association

Robert Klein
Statistician
Office of the Actuary
U.S. Department of Veterans Affairs

Pamela Larsen
Associate Dean/Director
University of North Carolina at
  Charlotte

Paul Lipkin
Chair
Council on Children with
  Disabilities
American Academy of Pediatrics

Don Lollar
Senior Research Scientist
Centers for Disease Control and
  Prevention

Elizabeth Lopez
Substance Abuse & Mental Health
  Services Administration
U.S. Department of Health and
  Human Services

Michael Manganiello
Senior Vice President, Government
  Relations
Christopher Reeve Foundation

Donna Martinez
Graduate Student
The George Washington University

Dennis Matthews
American Board of Physical
  Medicine and Rehabilitation

Michael McGeary
Study Director
Institute of Medicine

Merle McPherson
Director
Division of Services for Children
  with Special Needs
U.S. Department of Health and
  Human Services

J. Mark Melhorn
American Academy of Orthopedic
  Surgeons

John Melvin
Thomas Jefferson University

Justin Moore
Director
Congressional Affairs
American Physical Therapy
  Association

Charles Moseley
Director of Special Projects
National Association of State
  Directors of Developmental
  Disabilities Services

Margaret Nygren
Technical Assistance Director
Association of University Centers
  on Disability

Susan Palsbo
Principal Research Associate
Center for Health Policy, Research
  & Ethics

D.E.B. Potter
Senior Survey Statistician
Agency for Healthcare Research
  and Quality

Susan Prokop
Associate Advocacy Director
Paralyzed Veterans of America

Louis Quatrano
National Center for Medical
  Rehabilitation Research
National Institutes of Health

Anne P. Rohall
Director
Government Relations
National Association of Councils
    on Developmental Disabilities

Paddy Rossbach
President and CEO
Amputee Coalition of America

Peter Rzeszotarski
Acting Associate Director
Centers for Disease Control and
    Prevention

Judith Sangl
Health Scientist Administrator
Agency for Healthcare Research
    and Quality

Harvey Schwartz
Senior Adviser for Priority
    Populations
Agency for Healthcare Research
    and Quality

Arthur Sherwood
Science and Technology Advisor
National Institute on Disability and
    Rehabilitation Research
U.S. Department of Education

Nancy Shinowara
Program Director
National Center for Medical
    Rehabilitation Research
National Institute of Child Health
    and Human Development
National Institutes of Health

Elizabeth Skidmore
Assistant Professor
Department of Occupational
    Therapy
University of Pittsburgh

Frederick Somers
Executive Director
American Occupational Therapy
    Association

Karen Steinberg
Senior Science and Public Health
    Official (Acting)
Coordinating Center for Health
    Promotion
Centers for Disease Control and
    Prevention

Donald Stockford
Program Analyst
Veterans Health Administration
U.S. Department of Veterans
    Affairs

Kathy Sykes
Senior Adviser
Aging Initiative
U.S. Environmental Protection
    Agency

Kate Tiedeman
Intern
Aging Initiative
U.S. Environmental Protection
    Agency

Steven Tingus
Director
National Institute on Disability and
    Rehabilitation Research
U.S. Department of Education

Nancy White
President
Foundation of Physical Therapy

John Whyte
Director of Research
Moss Rehabilitation Research
Institute

Carolyn Zollar
Vice President
Government Relations and Policy
Development
American Medical Rehabilitation
Providers Association

Presenters

William A. Bauman
Director
Spinal Cord Damage Research
Center

Jay Bhattacharya
Assistant Professor of Medicine
Stanford University

Vicki A. Freedman
Professor
Department of Health Systems and
Policy
School of Public Health
University of Medicine and
Dentistry of New Jersey

Jack Guralnik
Acting Chief
Laboratory of Epidemiology,
Demography and Biometry
National Institute of Aging

June Kailes
Disability Policy Consultant
Associate Director
Adjunct Associate Professor
Center for Disability Issues and the
Health Professions
Western University of Health
Sciences

Bryan Kemp
Clinical Professor of Medicine and
Psychology
Director, Gerontology Program
University of California, Irvine
Director, Rehabilitation Research
and Training Center on Aging
with Disability
Rancho Los Amigos National
Rehabilitation Center

John G. Reiss
Chief, Division of Policy and
Program Affairs
Institute for Child Health Policy
Associate Professor of Pediatrics
and of Epidemiology and Health
Policy Research
University of Florida College of
Medicine

James H. Rimmer
Professor and Director
National Center on Physical
Activity and Disability and
Rehabilitation Engineering
Research Center on Recreational
Technologies and Exercise
Physiology
University of Illinois at Chicago

Tom Seekins
Director
RTC: Rural
Professor of Psychology
University of Montana

Rune J. Simeonsson
Professor of Education
Frank Porter Graham
Child Development Center
University of North Carolina–
Chapel Hill

Ruth E.K. Stein
Professor of Pediatrics and Vice
Chair
Department of Pediatrics
Albert Einstein College of Medicine

Margaret A. Turk
Professor
Physical Medicine & Rehabilitation
State University of New York
Upstate Medical Center

Michael Weinrich
Director
National Center for Medical
Rehabilitation Research
National Institute of Child Health
and Human Development

Gale Whiteneck
Director of Research
Craig Hospital

IOM Committee (as of workshop date)

Alan M. Jette, Committee Chair
Director
Health & Disability Research
Institute
Boston University

Elena Andresen
Professor and Chief
Epidemiology Division
Department of Health Services
Research, Management, and
Policy
University of Florida Health
Sciences Center

Dudley S. Childress
Professor of Biomedical
Engineering and Physical
Medicine and Rehabilitation
McCormick School of Engineering
and Feinberg School of
Medicine
Northwestern University

Vicki A. Freedman
Professor
Department of Health Systems and
Policy
School of Public Health
University of Medicine and
Dentistry of New Jersey

Patricia Hicks
Director
Continuity of Care Clinic
University of Texas Southwestern
Medical School
University of Texas Southwestern
Medical Center at Dallas

Lisa I. Iezzoni
Professor of Medicine
Harvard University and Beth Israel
Deaconess Medical Center

June Isaacson Kailes
Associate Director
Center for Disability Issues and the
  Health Professions
Western University of Health
  Sciences

Laura Mosqueda
Director of Geriatrics
Professor of Family Medicine
University of California, Irvine
  School of Medicine

P. Hunter Peckham
Donnell Professor of Biomedical
  Engineering and Orthopedics
Case Western Reserve University

James Marc Perrin
Professor of Pediatrics
Harvard Medical School and
  Massachusetts General Hospital

IOM Staff

Marilyn J. Field, Study Director

Afrah Ali, Senior Program
  Assistant

Andrew Pope, Director,
  Board on Health Sciences Policy

Linda G. Martin, Scholar in
  Residence

B

Conceptual Models of Disability: Past, Present, and Future

Gale Whiteneck*

In the last quarter century, the conceptualization of disability has progressed dramatically. Two World Health Organization (WHO) international classification systems serve as bookends to this period. The WHO *International Classification of Impairments, Disabilities, and Handicaps* (ICIDH),[1] published in 1980, suggested conceptual distinctions among three levels of performance—impairment at the organ level, disability at the person level, and handicap at the societal level. However, ICIDH sparked controversy by labeling the societal level as "handicap" and by failing to incorporate environmental factors. Twenty-one years later, WHO published its revision of ICIDH as the *International Classification of Functioning, Disability and Health* (ICF),[2] which replaced the three dimensions with more appropriate labels (body structure and function at the organ level, activity at the person level, and participation at the societal level) and recognized the importance of environmental factors with a new categorization system.

Between these two events, several advances articulated the significant role of the environment in the lives of people with disabilities. The Americans with Disabilities Act[3] established full participation in society as the goal for all people with disabilities and ensured their right to reasonable accommodation to achieve it. The National Institute on Disability and

---

*Gale Whiteneck, Ph.D., Director of Research, Craig Hospital, Englewood, Colorado. The analyses and views presented in this workshop paper are those of the author and not necessarily those of the Institute of Medicine Committee on Disability in America: A New Look.

Rehabilitation Research provided the new paradigm of disability that focused attention on the imperative of environmental modifications to improve the lives of people with disabilities.[4] The Institute of Medicine's (IOM's) book *Enabling America*[5] promoted the importance of environmental factors for people with disabilities. Researchers focused their attention on the development of participation and environmental measures, including the Craig Handicap Assessment and Reporting Technique,[6, 7] the Community Integration Questionnaire,[8] and the Craig Hospital Inventory of Environmental Factors.[9, 10]

Although the models theoretically incorporated the importance of environmental factors, little empirical evidence exists to support the theory. For example, spinal cord injury (SCI)-related research has linked impairment and disability to participation. Although the severity of the impairment had a strong relationship with the performance of activities of daily living, the research found no strong links between impairment or disability measures and participation.[11, 12] A meta-analysis conducted by Dijkers[13] concluded that participation was more strongly related to quality of life than to either impairment or disability.

MODELS OF DISABILITY

Society's and researchers' conceptualizations of disability have evolved over time. As noted in *Enabling America*[5] and on the basis of public policy at the time, "In the 1950s, impairment of a given severity was viewed as sufficient to result in disability in all circumstances; in contrast, the absence of impairment of that severity was thought to be sufficient grounds to deny disability benefits" (p. 63) Although the practice of rehabilitation certainly existed before then, it was not until the 1960s and the 1970s that conceptual frameworks for modeling disability appeared. These conceptual frameworks allowed greater scientific inquiry into both disability and rehabilitation.

In 1972, WHO, recognizing a need for better methods to evaluate health care, sought to expand the medical model of illness that provided the basis for its International Classification of Disease (ICD).[14] WHO recognized that ICD[14] suited the study of the outcomes of acute diseases and injuries that can be prevented or cured but that the medical model did a woefully inefficient job of detecting the consequences of nonacute diseases, particularly chronic and progressive or irreversible disorders. In 1980, WHO published ICIDH[1] as "a manual of classification relating to the consequences of disease." It extended the disease-related sequence of etiology, pathology, and manifestation with the illness-related sequence of disease, impairment, disability, and handicap. Although the original ICIDH model acknowledges a role of the environment by stating that "handicaps thus reflect interaction with and adaptation to the individual's surroundings," it has been criticized for its lack of an explicit recognition of the environmental role in its model.

Nagi[15] also recognized the process by which a pathology (e.g., arthritis) may lead to an impairment (e.g., limited joint range of motion), which may then result in a functional limitation (e.g., an inability to type), which ultimately may result in disability (e.g., an inability to work as a secretary). Possibly because of his attention to employment rather than health care services, Nagi noted that correlations among impairments, functional limitations, and social roles, such as employment, were poor. Unlike ICIDH, Nagi's model explicitly recognized that the environment could be studied separately from the individual and initiated research into environmental factors in the family, the community, and society that affect disability as an outcome. Fougeyrollas[19] further clarified the influence of environmental factors on social participation in a manner consistent with the Nagi approach.

Verbrugge and Jette[16] proposed an expanded model of the disablement process to account for behaviors and attributes that increase the risks of or that provide buffers to functional limitations and disability, elements not specified in Nagi's medical model. Relevant factors include both intraindividual characteristics (e.g., behavioral change and locus of control) and extraindividual characteristics (e.g., medical care, environmental barriers or adaptations, and instrumental support) that may operate at various points along the disablement trajectory.

IOM, in *Disability in America*,[17] derived its conceptual model of disability directly from Nagi and, in fact, defined disability "by the attributes and interactions of the individual and the environment" (p. 82). In the IOM model, risk factors exist not only within the individual but also in the physical and social environments, all of which theoretically affect the disability process. In the more recent IOM report, *Enabling America*,[5] the conceptual model was modified to emphasize that "the environment plays a critical role in determining whether each stage of disablement occurs and if transitions between the stages occur" (p. 64). The National Center for Medical Rehabilitation Research (NCMRR), in its research plan for the National Institutes of Health,[18] also emphasized the environment by use of a category of function called "societal limitations," which it defined as "restrictions attributable to social policy or barriers (structural or attitudinal) which limit fulfillment of roles or deny access to services and opportunities associated with full participation in society" (p. 25).

In addition to environmental factors, some researchers have argued that personal factors such as age, gender, and race also deserve separate consideration in disability theory. Personal factors may appear to be separate features of the individual distinct from a particular health condition or health state, yet they may influence the disability process. Such factors may also include variables such as habits, lifestyles, experiences, coping styles, and other psychological assets that may play a confounding role in the structural modeling of disability.[19]

WHO's ICF provides the most recent and, arguably, most comprehensive model of disability.[2] It revises the earlier ICIDH[1] by using less pejorative language (e.g., "participation" replaces "handicap" as a functional domain), explicitly incorporating environmental and personal factors as "contextual factors" that affect disability outcomes, and recognizing multiple levels and directions of potential causal relationships. Table B.1 summarizes key models of disability and illustrates the confusion attributable to the inconsistent terminology used to label conceptual domains.

ICF DOMAINS OF DISABILITY

WHO designed ICF[2] to achieve a better scientific understanding of health and health outcomes. ICF provides a common language of health to enable sharing of data among countries and health care providers. ICF describes broad health-related domains that can be transformed into a meaningful and consistent coding system. The ICF Model of Disability[2] is depicted in Figure B.1.

ICF has two parts: Part 1 covers functioning and disability, and Part 2 deals with contextual factors. Components of functioning and disability include body function and structure, activities, and participation. Components of contextual factors include environmental factors and personal factors. The model conceives these components as separate but related constructs with dynamic interactions between health conditions, like disease, disorders, and injuries, and contextual factors, such as personal and environmental factors.

Describing the model component body functions and structure, ICF refers to the "body" as the human organism. It includes not only physical aspects of the human body but mental functions as well. Body functions encompass the physiological and psychological functions of body systems. Body structures include the anatomical parts of the body, including the limbs and organs. ICF defines impairment as a problem in the body function or structure that results in a significant deviation or loss. Impairment does not always indicate the presence of disease and has a broader and more inclusive scope than disease. Impairments may cause other impairments; for example, impaired brain function may cause impaired cognitive function.

The ICF graphic model (Figure B.1) differentiates between the second and the third levels, activities and participation.[2] Activities refer to "the execution of a task or action by an individual," and participation refers to "involvement in a life situation." Examples of activities include listening, walking, and eating. Participation items describe roles that people perform,

TABLE B.1 Concepts and Terminology Used by Models of Disability

Model, Year	Origin	Organ Level	Person Level	Societal Level	Other Domains
Nagi, 1976[15]	Pathology	Impairment	Functional limitations	Disability	
WHO, 1980[1]	Disease	Impairment	Disability	Handicap	
IOM, 1991[17]	Pathology	Impairment	Functional limitations	Disability	
NCMRR, 1992[18]	Patho-Physiology	Impairment	Functional limitations	Disability	Societal limitations
IOM, 1997[5]	Pathology	Impairment	Functional limitations	Disability	Environmental factors quality of life
WHO, 2001[2]	Health Condition	Body structure and function	Activity	Participation	Environmental factors, personal factors

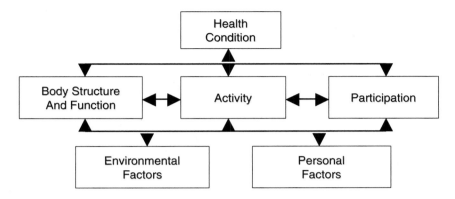

FIGURE B.1 ICF model of disability.[2]

such as forming relationships with others, caring for a household, or seeking and maintaining employment.

Although ICF depicts activities and participation separately in the graphic model, it uses one coding structure for both and covers the major areas of activity that one encounters throughout a life span. The list of domains includes learning and the application of knowledge, general tasks and demands; communication; mobility; self-care; domestic life; interpersonal interactions and relationships; major life areas; and community, social, and civic life. ICF defines difficulties as activity limitations or participation restrictions and measures them by comparing the performance of an individual with a health condition (a disease, injury, or disorder) with that of an individual without the condition. The difference between what one actually sees and what one expects to see provides a measure of the limitation.

One of two contextual components of ICF, environmental factors, includes the physical, social, and attitudinal environments, or the external factors of an individual's life. These factors can have either a negative influence ("barrier") or a positive influence ("facilitator") on a person's performance in society, on an individual's ability to carry out tasks, or on an individual's body function and structure. ICF organizes environmental factors into two levels: individual and societal. Individual environmental factors include the immediate environment of the individual, such as home and work: the physical or material features of the environment, as well as the individual's interaction with family, peers, acquaintances, and strangers. Societal factors include formal and informal services and systems in the community that affect a person's life. Societal factors encompass organizations and services related to work, community activities, government agencies, communication services, and transportation services.

Finally, ICF[2] identifies personal factors as "the particular background of an individual's life and living, and comprises features of the individual that are not part of health condition or health states" (p. 17). For example, these factors include gender, minority status, age, lifestyle, habits, upbringing, coping styles, education, profession, personality characteristics, marital status, and overall behavioral patterns. All of these factors may play a role in disability at any level, and although ICF does not classify these factors because of the large social and cultural variances that exist within them, it acknowledges their potential importance.

Although much progress has been made in refining disability models, categories of function, and the role of the environment,[1, 20, 21] only limited quantitative studies[22, 23, 24] have attempted to validate the models.

SUMMARY AND CRITIQUE OF ICF

This author's assessments of ICF compared with past models and the models of disability that are needed in the future can be summarized in the following title used in a recent presentation: "The ICF, one step forward, one step back, and a few steps yet to go for a complete model."[25] The one step forward was the inclusion of environmental factors; the one step back was the blurring of activities and participation; and the needed steps include the differentiation of activities and participation, the addition of quality of life to the model, elaboration of the impact of environmental factors, the development of personal factors, refinement of the graphic depiction of the model, definition of research strategies to better measure the domains of disability, and validation of the model.

Background on the Revision of ICF

ICF lists hundreds of people from scores of countries who were involved in the decade-long revision process. The author's comments here reflect a view of that process as gleaned from attendance at dozens of North American and international meetings. Although several cosmetic changes were made to ICIDH in the revision to ICF, substantive changes were also made. The cosmetic changes that occurred in the revision to ICF were the relabeling of the domains. That was necessary from the U.S. standpoint because the term "handicap" was completely unacceptable to the disability advocacy community because of its pejorative nature. ICF made an effort to use labels that were more neutral in tone, so "impairment" became "body structure and function," disability became "activity," and "handicap" became "participation." The underlying cause of all of these outcomes was relabeled "health condition," and there was recognition that this process was not a simple linear progression but included many interactions, so numerous arrows were added to the model. Finally, the label of the model was changed to the model of functioning and disability. That brought the model to a point where the same basic underlying concepts had simply been relabeled, but now a set of labels that would be acceptable in the United States and that were less negative toward people with disabilities was being used.

The Step Forward

The addition of environmental factors was the major step forward in this process, and among the U.S. delegation this was the highest priority. In fact, without that addition, the model would have remained unacceptable to disability advocacy groups and therefore would not have been used. The addition of environmental factors was the major part of adding broader contextual factors that included both environmental and personal factors. It took a few years for environmental factors to be incorporated into the draft model, and they seemed to slip out and periodically needed championing to keep them in. Eventually, they were maintained, and in the author's view, that was probably the major step forward in the conceptualization of disability outcomes.

The Step Backward

The loss of a clear distinction between activity and participation was the step backward. In the development of the category schemes and in the listing of the elements of the domains of activity and participation, there were disagreements. One school of thought was that everything is an activity and the issue is just one of the complexity of the activity. Therefore, for that group, the desire was to have a very long list of activities. From the U.S. perspective and the perspective of the delegations from other English-speaking countries, there was a desire to maintain the concept of participation in terms of performance as a member of society—working, going to school, parenting, and socializing—as a separate and distinct dimension. This was controversial. In the preliminary draft that was tested, a distinction between activity and participation was made; and a list of activities, as well as a list of participation, was made. Although there were disagreements about whether something was an activity or participation, a consensus on how to resolve these controversies was starting to develop among the delegations from the English-speaking countries. At the last minute, however, WHO decided to say that activity and participation both have the same elements. That resulted in one list of elements for the combined activity and participation domain—a decision that blurs the distinction between activity and participation.

The problem was further complicated by the last-minute introduction of two qualifiers to these dimensions—capacity and performance—with the implications that capacity was related to activity and that performance was related to participation. Furthermore, the suggestion that capacity should be measured in a uniform standard environment whereas participation should be measured in the real world also added confusion to the conceptual model.

SEVEN STEPS TO IMPROVE THE MODEL

It is the view of the author that seven steps are warranted to improve the present ICF Model of Disability. These steps represent conceptual clarifications and enhancements as well as research strategies that can be used to implement and validate the model. Both conceptual and empirical advances are needed to move the disability field forward. These advances are envisioned as iterative processes, in which the conceptual model guides research and empirical evidence informs theory, which culminate in a revised and validated Model of Disability (ICF-2). Continuing empirical work must proceed, without waiting for a perfect model, to inform theoretical perspectives. On the other hand, improved conceptualizations will guide the disability field. In the author's view, the primary role of ICF and its revisions are to guide and evaluate research, policy, and practice rather than to serve as a classification scheme. Although implementation of the proposed revisions will be a challenge, they will be worth the effort and will lead to a better theoretical understanding of disability, which, in turn, can improve the lives of people with disabilities.

Step 1:
Distinguishing Activity and Participation in the Next Model Revision

The blurring of activity and participation was a step backward that must be repaired. In the next revision of ICF, distinctions between activity and participation need to be clarified as the first step in improving the present model.

Several themes differentiate these two important concepts. First, and most importantly, activity is at the individual person level, whereas participation is at the societal level. Activities are more likely to be performed alone, whereas participation elements would more likely be performed with others. In some sense, activity is a simpler concept, whereas participation is a more complex process. Activity is related more closely to the extent of impairment, whereas participation is related more closely to perceived quality of life. Meta-analysis[13] demonstrates that the severity of the impairment is highly correlated with activities of daily living but is not strongly related to quality of life, whereas participation is more closely related to quality of life. Activity may be thought of as less environmentally dependent, whereas participation is more environmentally dependent. Although, conceptually, environmental factors play a role in both levels, it does seem clear that participation is the area that is the most influenced by the environment. Activity is embraced by the medical model of disability, whereas participation emerges from a social model of disability. The measurement of activity is a focus of rehabilitation, whereas the measurement of participation reflects the outcomes most important to individuals with disabilities, their family members, and society. Activity is more typically assessed in a rehabilitation setting, whereas participation should be assessed in the community setting. Activity is more often assessed by a clinician or professional, whereas participation is more often a self-report of the individual with a disability. Finally, in the current state of the science, all activity limitations cannot yet be eliminated, but theoretically, most participation restrictions can be eliminated. Although all disabilities cannot be cured, society is in a position, at least theoretically, to return people to active, productive lives that are well integrated into family and community life. Society is better prepared to maximize participation than to maximize activity.

Nagi made a strong conceptual basis for differentiating activities and participation in Appendix A of *Disability in America*,[2] in which he attempted to clarify the distinction between performance at the level of the person (which he called "functional limitations") and performance at the societal level (which he called "disability"). For Nagi, role performance was the defining concept at the societal level. He, like Parsons,[26] viewed "role performance" as an organized system of participation by an individual in a social system, whereas tasks are more specialized than roles and can be viewed as subsystems of roles. Nagi argued that activities of daily living are task behaviors that are parts of (but different from) role expectations inherent in a person's family, vocational, and social lives. Furthermore, Nagi suggested that tasks or activities were attributes or properties of individuals in isolation, whereas roles and participation were relational concepts requiring consideration of environmental factors in which the roles were performed. This early conceptual focus on roles as the defining characteristic of performance at the societal level may offer an effective way to differentiate activities and participation in ICF-2.

Step 2: Quality of Life, a Key Missing Component of ICF

ICF offers a comprehensive model of objective disability outcomes and provides rehabilitationists and researchers with a system for categorizing disability. However, it does not address the subjective perceptions and preferences of people with disabilities. It is for this reason that disability researchers have criticized ICF for lacking a subjective dimension and recommended augmentation of ICF with an additional dimension—quality of life[25]—as the second step in the revision of ICF.

Although WHO does not include the concept of quality of life in the ICF Model of Disability, it has recognized both the importance of the quality-of-life concept and its relationship to disability outcomes. WHO defined quality of life as "the perception of individuals of their position in life, in the context of the culture and value systems in which they live and in relation to their goals, expectations, standards, and concerns."[27] According to WHO, the determinants of quality of life include the consequences of disability, particularly handicap or participation.[1] On the basis of WHO documents, Barbotte and colleagues described quality of life as a wide-ranging concept "affected by people's social relationships, physical health, psychological state and level of independence, and by their relationship to salient features of their environment"[28] (p. 1048).

Quality of life, defined as a self-appraisal of subjective well-being or life satisfaction made by the person with a disability, might be acknowledged by the ICF WHO Model of Disability in one of three ways: (1) it could be added as a separate domain to the right of participation, indicating that the extent of quality of life is the ultimate outcome of the disability process; (2) it could be added as a qualifier to each of the present domains of ICF, indicating that satisfaction with participation, activities, and even body structures and functions is an important aspect of disability; or (3) it could be excluded from the model itself but acknowledged as a key life outcome influenced by the disability process. This author favors the first approach. The exclusion of quality of life from the model but acknowledgment of its importance fails to require that the subjective assessment of the individual with a disability be included in any comprehensive assessment of disability. The incorporation of a subjective satisfaction qualifier as part of each current domain adds conceptual confusion to each of the domains and fails to focus attention on a unique outcome of critical importance. Only the actual addition of a new quality-of-life domain acknowledges the validity of the subjective perceptions of people with disabilities and that those perceptions are distinct outcomes of the disability process.

Quality of life could be measured simply by using a standardized assessment of global life satisfaction[29] or an instrument that assesses satisfaction with domains of life;[30] but it should not be a composite measure of Health-Related Quality of Life (HRQOL), including impairment, activity limitation, participation restriction, and quality-of-life indicators, as is often the case with HRQOL measures.[31] The author suggests that the inclusion of a new quality-of-life domain is more important than the addition of a quality-of-life taxonomy with a coding system. Furthermore, the potential difficulty of adding a new domain and the complexity that it brings will be outweighed by the conceptual importance of the subjective assessment by the person with a disability. Quality of life was first recognized as an important domain by *Enabling America*, [5] and its addition to ICF is a critical revision.

Step 3: Elaborating the Complexity of Environmental Factors

The third step needed in the revision of ICF is elaboration of environmental factors. It was a tremendous step forward to acknowledge the role of environmental factors. The environmental factors research that has been done has given some insight into the relationship between environmental factors and participation. Conceptually, models have always suggested that the more barriers that people encounter, the lower their participation is and that barriers actually prevent people from participating in society. On the other hand, the theories suggest that the more facilitating the environment is, the more likely it is that people with disabilities will fully participate in society. In initial environmental research, most correlations between environmental barriers and participation were negative, as expected. However, it was a surprise to find a few positive correlations between some environmental factors and participation, indicating a more complex relationship. The data seemed to suggest that when people encounter barriers, their participation is less; but they also suggest that for those people who persevered and got out and involved in the community and fully participated, they also witnessed and perceived more environmental barriers. It is not a simple one-way relationship.

Only two disability studies have systematically examined environmental barriers and their relationship to other ICF concepts and quality of life: one in traumatic brain injury (TBI)[32] and one in SCI.[24] The TBI study surveyed 73 participants from one TBI model system program at their first anniversary of injury, with respondents reporting a greater impact from environmental barriers also reporting lower levels of participation and life satisfaction.[32]

The SCI study surveyed 2,726 participants from the 16 federally designated SCI model systems as they crossed their 1st, 5th, 10th, 15th, 20th, or 25th anniversary of injury. Environmental barriers accounted for only 4 percent of the variation in participation, but they accounted for 10 percent of the variation in quality of life. The SCI study supported the inclusion of environmental factors in models of disability, like ICF, but concluded that environmental factors had a stronger relationship to quality of life than they did to societal participation.[24] This last finding of the SCI study raises the pivotal question: do environmental factors directly influence participation, which in turn influences quality of life, or do environmental factors more directly influence quality of life? Environmental barriers may reduce participation, or the struggle to overcome barriers and fully participate may reduce quality of life. There is much to learn about the actual role of environmental factors in the disability process, and researchers need to develop some theory underlying the concept that helps explain under what conditions barriers actually mean that participation does not occur and under what conditions people move beyond those barriers and participate. Considerable theory building will be required to accomplish this third step in revising ICF.

Step 4: An Understanding and Taxonomy of Personal Factors

The fourth step needed to improve ICF is the development of personal factors. However, this step is controversial. The current conceptual model acknowledges that contextual factors, including both environmental and personal factors, play a major role in disability outcomes. Environmental factors are considered everything external to the individual—physical, attitudinal, and policy factors. Personal factors should be thought of as all of the factors that are internal to the individual but unrelated to the disability itself, including the preexisting conditions, demographic factors, and personal characteristics that existed before an impairment occurred or that are not directly related to the disabling process. Looking for demographic differences in disability outcomes is an area in which investigators are comfortable, but efforts to venture into the arena of personal factors beyond demographics have not been made. Psychological factors and personality factors are seldom examined, possibly for reasons of political correctness. The concern of advocacy groups is that if it begins to be suggested that motivation or compliance with treatment is an important factor in producing disability outcomes, then the field is precariously on the verge of once again suggesting that the problem lies with the individual instead of the environment. Advocacy groups would then once again challenge the medical model because it failed to consider environmental factors. Therefore, it is critical that people with disabilities and advocacy groups be fully involved in any development of a personal factors taxonomy. Furthermore, careful consideration will be needed when something that might seem to be a personal factor might better be viewed as psychological structure or function. However, eventually, to have a complete model that is able to predict a major portion of the variances in outcomes, personal factors will likely need to be included. Therefore, the development of a personal factors taxonomy with a better theoretical understanding of the significance of personal factors needs to be one of the steps in the ICF revision process.

Step 5: Refining a Graphic Representation of the Model

Neither the complex diagram of multiheaded arrows and boxes of ICF nor the "man on the mat" diagrams in *Enabling America* provide a clear depiction of the interaction of health conditions with contextual factors that produce disability outcomes. If a more compelling graphic depiction that clarified the nature of conceptual relationships in an intuitive manner could be developed, the more widespread adoption of the revised model would be more likely. Refining the graphic is therefore listed as the fifth step in revising the ICF.

Step 6: Developing Improved Measures of the Domains of Disability

The final two steps advocated for advancing the conceptual understanding of disability have more to do with the application of the model than its revision. Both current and future models of disability require extensive testing. The reliability and practicality of the taxonomy must be evaluated, but more importantly, the implied relationships among the concepts must be assessed. A prerequisite of that task is the availability of psychometrically sound measures of the ICF concepts. Although many measures of impairment and activities of daily living have been developed, the measurement of participation is a relatively new field and the measurement of environmental factors is in its infancy. Considerable psychometric evaluation of existing and newly developed instruments is needed to reach a consensus on standardized methods of quantifying each of the domains of the disability. Major surveys need to incorporate reliable and valid measures specifically designed to assess the conceptual domains of ICF rather than simply trying to retrofit existing survey questions to the ICF taxonomy by developing "crosswalks" to ICF codes.

Step 7: Validate the Model

Once valid and reliable tools are developed, they can be applied in multivariate analyses to determine the strength of relationships among ICF concepts. Replication of such work with multiple populations with different impairments will be needed. The development of a research strategy to tackle this problem would be a significant step and contribution to the field, but full validation of the model also requires the use of the model to guide interventions to improve the lives of people with disabilities. Therefore, the final step includes the design, implementation, and rigorous evaluation of interventions based on the conceptual model. The ultimate test of a model is whether it facilitates effective interventions. The revised conceptual model, in combination with the empirical tests of the model, should provide the information necessary to direct effective interventions.

CONCLUSIONS

As IOM begins the process of reconsidering its seminal works *Disability in America* and *Enabling America*, published nearly 15 and 10 years ago, respectively, clear advances have occurred in the conceptualization of disability, but more work is needed in clarifying concepts. WHO's ICF has incorporated a major concept advocated by *Enabling America*—environmental factors—and ICF, as the currently accepted international model, should be the starting point for advocating future conceptual revisions. Seven steps have been outlined to improve the ICF conceptualization, including the differentiation of activities and participation, the addition of quality of life to the model, elaboration of the impact of environmental factors, the development of personal factors, refinement of the graphic depiction of the model, definition of research strategies to better measure the domains of the model, and validation of the model by testing the interrelationships among its concepts and deriving interventions to improve the lives of people with disabilities.

REFERENCES

1. World Health Organization. *International Classification of Impairments, Disabilities and Handicaps: a Manual of Classification Relating to the Consequences of Disease.* Geneva, Switzerland: World Health Organization; 1980.
2. World Health Organization. *International Classification of Functioning, Disability, and Health.* Geneva, Switzerland: World Health Organization; 2001.
3. The Americans with Disabilities Act. P.L. 101-336. 1990.
4. National Institute on Disability and Rehabilitation Research. National Institute on Disability and Rehabilitation Research (NIDRR) Long Range Plan for Fiscal Years 1999-2003. Web Page. Available at http://www.ncddr.org/new/announcements/nidrr_lrp/index.html. Last accessed October 18, 2005.
5. Institute of Medicine. *Enabling America: Assessing the Role of Rehabilitation Science and Engineering.* Washington, DC: National Academy Press; 1997.
6. Whiteneck GG, Charlifue SW, Gerhart KA, Overholser JD, Richardson GN. Quantifying handicap: a new measure of long-term rehabilitation outcomes. *Archives of Physical Medicine and Rehabilitation* 1992; 73:519–526.
7. Whiteneck G, Brooks C, Charlifue S, et al. *Guide for Use of CHART: Craig Hospital Assessment and Reporting Technique.* Englewood, CO: Craig Hospital; 1992.
8. Willer B, Rosenthal M, Kreutzer J, Gordan W, Rempel R. Assessment of community integration following rehabilitation for traumatic brain injury. *Journal of Head Trauma and Rehabilitation* 1993; 8:75–87.
9. Craig Hospital Research Department; *Craig Hospital Inventory of Environmental Factors (CHIEF) Manual*, Version 3.0. Englewood, CO: Craig Hospital; 2001.

10. Whiteneck G, Harrison-Felix C, Mellick D, Brooks C, Charlifue S, Gerhart K. Quantifying environmental factors: a measure of physical, attitudinal, service, productivity and policy barriers. *Archives of Physical Medicine and Rehabilitation* 2004; 85:1324–1335.

11. Whiteneck G. Outcome analysis in spinal cord injury rehabilitation. *In: Rehabilitation Outcomes: Analysis and Measurement*. Fuhrer MJ, ed. Baltimore, MD: Paul H. Brookes Publishing Co.; 1987:221–231.

12. Whiteneck G. Outcome evaluation and spinal cord injury. *NeuroRehabilitation* 1992; 2:31–41.

13. Dijkers M. Quality of life after spinal cord injury: a meta analysis of the effects of disablement components. *Spinal Cord* 1997; 35:829–840.

14. World Health Organization. *International Classification of Disease*, 9th Revision. *Clinical Modifications*. Ann Arbor, MI: Commission of Professional and Hospital Activities; 1986.

15. Nagi SZ. An epidemiology of disability among adults in the United States. *The Milbank Memorial Fund Quarterly* 1976; 54:439–467.

16. Verbrugge LM, Jette AM. The disablement process. *Social Science & Medicine* 1994; 38:1–14.

17. Pope A, Tarlov A. *Disability in America: Toward a National Agenda for Prevention*. Washington, DC: National Academy Press; 1991.

18. National Institutes of Health. *Research Plan for the National Center for Medical Rehabilitation Research*. NIH Publication 93-3509. Washington, DC: U.S. Department of Health and Human Services; 1993.

19. Fougeyrollas P. Documenting environmental factors for preventing the handicap creation process: Quebec contributions relating to ICIDH and social participation of people with functional differences. *Disability and Rehabilitation* 1995; 17:145–153.

20. Fougeyrollas P. Explanatory models of the consequences of disease and trauma: the handicap creation process. *ICIDH, International Network* 1993:6.

21. Whiteneck G, Fougeyrolles P, Gerhart G. Elaborating the model disablement. *In: Assessing Medical Rehabilitation Practices: the Promise of Outcomes Research*. Fuher M ed. Baltimore, MD: Paul H. Brookes Publishing Co.; 1997:91–102.

22. Heinemann A, Whiteneck G. Relationships among impairment, disability, and life satisfaction in persons with traumatic brain injury. *Journal of Head Trauma Rehabilitation* 1995; 10:54–63.

23. Hall MK, Hamilton BB, Gordon WA, Zasler N.D. Characteristics and comparisons of functional assessment indices: Disability Rating Scale, Functional Independence Measure, and Functional Assessment Measure. *Journal of Head Trauma Rehabilitation* 1993; 8:60–74.

24. Whiteneck G, Mead M, Dijkers M, Tate D, Bushnik T, Forchheimer M. Environmental factors and their role in participation and life satisfaction after spinal cord injury. *Archives of Physical Medicine and Rehabilitation* 2004; 85(11):1793–1803.

25. Whiteneck G. The ICF: one step forward, one step back, and a few steps to go to a complete model. Presentation to conference on State of the Science: Outcome Research in Post-Acute Care. April 24-25, 2003, Washington, DC. Organized by Boston University. Web Page. Available at http://www.bu.edu/cre/webcast/test_whiteneck.doc. Last accessed October 18, 2005.

26. Parsons, T. Definitions of health and illness in the light of American values and social structure. *In: Patients, Physicians and Illness*. Jaco EG, ed. Glencoe, IL: Free Press; 1958.

27. World Health Organization. Study protocol for the World Health Organization project to develop a quality of life assessment instrument: WHOQOL. *Quality of Life Research* 1993; 2:153–159.

28. Barbotte E, Guillemin F, Chau N. Prevalence of impairments, disabilities, handicaps, and quality of life in general population: a review of recent literature. *Bulletin of the World Health Organization* 2001; 79(11):1047–1055.

29. Diener E, Emmons R, Larsen J, Griffin S. The Satisfaction with Life Scale. *Journal of Personality Assessment* 1985; 49(1):71–75.

30. Flanagan J. A research approach to improving our quality of life. *American Psychologist* 1978; 33:138–147.

31. Ware J, Sherbourne C. The MOS 36-item short-form health survey (SF-36). I. Conceptual framework and item selection. *Medical Care* 1992; 30:473–483.

32. Whiteneck G, Gerhart K, Cusick C. Identifying environmental factors that influence the outcomes of people with traumatic brain injury. *Journal of Head Trauma Rehabilitation* 2004; 19(3):191–204.

C

Defining and Classifying Disability in Children

*Rune J. Simeonsson**

"during the third or fourth month, the most important acquisition being the power of balancing the head on the shoulders; the absence of this power at this stage was one of the earliest signs of mental deficiency"
(Forsyth, 1915, p. 535).

Defining and measuring disability in the first two decades of life has been a uniquely challenging task. From infancy to adolescence, it is a period marked by dynamic changes in body structures and functions; the acquisition of physical and mental skills; and progressive steps toward independence of movement, thought, and behavior. In contrast to the relatively stable characteristics of the adult, the evolving characteristics of the child represent a moving target, complicating the task of assessing function and distinguishing significant limitations from variations in normal developmental processes. The younger and less mature that the child is, the greater the challenge has been to define disability.

In the history of childhood disability (Schalick, 2000), earlier approaches to defining disability took the form of observing physical signs (Down, 1887) or noting discrepancies in the appearance of basic maturational skills (Forsyth, 1915). These approaches are still followed today as strategies for the identification of developmental problems of infants and young children, although contemporary determination of disability is now often linked to the documentation of diagnosed conditions, such as trisomy 21. As the child develops, observation and assessment are increasingly used as documentation strate-

*Rune J. Simeonsson, Ph.D., M.S.P.H., Professor of Education and Research Professor of Psychology, University of North Carolina at Chapel Hill and Adjunct Professor of Medical Psychology, Department of Psychiatry, Duke University. The analyses and views presented in this workshop paper are those of the author and not necessarily those of the Institute of Medicine Committee on Disability in America: A New Look.

gies, but variability in the nature and rate of development continues to be a source of confounding in the identification of disability (Simeonsson and Rosenthal, 2001). The lack of theory and the lack of consistent concepts of disability in childhood have resulted in identification and classification approaches that have been idiosyncratic to disciplines or service systems and taken the form of diagnoses, syndromes, or categories.

Although the definition and classification of disability in children are issues of current significance, they are not new problems. Concerns about diagnoses, categorical assignment, and the associated labeling of children with disabilities prompted a request for a coherent classification system in the early 1970s by then Secretary of Health, Education and Welfare Elliot Richardson (Hobbs, 1975a). In addition to the problem of labeling and its impact on children, the task of the project was also to address the inappropriate use of psychometric instruments and classification practices in the determination of disability in children from minority groups. The project resulted in two publications, with the first, *Issues in the Classification of Children* (Hobbs, 1975a), summarizing problems and challenges. In the second book, *The Futures of Children*, Hobbs (1975b) recommended a functional basis for the classification of children's disabilities. The functional approach recommended by Hobbs was not realized, and the categorical basis for determining the eligibility of children for funding and services continues to raise concerns in the context of fragmented and incomplete services (Hughes et al., 1996; Newacheck et al., 1998).

Although the terminology for the concerns defined in the 1970s may have changed, many of the problems raised at that time remain the same today, requiring revisiting of the identification and the classification issues three decades later. The purpose of this paper is to (1) review concepts of development and disability; (2) present models and representative data on childhood disability; (3) describe current issues; and (4) identify emerging issues to advance the definition, measurement, and classification of disability in childhood.

CONCEPTS OF DEVELOPMENT AND DISABILITY

Concepts of Atypical Development

Although there is no universal standard for defining childhood disability, a number of concepts have framed disability related to atypical development. In reviewing the research on different outcomes for children who have experienced significant developmental risk factors, Sameroff and Chandler (1975) described main-effect, interactional, and transactional models to capture the evolving findings on the roles of biological and environmental factors in child development. In the main-effect model, a nurturist view posited that a good environment could compensate for a poor biological state, whereas in the nativist view, the biological state (good or poor) determined the outcome. The main-effect model was seen as static, as it failed to account for interactive effects on development. The interactive model of developmental outcome posited intermediate outcomes. However, recognition of the ongoing reciprocal influences of environment on the child and the child on the environment led to the proposal of a transactional model to account for different outcomes of development. The transactional model has been drawn upon widely as a framework for designing and evaluating interventions for children with disabilities and their families.

An important question pertaining to disability in childhood has focused on whether atypical development represents qualitative differences or quantitative lags in development. This question has been addressed in contributions by Zigler (1969) and Inhelder (1966, 1968). Although both contributions were framed with reference to children with mental retardation, the main premise seems applicable to children with any disability. Zigler (1969) proposed that the cognitive development of children with mental retardation that was not organic in origin was similar in structure and followed a similar sequence to that of children without disabilities. Within the framework of Piaget's theory of cognitive development, Inhelder (1966, 1968) advanced a similar concept of an invariant sequence to describe the delayed rate of cognitive development in individuals with mental retardation. Mental retardation was characterized by a delayed progression through stages of development and an ultimate failure to achieve the ability to perform formal operations at maturity, representing a "false equilibrium," that is, an incomplete level of cognitive development. The severity of mental retardation corresponded to fixation at lower stages of cognitive development.

As noted above, although the rate of development of children with disabilities may differ from that of children without disabilities, the general assumption is that the sequence and structure of development in children with disabilities are similar to that of all children. Furthermore, children with disabilities, as all children, are assumed to be characterized by individual differences. Theory as well as extensive research has supported this premise and formed the basis for conceptualizations of variations in development. It may be useful to consider three developmental perspectives on disability: (1) the continuum of reproductive casualty, (2) the continuum of care-taking casualty, and (3) the continuum of central nervous system (CNS) dysfunction.

The Continuum of Reproductive Casualty

Almost 40 years ago, Pasamanick and Knobloch (1966) became intrigued with the variations in the developmental outcomes of children who had experienced pre- and perinatal complications. On the basis of a systematic examination of the developmental consequences of pregnancy and delivery complications, they advanced the concept of a continuum of reproductive casualty to define the range of possible outcomes due to insult in the prenatal period. This range of outcomes was proposed to reflect the contributions of three factors: the nature, the extent, and the developmental timing of the insult. The result of complications at one end of the continuum was nonsurvival, whereas the complications at the other end of the continuum were negligible. For infants who survived the complications, "there must remain a fraction so injured who do not die, but depending on the degree and location of the trauma, go on to develop a series of disorders extending from cerebral palsy, epilepsy and mental deficiency, through all types of behavioral and learning disabilities, resulting from lesser degrees of damage sufficient to disorganized behavior development and lower thresholds to stress" (Pasamanick and Knobloch, 1966, p. 7).

Central to the concept of the continuum of reproductive casualty was the assumption that the range of outcomes expressed in different manifestations of disability, such as mental retardation, cerebral palsy, and learning disability, reflected the differential effects of complications on common developmental processes (Baum, 1977; Ounsted, 1987). This concept has been used to interpret the long-term outcomes for low-birth-weight children (Forfar et al., 1994) and for findings that associate obstetric complications with conditions , such as mental retardation, autism, learning disabilities, and disorders resulting from organic conditions or toxic exposures (Eaton et al., 2001). By defining disability in terms of the various outcomes of prenatal complications, the continuum of reproductive casualty can be seen as a precursor of later conceptualizations in which disability is seen as universal with problems manifested on a continuum.

The Continuum of Caretaking Casualty

After the introduction of the concept of the continuum of reproductive casualty, there was a growing recognition that the outcomes for children experiencing pre- and perinatal complications were influenced by a complex of factors. Baum (1977) pointed out that the outcomes of infants experiencing significant perinatal insults were not consistent with the reproductive casualty continuum hypothesis and recommended that more attention needed to be paid to the role of the postnatal environment on developmental outcomes. Of particular interest was recognition of the impact of environmental factors on the developing child beyond the pre- and perinatal period with the potential to account for developmental outcomes (Roosa et al., 1982). On the one hand were studies demonstrating that the outcomes for children with prenatal or birth complications could be positively modified by environmental interventions. On the other hand were findings showing that the development of children with uneventful fetal histories could be seriously delayed or distorted by certain caregiving histories. The caregiving environment thus became a factor of significant interest as a variable affecting the developmental outcomes of children.

This emphasis on the caregiver's role in influencing outcome was central to the articulation of the concept of the continuum of caretaking casualty by Sameroff and Chandler (1975). The major premise of this concept is that developmental outcome is not defined by pre- or perinatal factors alone but is a product of continuing transactions between the child and the stimulation and nurture provided by the caregiver in the child's development. Similar to the concept of the continuum of reproductive casualty, the concept of the continuum of caretaking casualty proposes that the developmental outcomes of children are expressed as a range of manifestations rather than as discrete entities. The utility of this concept can be illustrated in a study of the affective development of young children reared in different caregiving environments (Smyke et al., 2002). Consistent with the concept, children experiencing greater social deprivation manifested greater disturbances. The concept of caretaking casualty thus extends the continuum of reproductive casualty and defines differences in children with disabilities as developmental expressions of processes occurring in the prenatal period as well as the postnatal period.

The Continuum of CNS Dysfunction

A third concept advanced to define disability in childhood is the continuum of CNS dysfunction. Whereas the previous two concepts were linked in terms of their development, the continuum of CNS dysfunction was advanced without a link to the others. Capute and Palmer (1980) used the term to emphasize the associated deficits that stem from a common underlying dysfunction of the CNS. For optimal assessment and treatment of the developmentally disabled child, both the spectrum of expressed disability and the underlying dysfunction need to be recognized (Capute et al., 1981). In this model, specific conditions associated with disability are grouped under the three major conditions of cerebral palsy, mental retardation, and communicative disorders. Cerebral palsy is considered prototypic of developmental disabilities, as individuals with this condition often have cognitive as well as communicative deficits. Communicative deficits were defined to include both central dysfunctions (language disorder, learning disability, or autism) and peripheral dysfunctions (hearing or visual impairment). Distinguishing between the spectrum of disabilities and the underlying dysfunction is important for the detection and the diagnosis of disabilities in children.

Two associated concepts are advanced in an elaboration of the con-

TABLE C-1   Complementary Contributions of Three Continuum
Concepts to Defining Disability in Childhood

Continuum	Disability as Developmental Outcome	Complementary Contribution
Continuum of reproductive casualty	Range of developmental outcomes as a function of nature and timing of pre- or perinatal insult	Disability as a variable expression of prenatal and perinatal factors
Continuum of caretaking casualty	Range of developmental outcomes as a function of transactions between child and postnatal environment	Disability as variable expression of postnatal experiences
Continuum of CNS dysfunction	Range of developmental outcomes as a function of the location, nature, and severity of the underlying CNS dysfunction	Disability as variable expression of motor-sensory and central-peripheral dysfunction

tinuum of CNS dysfunction: deviancy and dissociation. Both are proposed
to facilitate the identification of problems and atypical development. Deviancy refers to deviations of a child's abilities from normal values within a
certain domain. The dissociation phenomenon refers to discrepancies in
level of functioning from one domain to another, for example stronger
motor skills but weaker language skills or stronger mental skills but weaker
motor skills. Recognition of the deviancy phenomenon may thus contribute
to the detection of a child whose behavior is atypical and whose subsequent
development needs careful monitoring. Sensitivity to the dissociation phenomenon could contribute to the documentation of a child's relative
strengths and deficits. This is evident in children with motor impairments,
for example, whose language abilities are often advanced relative to their
motor abilities.

In summary, the continuum of outcomes attributed to reproductive or
caretaking complications, or CNS dysfunction have contributed to conceptualizations of disabilities based on a model of child-environment interactions. Specifically, the three continuum concepts make this contribution
by emphasizing the variability of common developmental processes (Table
C-1). Their contributions advance the developmental basis for conceptualizing the dimensions of childhood disability.

These concepts provide an alternative to the medical model, which focuses on symptoms of health conditions within the child. The premise of a continuum of outcomes supports a functional model that encompasses commonalities and variations in development across major domains. These developmental domains reflect the manner in which the child actively explores and acts upon the physical and the social environments. The domains include cognition, communication, social development, and behavior.

MODELS OF DISABILITY IN CHILDREN

Medical Model

Although they may not be consistently defined, medical, social, and functional models have generally framed definitional, measurement, and classification issues related to disability in adults. In the absence of a specific model for defining disability in childhood, these have also been applied in considering disability of children and youth.

Reference to the medical model implies that the locus of the disability is in the person (Marks, 1997) and that disability is defined by the manifestation of a health condition in the form of anomalies or impairment of physical or mental structures or function. Documentation of disability usually takes the form of recording the diagnoses, syndromes, or signs or symptoms that meet the criteria for assignment to a category. In health, mental health and health related settings, codes from the International Classification of Diseases, 9th Revision (ICD-9) and the Diagnostic and Statistical Manual of Mental Disorders, Fourth Edition, Text Revision (DSM-IV-TR) are likely to be the basis for determining a child's eligibility for services and support. In education, assignment to 1 of 13 categories under Part C of the Individuals with Disabilities Education Improvement Act (IDEA; P.L. 94-142) defines eligibility for special education services. These categories were put in place in 1976 with the establishment of special education under P.L. 94-142 and reflect a medical model because the categories either are diagnosed conditions (e.g., mental retardation, autism, traumatic brain injury [TBI], and learning disabilities) or specify criteria based on physical or mental impairments (e.g., auditory and visual impairments and severe emotional disturbance). It should be noted, however, that the categorical terms are specific to the field of education and do not necessarily correspond to the diagnoses defined by ICD-9 or DSM-IV-TR classifications. The categories reflect a medical model perspective and were designated as "handicaps" in the original legislation and then as "disabilities" in the 1991 reauthorization of IDEA. The autism category was added in 1991, and the category for TBI was added in 1997.

Interestingly, attention deficit-hyperactivity disorder (ADHD), a highly prevalent childhood condition, does not constitute a formal IDEA category.

To be served under IDEA, children with ADHD must qualify under the category of other health impairment. The idiosyncratic nature of the 13 categories is further illustrated by the fact that children who are deaf and blind are assigned to the deaf-blind category, whereas children with other co-occuring conditions are assigned to the category of "multiple disabilities." The fact that states can exercise discretion in measurement approaches to determine eligibility for assignment to a category lowers the specificity of information about the characteristics of the children in that category and raises questions about the aggregation of data by categories. However, as the federal government requires the states to report annually on the numbers of students served in special education under these categories, the resulting data do provide estimates of the prevalence of childhood disability. An analysis of ten-year data (www.IDEAdata.org) indicates that population prevalence rates for all children served in special education ages 3 to 21 increased from 7.44 to 8.56 percent from 1993 to 2003. Limiting the analysis to the 6- to 21-year-old group or 6- to 11-year-old group revealed increasing rates over the decade from 8.21 to 9.05 percent and 10.86 to 11.23 percent, respectively.

An analysis of the prevalence rates by disability categories for students 6 to 21 years of age reveals that the five most prevalent categories in 2003 were learning disabilities (4.28 percent), speech and language impairments (1.70 percent), mental retardation (0.87 percent), emotional disturbance (0.73 percent), and other health impairment (0.73 percent). The prevalence rate for each of the remaining categories was 0.2 percent or less. Although the rates for most categories have remained relatively stable from 1993 to 2003, there is a gradual decline in the rate for mental retardation and relatively marked increases in the rates for other health impaired (0.14 to 0.68 percent), autism (0.03 to 0.21 percent) and for developmental delay from 1997 to 2003 (0.01 to 0.10 percent).

Social Model

The emergence of the disability movement has been characterized by definitions of disability from the perspective of individuals with disabilities (Kaplan, 2000). A major reaction to the medical model resulted in the articulation of a social perspective on disability, the social model in Britain, and the minority group model in the United States. The basic assumption of these models was a rejection of seeing disability as a characteristic within the person and seeing it instead as a social construction defined by discrimination and exclusion by mainstream social environment (Marks, 1997). The emphasis on environmental barriers and the denial of human rights in the social model of disability has served as a powerful premise for political action and advocacy. Although the social model has contributed significantly to the formulation of inclusive policies and practices for environmental access for adults, its influence on policies and practices involving children is less obvious.

Munn (1997) has maintained that a weakness of the social model is that it failed to adequately account for children with disabilities, who are a minority within the minority of individuals with disabilities. Their minority status is defined by the fact that "disabled children are twice ignored and they are also twice vulnerable to the lack of resource, the stigma and stress of disability, together with the strain on their already compromised development and family relations" Munn (1997, p. 484). Munn thus argues for a movement away from categorization based on physical criteria and the incorporation of a developmental emphasis in the minority group model. The concepts of least-restrictive environments and full inclusion in placements for special education students are consistent with the social-minority group model.

In a somewhat different context, Landsman (2005) draws on the social model in interpreting the nurturing experience of mothers of children newly diagnosed with disabilities. Over time, mothers replaced their problem-oriented focus based on the medical model with a social model focused on integration and acceptance of their children.

Functional Model

Although "functional model" may not be a term that has been formalized or used with the same level of consensus as the medical and social models, it seems appropriate to use the term in reference to a number of contributions to research and practice that have defined disability as the basis of functional limitations. A variety of contributions began to emerge in the last decade, advocating alternative ways of conceptualizing and measuring disability in childhood. In a line of research, Stein and colleagues (Stein et al., 1993; Westbrook et al., 1998; Stein and Silver, 1999; Stein and Silver, 2002) examined the utility of a noncategorical approach to the identification of children with chronic conditions and disabilities. Based on the language of the Americans with Disabilities Act (P.L. 101-336), three criteria for the definition of disabling or chronic conditions in childhood were specified. A disability was defined on the basis of the fact that it (1) was a consequence of an ongoing health condition, (2) was manifested in functional limitations or dependence on compensatory mechanisms or the use of services or care beyond usual or normal levels for the age group, and (3) lasted or was expected to last 12 months or more. By use of a random sample of households in a national data set, a comparative analysis identified 9 percent as having a disability on the basis of functional limitations, 10 percent as having a disability on the basis of dependence on compensatory devices, and 13 percent as having a disability on the basis of the use of services or care beyond the norm for the child's age. Overall, 18 percent of children under the age of 18 years were identified as having a disability (Westbrook et al., 1998).

In another study with data from the 1994 National Health Interview Survey (NHIS), 9.6, 5.1, and 10.6 percent of children were identified respectively on the basis of having functional limitations, relying on compensatory resources, and using services or care beyond levels usual or normal for their age group (Stein and Silver, 1999). The overall proportion of the sample identified to have at least one of these characteristics was 14.8 percent.

Also using the 1994 NIHS data set, Hogan et al. (1997) generated prevalence estimates of disability in childhood based on indicators of functional limitations in mobility, self-care, communication, and learning ability. Analyses based on data for school-aged children between 5 and 17 years of age identified 10.6 percent with limitations in learning, 5.5 percent with communication limitations, 1.3 percent with limitations in mobility, and 0.9 percent with limitations in self-care. Socioeconomic differences were associated with higher rates of disabilities in children. Other demographic factors associated with higher rates of disability were found to include male gender and being a child of school age (Mudrick, 2002).

In a comprehensive analysis of the 1994-1995 NHIS Disability Supplement (NHIS-D), Fedeyko and Lollar (2003) assigned 42 of the NHIS-D questions to one of eight Activity and Participation domains used in the World Health Organization's International Classification of Functioning, Disability and Health (ICF) (WHO, 2001). The results revealed that 12.1 percent of 5- to 17-year-olds reported a limitation compared to 17.2 percent for those 18 to 64 years of age. In an analysis of limitations for 5- to 17-year-olds by domains, 1.3 percent reported sensory limitations, less than 1 percent reported movement and mobility limitations, 4.8 percent reported communication limitations, however, 9.4 percent reported learning limitations.

The concept of functional limitations has also been applied in epidemiological studies to document the prevalence of mental health problems in children and youth. As has been true for other disabilities, definitions of mental illness and emotional disturbance vary in terms of the criteria for the nature and the severity of the conditions. Such variability of definitions in the two primary settings of mental health and education complicates both the identification of children needing help and the coordination of services for them.

In recognition of the impact of such definitional variability on the estimation of prevalence, Narrow et al. (1998) used an epidemiological survey to compare three federal definitions of severe mental illness (one education definition and two mental health definitions) in children and youth between 9 and 17 years of age. The term serious emotional disturbance (SED) was used in the education definition based on IDEA and in a mental health definition advanced by the Alcohol, Drug Abuse and Mental Health Administration Reorganization Act of 1992 (P.L. 102-321). These two definitions differed from the other mental health definition in that they required documentation of functional limitations, in addition to a formal diagnosis of the disorder. The results revealed a range in the proportion of children whose conditions met the criteria of severe mental illness or SED, with 3.0 percent meeting the criteria for diagnosed disorders, 11.8 percent meeting the criteria for the IDEA-based definition, and from 12.1 to 22.6 percent meeting the criteria for the mental health-based SED definition.

The prevalence of SED was also examined in two studies involving the Great Smoky Mountains Study of Youth, which monitored 9-, 11-, and 13-year-old children over a period of 8 years. In the first study, the proportion of children with an SED identified on the basis of any diagnosed mental health disorder was 20.3 percent, whereas the proportion identified on the basis of an SED definition was 4 to 8 percent (Costello et al., 1996). A subsequent follow-up study found a prevalence of 13.3 percent of any diagnosed disorder, whereas the prevalence of SED was 6.8 percent (Costello et al., 2005).

These findings and those of Narrow et al. (1998) yield population prevalence rates of SED in children that are significantly higher (4 to 11.8 percent) than the rates in special education under IDEA (0.73 percent). Prevalence rates much closer to those reported by IDEA were found by Halfon and Newacheck (1999) in an analysis of the 1992 and 1994 NHIS data sets. For children under 18 years of age, the prevalence of disability associated with a mental health condition was 2.13 percent. Of those children, 0.1 percent were characterized by severe disability, 1.92 percent were characterized by moderate disability, and 0.1 percent were characterized by mild disability.

The findings from the studies described above demonstrate that definitions play an important role in estimating the prevalence of disability associated with mental health conditions in children. They also illustrate the importance of distinguishing between the documentation of underlying health conditions and the documentation of disability defined by the manifestation of functional limitations.

CURRENT ISSUES

As noted earlier in this paper, there is no common, agreed-upon model of childhood disability. Instead, a variety of models, concepts, and definitions have been employed to describe the sources, nature, and consequences of atypical development in terms of disability and chronic conditions. Available prevalence estimates vary as a function of the definitions chosen by different researchers and research sponsors. A significant consequence of this variability is an inadequate epidemiology of disability in childhood. Other factors also contribute to the current lack of an adequate epidemiology of disability in childhood, for example, variability in the selection of age groups for study and inconsistent criteria for the labeling and classification of disabilities.

As illustrated in the studies described above (Stein and Silver, 1999; Westbrook et al., 1998), the overall prevalence of disability and chronic conditions among children under 18 years of age have been estimated as high as 18 percent. Both studies used national data sets, with the findings reported by Stein and Silver (1999) based on data from the 1994 NHIS. In other studies that have used the 1992 or 1994 NHIS data set with different definitions of disability, the prevalence of disability among 5- to 17-year-olds was estimated to be 7.5 percent (LaPlante and Carlson, 1995), 6.5 percent (Newacheck and Halfon, 1998) and 12.1 percent (Fedeyko and Lollar, 2003) and for children under 18 years of age, 13 to 17 percent (Stein and Silver, 2002). These population prevalence figures are from 30 percent to almost 100 percent higher than the prevalence (9.05 percent) of school age children, 6 to 21 years of age, who are served in special education based on categorical assignment.

The variability of the estimates can be attributed to at least two sources: how disability was defined and the grouping of children by age for analyses. The noncategorical definition of Stein and colleagues focused on the identification of children for whom the consequences of a health condition manifested as dependence on compensatory mechanisms, functional limitations in activities, or an extensive need for services or care. The estimates provided by LaPlante and Carlson (1995) and Newacheck and Halfon (1998) were based on the severity of limitation in the major activities of engaging in play (children under 5 years of age) or attending school (children from 5 to 17 years of age) whereas the results provided by Fedeyko and Lollar (2003) did not take degree of limitation into account.

The second source of variability contributing to an inadequate epidemiology of childhood disability is inconsistency in the identification of age groups for analysis. In the studies, described above, that used the NHIS data sets, for example, data are reported for 13 different age groups. LaPlante and Carlson (1995) report their findings by age group for children under 5, 5 to 13, and 14 to 17 years of age and overall for those 5 through 17 years of age. In Newacheck and Halfon's (1998) study, the age groups are under 6, 6 to 11, and 12 to 17 years and overall for children under 18 years of age. Stein and Silver (1999) report their findings for the age groups of under 3, 4 to 6, 7 to 11, and 12 years old and older and overall for children under 18 years of age. The combination of definitional differences and the overlap of age groups across studies complicate the interpretation and use of epidemiological studies of disability in children at a national level.

Another issue contributing to problems in estimating disability in children and youth is the lack of a common standard for naming and classifying disabilities and chronic conditions. The approaches used to name and classify disabilities in children vary as a function of the disciplines or the agencies providing services to children. Thus, even though the nature of the child's disability or chronic condition is the same across different settings, disciplines and agencies use different criteria and systems to define and classify the child's condition. In health and mental health settings, children are assigned diagnoses on the basis of the definitions in ICD-9 and DSM-IV-TR (First and Pincus, 2002). Increasingly, syndromes are also being used to define children with disabilities in clinical as well as research contexts. In educational settings, children with disabilities are assigned to 1 of 13 IDEA categories that are based on underlying impairments. For children who are under 18 years of age and who are in contact with the Social Security System, eligibility for supplemental support is based on satisfying three elements of the definition of disability: (1) a medically determinable physical or mental impairment (2) that results in marked and severe functional limitations and (3) that has lasted or that is expected to last a year or to result in death. Determination of whether the child's condition satisfies the definition of disability is based on the correspondence of the child's manifested problems with the conditions in the List of Impairments (SSA, 2005).

The List of Impairments constitutes a classification of functional limitations as well as diagnosed diseases and disorders across 15 sections, ranging from growth impairments to the immune system (SSA, 2005). A review of the definitional approaches associated with these programs in health, education, and social services reveals that although all approaches are based on a medical model, there is no direct correspondence between the definitional approaches and the definitions or the associated systems for the classification of disabilities. As many of the children with disabilities and chronic conditions will be in contact with all three of these settings, the lack of a common standard and language of disability complicates the derivation of data regarding needs and services. It also limits interdisciplinary and interagency communication and planning of integrated services.

Inconsistency in the naming of identified populations is a fourth issue characterizing current policy and practice related to children with disabilities. At the broadest level this issue is reflected in the overlap of populations described by the terms "disability" and "chronic conditions" in prevalence studies. The premise that disability is chronic and often associated with an observed or inferred underlying health condition is accepted. At issue is the fact that the terms chronic conditions and disability do differ (Aron et al., 1996) and should be differentiated with reference to inclusion and exclusion criteria.

The categories under IDEA illustrate the lack of consistent criteria for defining disability. Under IDEA, disabilities are defined as conditions such as mental retardation, hearing or vision impairment, learning disabilities, autism, and traumatic brain injury; children having these conditions are eligible for special education. With the exception of the category of developmental delay (available for use with children up to the age of 9 years), the remaining categories require evidence that the child has "a condition." The criteria for documenting that a child has a condition, however, are not based on a common dimension but vary from condition to condition. Thus, the criteria for mental retardation are based on measured intelligence, for traumatic brain injury the focus is on etiology, and for autism the focus is on symptoms consistent with a diagnosis.

The criteria used to document learning disabilities in special education have changed over time, with the criteria in the 2004 reauthorization of IDEA reflecting a shift from the documentation of a significant discrepancy between intelligence and achievement to evidence of significant limitations in language use. A final illustration of inconsistencies in IDEA categories is that of "other health impairment." Although chronic disease conditions meet the criteria for this category, it is not clear on what basis children with problems of attention and activity (ADHD) are eligible for special education under this category.

The issue of variable criteria for defining disability is also illustrated in the List of Impairments (Part B) for disability evaluation under Social Security. As noted earlier in this paper, the List of Impairments consists of 15 sections that encompass body systems, physical and mental disorders, as well as a loss or limitations of function. The criteria for defining disability differ depending on whether the identified condition is a disorder, a disease, or limitations of function.

EMERGING ISSUES

As stated at the beginning of this paper, concerns about the definition, measurement, and classification of disability in childhood are not new. The broad issues raised in the project on the classification of children in 1975 are consistent with those now being faced three decades later. These issues focused on the need for a comprehensive approach that includes the spectrum of disabling conditions, that recognizes the influence of environmental factors on development and disablement (Verbrugge and Jette, 1994), and that places emphasis on functioning rather than diagnoses as the basis for defining disability (Lollar and Simeonsson, 2005). The review of concepts and models in this paper has illustrated a number of contributions that support the use of such a comprehensive approach. The transactional model has reinforced the significance of the child-environment interaction in defining developmental outcomes. The concepts positing a continuum of outcomes attributed to reproductive casualty, caretaking casualty, and CNS dysfunction are consistent with childhood disability expressed as dimensional rather than discrete entities. Furthermore, although the medical model is still pervasive in defining disability through the use of health classifications (ICD-9 and DSM-IV) and disability categories (IDEA), there is a growing reliance on the estimation of the prevalence of functional limitations in national surveys. Although there is variability in the prevalence data derived from such surveys, they illustrate the use of functional data in estimating the prevalence of disability in childhood.

A central issue is the need for a comprehensive approach that is inclusive of the manifestations of disability in children. The differentiation of underlying health conditions from limitations in the performance of activities has increasingly been recognized as the basis for defining disability. With the publication of the ICF, a framework and classification is available for documenting disability (see discussion in Appendix B). ICF draws on a biopsychosocial framework in its portrayal of human function across the dimensions of Body Structures and Function, Activities, and Participation in life roles. Environmental Factors are recognized as having an ongoing role in mediating a person's performance of activities and participation in major life areas. ICF formalizes the functional model of disability by defining the dimensions of universal, human characteristics, providing a standard taxonomy for the documentation of disability in terms of impairments of function, activity limitations, and participation restrictions.

The content of the main volume of ICF, however, was not sufficiently sensitive to the developmental aspects of functioning in children, particularly young children (Simeonsson et al., 2003). A derived version of ICF for children and youth (ICF-CY) has been under development, with publication expected by WHO in 2006. A primary focus in the development of the ICF-CY has been content that captures the activities of the developing child in the home, school, and community environments (Simeonsson et al., 2003). This has been done by extending the coverage of the main ICF volume through the expansion of content and the provision of increased detail.

The person-environment focus of the transactional model of developmental outcome (Sameroff and Chandler, 1975) is consistent with the biopsychosocial perspective of ICF-CY, which emphasizes the ongoing influence of the environment on the child's functioning. New codes in the ICF-CY have been added for Body Functions and Structures, Activities, Participation, and Environmental Factors to capture the growth and development of infants, toddlers, children, and adolescents. These new codes represent significant areas of development and include sensory exploration, self-regulation, symbolic and social play, communication, learning, and meeting task demands.

The dimensional framework of ICF-CY offers a structure that can be used to define disability in terms of functional limitations in children's performance of activities and participation in major life roles appropriate for their age. Three applications of ICF-CY are proposed below to address the issues on variability in defining childhood disability raised in this paper.

A first recommendation is that functional limitations be defined by the IFC-CY domain of Activities and Participation. This would involve the identification of a limited number of codes in a set that represent key indicators of child functioning, such as communication, mobility, and learning. One or more codes from a given set could be used in surveys or in screening or assessment instruments to ensure consistent measurement of the particular indicator or area of functioning. This approach has been used in medicine to generate core sets; however, the focus in these applications has been to identify a limited set of codes associated with a specific disease entity (Grill et al., 2005). In this proposed application for the documentation of disability in childhood, the focus is on core sets associated with developmental indicators.

A second recommendation is to establish standard age groups for use in the analysis and reporting of data to improve the comparability of prevalence estimates across different assessments. The age groups currently used to report special education data (0 to 2, 3 to 5, 6 to 11, and 12 to 17 years of age) are recommended for adoption as standards for all studies, as they are (1) consistent with the stage divisions of developmental theories, (2) compatible with the age groupings of existing programs and services for children, and (3) already well established in education. Table C-2 illustrates identification of potential ICF-CY codes by age groups for key indicators, similar to those reported in the studies reviewed in this paper. In practice, identification of best codes would require the selection on the basis of research findings.

A third recommendation is that children's health conditions be documented by codes from the domains of Body Functions and Body Structures. This would avoid the heterogeneity of current classification practice in which underlying health conditions are documented by syndromes, categories, or disease entities. The use of codes from ICF domains would promote a standard basis for documentation as well as clarify the information provided by syndromes and diseases entities.

Related to the above recommendations for use of ICF codes in documenting health conditions and functional limitations of children is the need to use a common qualifier for the severity of disability across survey, clini-

TABLE C-2 Examples of ICF Activities and Participation Codes for Key Indicators

Activity	Codes for the following age groups				
	0–2 yr	3–5 yr	6–11 yr	12–17 yr	
Mobility	d420, transferring oneself	d455, moving around	d470, using transportation	d470, using transportation	
Communication	d315, receiving nonverbal messages	d330, speaking	d350, conversation	D355, discussion	
Self-care	d550, eating	d530, toileting	d540, dressing	d570, looking after ones health	
Learning	d120, other purposeful sensing	d140, learning to read	d175, solving problems	d177, making decisions	
Social interactions	d7601, child-parent relationships	d710, basic interpersonal relationships	d750, informal social relationships	d740, formal relationships	

cal, and research applications. Although the variability found in current prevalence data is no doubt attributable to different definitions used in surveys and service reports, the use of a severity qualifier in some studies and not others is also likely to be a significant source of variability. The adoption of a common qualifier for severity is important to enhance the comparability of data gathered in different surveys. It should also improve correspondence of survey data with documentation provided in the context of systems such as, health services, social security and special education. Although this recommendation has been proposed in the context of the ICF, its consideration is not contingent upon the use of the ICF but is applicable for any form of documentation.

Another area of potential application is the use of the ICF-CY taxonomy for the alignment of content for a new generation of developmentally appropriate instruments. Finally, ICF-CY may serve as a reference for the identification of concise indicators for surveys (McDougall and Miller, 2003; Hutchison and Gordon, 2005).

Adoption of ICF-CY as the standard for defining and classifying disability can serve as a unifying mechanism and a common language for the provision of services for children and youth everywhere. In the continuing effort to improve policy and practice on behalf of children with disabilities, the admonition stated by Hobbs thirty years ago is still timely: "classification is serious business. Classification can profoundly affect what happens to a child. It can open doors to services and experiences the child needs to grow in competence, to become a person sure of his worth, and appreciate the worth of others, to live with zest and to know joy" (Hobbs, 1975b, p.1).

REFERENCES

Aron, L.Y., Loprest, P.J., and Steuberle, C.E. (1996). *Serving Children with Disabilities: A Systematic Look at the Programs.* Washington, DC: Urban Press.

Baum, J.D. (1977). The continuum of caretaking casualty. *Developmental Medicine & Child Neurology* 19(4):543–544.

Capute, A.J. and Palmer, F.B. (1980). A pediatric overview of the spectrum of developmental disabilities. *Journal of Developmental and Behavioral Pediatrics* 1:66–69.

Capute, A.J., Shapiro, B.K., and Palmer, F.B. (1981). Spectrum of developmental disabilities: continuum of motor dysfunction. *Orthopedic Clinics of North America* 12(1):3–22.

Costello, E.J., Angold, A., Burns, B.J., Erkanli, A., Stangl, D.K., and Tweed, D.L. (1996). The Great Smoky Mountains Study of Youth. Functional impairment and serious emotional disturbance. *Archives of General Psychiatry* 53(12):1137–1143.

Costello, J., Mustillo, S., Erkanli, A., Keeler, G., and Angold, A. (2005). Prevalence and development of psychiatric disorders in childhood and adolescence. *Archives of General Psychiatry* 60:837–844.

Down, J.L. (1887). Abstracts of the Lettsomian lectures on some of the mental affections of childhood and youth. *British Medical Journal* 8:49–50.

Eaton, W.W., Mortensen, P.B., Thomsen, P.H., and Frydenberg, M. (2001). Obstetric complications and risk for severe psychopathology in childhood. *Journal of Autism and Developmental Disorders* 31(3):279–285.

Fedeyko, H. J. and Lollar, D.J. (2003). Classifying disability data: a fresh, integrative perspective. In B.M. Altman, S.N. Barnartt, G.E. Hendershot and S.A. Larson (Eds.) Using survey data to study disability: results from the National Health Interview Survey on Disability. *Research in Social Science and Disability* 3:55–72.

First, M.B. and Pincus, H.A. (2002). The DSM-IV text revision: rationale and potential impact on clinical practice. *Psychiatric Services.* 53(3):288–292.

Forfar, J.O., Hume, R., McPhail, F.M., Maxwell, S.M., Wilkinson, E.M., Lin, J.P., and Brown, J.K. (1994). *Developmental Medicine & Child Neurology* 36(12):1037–1048.

Forsyth, D. (1915). The development of children. *British Medical Journal.* March 20, pg. 535.

Grill, E., Ewert, T., Chatterji, S., Kostanjsek, N., and Stucki, G. (2005). ICF core sets development for the acute hospital and early post-acute rehabilitation facilities. *Disability and Rehabilitation* 27(7–8):361–366.

Halfon, N. and Newacheck, P. (1999). Prevalence and impact of parent reported disabling mental health conditions among U.S. children. *Journal of the American Academy of Child and Adolescent Psychiatry* 38(5):600–609.

Hobbs, N., ed. (1975a). *Issues in the Classification of Children.* San Francisco, CA: Jossey Bass.

Hobbs, N. (1975b). *The Futures of Children.* San Francisco, CA: Jossey Bass.

Hogan, D.P., Msall, M.E., Rogers, M.L., and Aver, R.C. (1997). Improved disability estimates of functional limitations among American children aged 5–17. *Maternal Child Health Journal* 1(4):203–216.

Hughes, D., Halfon, N., Brindis, C., and Newacheck, P. (1996). Improving children's access to health care: the role of decategorization. *Bulletin of the New York Academy of Medicine* 73:237–254.

Hutchison, T., and Gordon, D. (2005). Ascertaining the prevalence of childhood disability. *Child: Care Health and Development* 31(1):99–107.

Inhelder, B. (1966). Cognitive development and its contributions to the diagnosis of some phenomena of mental deficiency. *Merrill Palmer Quarterly* 11:299–311.

Inhelder, B. (1968). *The Diagnosis of Reasoning in the Mentally Retarded.* New York: John Day.

Kaplan, D. (2000). The definition of disability: perspective of the disability community. *Journal of Health Care Law and Policy* 3(2):352–364.

Landsman, G. (2005). Mothers and models of disability. *Journal of Medical Humanities* 26(2/3):121–139.

LaPlante, M. and Carlson, D. (1995). *Disability in the United States. Prevalence and Causes, 1992.* Report of the Disability Statistics Rehabilitation Research and Training Center. Washington, DC: National Institute on Disability and Rehabilitation Research.

Lollar, D.J. and Simeonsson, R.J. (2005). Diagnosis to function: classification for children and youths. *Journal of Developmental and Behavioral Pediatrics.* 26(4):3323–330.

Marks, D. (1997). Models of disability. *Disability and Rehabilitation* 19(3):85–91.

McDougall, J. and Miller, L.T (2003). Measuring chronic health condition and disability as distinct concepts in national surveys of school-aged children in Canada: a comprehensive review with recommendations based on the ICD-10 and ICF. *Disability and Rehabilitation* 25(16):922–939.

Mudrick, N.R. (2002). The prevalence of disability among children: paradigms and estimates. *Physical Medicine and Rehabilitation Clinics of North America.* 13:775–792.

Munn, P. (1997). Models of disability for children. *Disability and Rehabilitation* 19(11):484–486.

Narrow, W.E., Regier, D.A., Goodman, S.H., Rae, D.S., Roper, M.T., Bourdon, K.H., Hoven, C., and Moore, R. (1998). A comparison of federal definitions of severe mental illness among children and adolescents in four communities. *Psychiatric Services* 49(12):1601–1608.

Newacheck, P. and Halfon, N. (1998). Prevalence and impact of disabling chronic conditions in childhood. *American Journal of Public Health* 88(4):600–607.

Newacheck, P., Halfon, N., Brindis, C.D., and Hughes, D.C. (1998). Evaluating community efforts to decategorize and integrate financing of children's health services. *Milbank Quarterly* 76(2):57–73.

Ounsted, M. (1987). Cause, continua and other concepts. I. The "continuum of reproductive casualty." *Paediatric & Perinatal Epidemiology* 1(1):4–7.

Pasamanick, B., and Knobloch, H. (1966). Retrospective studies on the epidemiology of reproductive casualty: old and new. *Merrill-Palmer Quarterly* 12:7-26.

Roosa, M.W., Fitzgerald, H.E., and Carlson, N.A. (1982). Teenage parenting and child development: a literature review. *Infant Mental Health Journal* 3(1):4–18.

Sameroff, A.J. and Chandler, M.J. (1975). Reproductive risk and the continuum of caretaking casualty. In F.D. Horowitz, M. Hetherington, S. Scarr-Salapatek, and G. Siegel, eds. *Review of Child Development Research*. 4:187–244. Chicago: University of Chicago Press.

Schalick, W.O. (2000). Children, disability and rehabilitation in history. *Pediatric Rehabilitation* 4(2):91–95.

Simeonsson, R.J. and Rosenthal, S.L. (2001). Developmental models and clinical practice. In C. E. Walker and M. C. Roberts, Eds. *Handbook of Clinical Child Psychology*, 3rd ed. New York: Wiley.

Simeonsson, R.J., Lollar, D., Hollowell, J., and Adams, M. (2000). Revision of the International Classification of Impairments, Disabilities and Handicaps: developmental issues. *Journal of Clinical Epidemiology* 53:113–124.

Simeonsson, R.J., Leonardi, M., Bjorck-Akesson, E., Hollenweger, J., and Lollar, D. (2003). Applying the International Classification of Functioning Disability and Health to measure childhood disability. *Disability & Rehabilitation* 25(11–12):602–610.

Smyke, A.T., Dumitrescu, B.A., and Zeanah, C.H. (2002). Attachment disturbances in young children. I. The continuum of caretaking casualty. *Journal of the American Academy of Child & Adolescent Psychiatry* 41(8):972–982.

SSA (Social Security Administration). (2005). *Disability Evaluation under Social Security*. Office of Disability Programs, Social Security Administration. Washington, DC: Social Security Administration.

Stein, R.E. and Silver, E.J. (1999). Operationalizing a conceptually based noncategorical definition: a first look at US children with chronic conditions. *Archives of Pediatric and Adolescent Medicine* 153 (1):68–74.

Stein, R.E. and Silver, E.J. (2002). Comparing different definitions of chronic conditions in a national data set. *Ambulatory Pediatrics* 2(1):63–70.

Stein, R.E., Bauman, L.J., Westborrok, L.E., Coupey, S.M. and Ireys, H.T. (1993). Framework for identifying children who have chronic conditions: the case for a new definition (special article). *J. Pediatrics* 122:342–347.

Verbrugge, L. and Jette, A. (1994). The disablement process. *Social Science and Medicine* 38(1):1–14.

Wells, T. and Hogan, D. (2003). Developing concise measures of childhood activity limitations. *Maternal and Child Health Journal* 7(2):115–126.

Westbrook, L.E., Silver, E.J., and Stein, R. E. K. (1998). Implications for estimates of disability in children: a comparison of definitional components. *Pediatrics* 101(6):1025–1030.

WHO (World Health Organization) (2001). *International Classification of Functioning, Disability and Health*. Geneva, Switzerland: World Health Organization.

Zigler, E. (1969). Developmental versus difference theories of retardation and the problem of motivation. *American Journal of Mental Deficiency* 73:536–556.

D

How Does the Environment Influence Disability? Examining the Evidence

*Julie J. Keysor**

How the environment influences disability is a crucial clinical and policy question. If facilitative environments decrease disability, then policies and clinical interventions could be implemented to support the environmental elements that are conducive to minimizing disability and optimizing participation in daily life activities. Recent conceptual frameworks of disability highlight the important role of the environment in the disablement process; that is, people are believed to interact with their environments to produce disabilities (IOM, 1997; Teel et al., 1997). Thus, the environment is identified as a contextual factor in the process of disablement (Letts et al., 1994; Fougeyrollas, 1995; WHO, 2000). Yet, there are many research questions that pertain to the proposed theoretical frameworks. If the environment does influence disability, how does it do so? Which environmental domains influence disability? Which facilitators and barriers influence disability?

This paper addresses these questions by examining the empirical evidence. First, recent environmental measurement approaches are reviewed

*Julie J. Keysor, Ph.D., P.T. Assistant Professor, Department of Physical Therapy and Athletic Training, Sargent College of Health and Rehabilitative Sciences, Boston University. This work was supported by National Institute on Disability and Rehabilitation Research Grant H133B990005-01, National Institute of Child Health and Human Development Grant 5 K12 HD043444-02, and an Arthritis Foundation Arthritis Investigator Award. The analyses and views presented in this workshop paper are those of the author and not necessarily those of the Institute of Medicine Committee on Disability in America: A New Look.

and critiqued. Second, the evidence on the environment-disability link among adults with mobility limitations is examined. Third, challenges to this area of research are discussed. A thorough review covering all areas of disability is beyond the scope of this paper. Instead, the focus is on the environment-disability link in adults with mobility limitations. Other important areas of the environment-disability link among children and individuals with hearing, visual, or learning impairments are not discussed here.

ENVIRONMENT MEASUREMENT APPROACHES

Researchers face several formidable challenges when they pursue environmental assessments. The first challenge is conceptual. To study the complex interplay between environmental factors and disability, researchers need to know how to identify and measure the environmental factors that are relevant to individuals. Fougeyrollas (1995) suggests that the organization and context of society contain social, cultural, and physical dimensions. Factors in these dimensions can become obstacles or supports to individual functioning. The taxonomy of environmental factors of Fougeyrollas and colleagues (1991) includes socioeconomic organization (e.g., family structure, political systems, and economic systems), social roles (e.g., law, values, and attitudes), nature (e.g., geography, climate, and time), and development (e.g., architecture, land development, and technology).

The *International Classification of Functioning, Disability and Health* (ICF), on the other hand, specifies five environmental domains: products and technology; natural environment and human-made changes; support and relationships; attitudes; and services, systems, and policies (WHO, 2000). The Craig Hospital Inventory of Environmental Factors (CHIEF) assesses five domains that are similar to those used in the ICF taxonomy: (1) attitudes and support, (2) services and assistance, (3) physical and architectural, (4) policies, and (5) work and school (Whiteneck et al., 2004c). Shumway-Cook and colleagues (2002, 2003), in contrast, focus on the physical domain of the environment and identify eight dimensions: (1) temporal, (2) physical load, (3) terrain, (4) postural transitions, (5) distance, (6) density, (7) attentional demands, and (8) ambient conditions. To date there is no consensus on which environmental domains or which elements of the domains should be measured to study the importance of the environment in the lives of people with disabilities.

The second challenge is one of measurement, with three general approaches currently being used. The first approach assesses an individual's perceptions of the degree to which environmental factors influence his or her participation in daily life. Four instruments assess the environment in this manner: (1) CHIEF (Whiteneck et al., 2004c); (2) the Measure of the Quality of the Environment (Fougeyrollas et al., 1997); (3) the Facilitators and Barriers to Participation for People with Mobility Impairments and Limitations (Gray et al., 2005); and (4) Fange and Iwarsson's (1999) self-assessment of the physical housing environment.

CHIEF is a 24-item self-report instrument that assesses the frequency with which people encounter environmental barriers related to attitudes and support, services and assistance, physical and architectural domains, policies, and work and school and the impact of each environmental factor on daily life, as perceived by the individual (Whiteneck et al., 2004c). The respondents are asked to indicate how often various barriers in the environment have been a problem over the past 12 months. If environmental factors have been a problem, the respondents are asked to indicate whether the factor has been a big or a little problem. The reliability and validity of the instrument are acceptable for measurement of the effects of all domains.

The Measure of the Quality of the Environment is a 72-item self-report instrument that assesses the extent to which various barriers and facilitators of the environment influence peoples' daily lives in six domains: (1) support and the attitudes of family and friends; (2) income, job, and income security; (3) governmental and public services; (4) the physical environment and accessibility; (5) technology; and (6) equal opportunity and political directions (Fougeyrollas et al., 1997).

The Facilitators and Barriers to Participation for People with Mobility Impairments and Limitations is also a self-report instrument that assesses the perceived accessibility of elements of the home and community environments (Gray et al., 2005). Fange and Iwarsson (1999) take a similar approach in their recently developed self-report assessment of the physical housing environment. The 31-item instrument assesses eight dimensions of the physical environment, including (1) overall satisfaction with housing conditions, (2) suitability, (3) security and safety, (4) importance, (5) privacy, (6) social contacts, (7) flexibility, and (8) accessibility. The reliability and content validity of the instrument are acceptable (Fange and Iwarsson, 1999).

Instruments like those reviewed above are important for identifying relevant environmental domains as well as important barriers and facilitators. However, a perception of an environmental impact is not direct evidence of its actual influence on a person's level of participation. A person's perception of the impact that the environment has on his or her participation may be strongly correlated with his or her participation, thereby resulting in inflated measures of effect. Thus, measurement of a person's perception of environmental barriers does not allow the researcher to examine empirically whether the presence or the absence of such a factor in a person's environment is directly associated with variation in a person's level of participation. A more direct measure of the actual environment is needed. To examine how environmental factors affect peoples' involvement in daily activities, the extent to which a person's environment contains elements that could facilitate or restrict participation needs to be characterized and correlated with the level of disability.

Two approaches described in the current literature attempt to characterize the elements of people's environments. One approach, developed by Shumway-Cook and colleagues (Shumway-Cook et al., 2003), assesses the extent to which people avoid and encounter barriers and facilitators in the physical environment by using the self-report Environmental Components of Mobility Questionnaire. The questionnaire assesses eight dimensions of the physical environment: (1) temporal, (2) physical load, (3) terrain, (4) postural transitions, (5) distance, (6) density, (7) attentional demands, and (8) ambient conditions. Shumway-Cook and colleagues' self-report approach has been shown to be reliable (Shumway-Cook et al., 2003); however, the limitation of this approach is that asking people to ascertain the extent to which they avoid or encounter barriers may not necessarily correspond to the factors that are in their environments. For example, if someone with mobility limitations is unable to negotiate stairs, he or she may state that he or she avoids stairs, but the person's environment may not have stairs. In addition, whether people avoid aspects of their environment is likely to be confounded by function; people will avoid stairs if they are unable to negotiate stairs.

Shumway-Cook and colleagues developed an observational approach that corresponds to the Environmental Components of Mobility Questionnaire in which specific factors of the environment comprising the physical domain are assessed independently of a person's level of participation (Shumway-Cook et al., 2002). The administration of the measure involves a structured observational encounter between a researcher and a participant; that is, a researcher observes and videotapes the participant as he or she performs community mobility activities, such as going to a grocery store or seeing a health care provider. Although this approach provides the investigator with an independent assessment of environmental factors, the limitations are the protocol's cost and the time that it takes to administer it. Although it has attractive features, the protocol of Shumway-Cook et al. is not feasible in large-scale field studies, in which feasibility, study costs, and participant burden are paramount concerns.

Another means of characterization of the environment is description of the actual elements of the environment. This measurement approach is taken by Keysor and colleagues (2005) in the Home and Community Environment (HACE) instrument. HACE is a 36-item instrument that assesses barriers and facilitators in six conceptual domains: (1) home mobility, (2) community mobility, (3) basic mobility devices, (4) communication devices, (5) transportation factors, and (6) attitudes (Keysor et al., 2005). The home mobility domain assesses the extent to which people have barriers in the home, such as the number of steps at the main entrance or the number of stairs inside the home. Facilitators are also assessed, including ramps, elevators, and chairlifts. The community mobility domain assesses the extent to which a person's community has barriers such as uneven sidewalks and curbs without curb cuts. Basic mobility devices, communication devices, and transportation facilitators are assessed to indicate whether the respondent has a mobility or communication device and the type of transportation, irrespective of its use. Reliability was acceptable for all subscales. This approach allows the person to characterize the environment irrespective of his or her level of participation or functional ability. The investigators found, however, that participants were unable to characterize environmental domains related to policies and services. Thus, it is questionable whether participants can validly characterize the availability of services and policies for individuals with limitations in daily activities, which is a potential limitation to this assessment approach.

Taking a similar approach of characterizing the environment but focusing on the home environment, Freedman and Agree (2005) report on a new instrument that can be used to assess the "existence," "acquisition," and "use" of environmental modifications and assistive technologies. The self-report survey covers five general areas: (1) the home environment, (2) mobility and other devices, (3) the effectiveness of features and devices, (4) the presence of computers and telephones, and (5) residual activity of daily living and instrumental activity of daily living. The reliability and validity of the instrument are acceptable (Freedman and Agree, 2005). The Enabler is another instrument that characterizes the environment irrespective of the level of function (Iwarsson, 1997). This instrument is completed by a trained professional. The level of functional impairment and the presence of barriers in the home and community environment are assessed, and a combined score indicates the degree of accessibility problems.

In summary, a new generation of instruments that can be used to assess the environment has been developed over the past several years. Researchers appear to take three general approaches, with each approach having strengths and weaknesses (Table D-1).

THE EVIDENCE: THE DISABILITY-ENVIRONMENT LINK

Medline and the Cumulative Index of Nursing and Allied Health Literature were reviewed to identify research articles examining the environment-disability link among adults with mobility limitations. "Environment," "environmental," "technology," and "device" were referenced to title searches and cross-referenced with the terms "disability," "disablement," "handicap," and "participation." Research articles pertaining to the role of the environment on disability among adults with mobility limita-

TABLE D-1 Comparison of Approaches for Measurement of the Environment

Approach	Description	Strengths	Weaknesses
Determination of perceived impact	Self-report assessment of the degree to which the environment influences participation; includes accessibility	Seems to be a reliable approach for people to self-report barriers and facilitators	May create a statistical bias: artificially correlated with disability (participation) Perceived barriers or facilitators may not be actual elements of the individual's environment
Determination of barriers encountered or avoided (perceived or actual)	Self-report and observational approach that assesses the extent to which barriers are avoided	Self-report and observational methods seem to be reliable	A time-consuming observational method that is not feasible for large epidemiological studies; assessment is confounded by functional ability
Characterization of the environment	Self-report or observational assessment of actual elements of the environment	Representation of the environment irrespective of level of function or disability	Some domains or aspects of the environment may be difficult to reliably self-report; observational methods are time-consuming and not feasible for use in large epidemiological studies

tions, including stroke, arthritis, spinal cord injuries, and general aging, were reviewed.

Several studies show that individuals with mobility limitations report the presence of barriers and facilitators in their environment that restrict participation. Barriers are reported in the built environment domain, as well as in the domains of social attitudes, social institutions, cultural norms, and technology (Meyers et al., 2002; Noreau et al., 2002; Gray et al., 2003; Whiteneck et al., 2004a). On the other hand, individuals with mobility limitations report that important facilitators in the environment are the positive attitudes of individuals in the community; social support; and the availability of technology, devices, and products and accessible transportation (Meyers et al., 2002; Noreau et al., 2002; Gray et al., 2003).

Individuals with mobility limitations may also avoid physical barriers in the community. Shumway-Cook and colleagues (2003) showed that people with mobility limitations were more likely to report that they avoided long-distance ambulation, crossing streets with traffic lights, crossing busy streets, using stairs and escalators, walking on curbs or uneven surfaces, and going out in icy conditions. There were no differences between individuals with mobility limitations and individuals without mobility limitations in the rates of going outside when it was dark, snowing, very hot or cold, wet or noisy. However, when actual behavior was observed, there were fewer differences between individuals with mobility limitations and those without (Shumway-Cook et al., 2002). Individuals with mobility limitations were more likely than age-matched individuals without mobility limitations to use the elevator and were less likely to ascend two flights of stairs or walk on uneven surfaces. However, there were no differences between the two groups in the average distance walked; the rate of crossing streets with traffic lights; or the temperature, light conditions, and level of precipitation during a walk.

Although this descriptive approach shows that people with mobility limitations do perceive that aspects of their environment limit or enhance their participation, it does not provide strong evidence showing how the environment influences disability. To address this question, the environment needs to be correlated with measures of disability. Surprisingly, only a few published studies have assessed the effects of the environment on disability outcomes. The few studies that have been published in the literature are reviewed below.

Three studies of adults with mobility limitations showed a small but significant association of the environment on disability. Whiteneck and colleagues (2004a), in a large population-based study of 2,726 individuals with spinal cord injuries, correlated the results obtained with CHIEF environment scales with measures of participation and life satisfaction. The CHIEF environment scales (i.e., physical-structural, services-assistance, and attitudinal-support) showed a small but significant association with the total Craig Handicap Assessment and Reporting Technique (CHART) score, although the CHIEF environment scales accounted for only 4 percent of the variance in participation. Demographics, injury-related factors, and activity limitations each accounted for approximately 20 percent of the variance in participation. Similar patterns emerged when the findings obtained with the individual CHIEF subscales were correlated with those obtained with the CHART subscales. Physical and structural barriers were weakly correlated with physical independence, mobility, and occupation; services and assistance were weekly associated with physical independence, cognitive independence, mobility, occupation, and social integration; and the attitudinal domain and support were associated with physical independence and cognitive independence. The CHIEF subscales were more strongly associated with life satisfaction, accounting for approximately 10 percent of the variance in life satisfaction.

Similar findings have been reported in other studies (Badley et al., 1998; Rochette et al., 2001). Badley and colleagues (1998), in a cross-sectional population-based study of 16,017 individuals with self-reported, arthritis-associated disability, reported that modifications to the kitchen were associated with less dependence in external household activities and domestic activities of daily living, whereas a modified bathroom, as well as a cane and other moving aids, was associated with more disability in domestic and personal care activities of daily living. The environmental factors explained 8 percent of the variance in dependence in daily activities (i.e., disability), with functional limitation explaining more than 40 percent of the variance in disability. However, the combination of functional limitation and environmental barriers explained a larger amount of the variance in disability than the combination of functional impairment and personal or sensory factors. In a cross-sectional study of 51 stroke patients selected from a rehabilitation unit, Rochette and colleagues (2001) showed that environmental barriers explained 6 percent of the variance in disability, as measured by the Assessment of Life Habits.

One study showed that individuals with spinal cord injuries believed that the biggest factor limiting their daily life activities was related to technology. In a cross-sectional study of 70 individuals with spinal cord injuries who used a wheelchair, Chaves and colleagues (2004) found that limitation due to one's wheelchair was most strongly correlated with perceived participation limitations, followed by the environment and physical impairments.

Stronger evidence on the impact of the environment on disability will come from prospective studies. No published prospective studies met the search criteria established for this paper. However, the author and colleagues recently conducted a 12-month longitudinal study of adults who were discharged from the acute-care hospital setting with a diagnosis of neurological disorder, lower-extremity orthopedic trauma, or medically complex conditions (Jette et al., in press). Data for 345 participants who completed 1-month and 6-month interviews were analyzed to examine the impact that the environment had on disability. HACE was used to assess home and environmental barriers and facilitators (Keysor et al., 2005), the Medical Outcomes Study-Social Support was used to assess social support (Sherbourne and Stewart, 1991), and the Participation Measure for Post-Acute Care was used to measure disability (Gandek et al., in press). In multivariate analyses that adjusted for age, sex, educational attainment, race, disease severity, physical and mobility activities, and applied cognition, it was found that at 1 month greater numbers of community mobility barriers were statistically significantly associated with more community disability, with transportation facilitators approaching statistical significance. On the other hand, more home mobility barriers were associated with less social and home participation, whereas more community barriers, more mobility technology facilitators, and more social support were associated with more social and home participation. With the exception of social support, however, environmental barriers and facilitators were not predictive of community participation and social and home participation at 6 months (Keysor et al., submitted for publication).

The strongest evidence of the environment-disability link comes from an 18-month prospective randomized controlled trial conducted by Mann and colleagues (1999). One hundred four community-dwelling elderly people were randomized either to a treatment group that received resources for assistive technology (e.g., a walker or a wheelchair) or environmental modifications (e.g., the addition of ramps or the removal of scatter rugs) that were evaluated as being necessary by trained clinicians or to a control group of individuals who received the usual care for their conditions. There were no differences in disability between the treatment and the control groups, as measured by CHART. However, the treatment group had significantly less decline in function over the 18-month period and lower health care costs related to institutionalized care.

On the other hand, Whiteneck and colleagues (2004b), in a study of 73 individuals with traumatic brain injuries, found that the environment was an important determinant of participation. Transportation, the surroundings, government policies, attitudes, and the natural environment were perceived to have the most impact on people's lives. The total CHIEF score and the subscales of attitudes and services, which represent the impacts of environmental barriers, were associated with more disability, as measured by the overall CHART score. More physical and policy barriers, as measured by two subscales of CHIEF, were associated with the mobility and occupation subscales of CHART. More barriers in attitudes and services were associated with less cognitive independence.

SUMMARY AND CRITIQUE OF CURRENT EMPIRICAL EVIDENCE

Research on how the environment influences disability has been limited. The majority of studies have small sample sizes; and many studies draw samples from a convenience clinical population, thereby limiting the generalizability of the findings of the studies. The study designs are cross-sectional, thereby limiting the causal inferences of the effects of the environment on restricting or enhancing participation that can be made. Lastly, the majority of study samples comprise individuals whose primary mode of locomotion is a wheelchair, so little or nothing is known about the impact of the environment on other populations.

The studies that have been published have provided evidence that individuals with mobility limitations perceive that particular barriers and facilitators of the environment—particularly in the physical and social domains—restrict or enhance their participation in life activities. In addition, individuals with mobility limitations seem to avoid physical barriers in the community, although their actual behavior patterns may differ from self-reported perceptions.

Despite the findings that people with mobility limitations report the presence of barriers in their environment, it is not clear how the environment influences disability. A few studies have reported a small association of the environment with disability, but this explains less than 10 percent of the variance in disability (Badley et al., 1998; Rochette et al., 2001; Whiteneck et al., 2004a). On the other hand, one study of individuals with traumatic brain injuries showed a stronger association of the environment with disability (Whiteneck et al., 2004b), a finding that could suggest that the environment-disability link could be dependent on the specific type of disability.

FUTURE CHALLENGES

Researchers in the field of environment-disability face several challenges in the upcoming years. The first challenge pertains to measurement. Further work is needed on conceptualizing the domains of the environment that are relevant to disability as well as what elements of each domain need to be assessed—particularly in relation to the social, political, and attitudinal domains of the environment. Additional work is also needed to illuminate the best measurement approach for assessment of the environment in a manner that can be used to examine whether and how the environment influences disability. Does assessment of the perceived impact of the environment bias associations with participation; that is, is the perceived impact of the environment artificially correlated with participation? Is ascertainment of characteristics of the environment irrespective of disability a better approach to examination of the impact of the environment on disability? On the other hand, as Fange and Iwarsson (1999) advocate, should both approaches be used? Can participants reliably self-report characteristics of their environment? Are the measures valid? Lastly, can the diverse domains of the environment be assessed in a parsimonious manner to minimize respondent burden?

The second challenge pertains to disentangling the causal relationship of the environment on disability. The evidence to date shows that some environments that are more facilitative are associated with less disability, whereas other environments that are facilitative are associated with more disability. This finding may reflect a human adaptation process, with people modifying their environment because of their health status. It is likely that people adapt to their environment—i.e., they change how they accomplish activities. In addition, people may adapt or change their environment to meet their needs. This element of human adaptation poses particular challenges for understanding how the environment influences disability. Prospective longitudinal studies are needed to develop evidence of whether the changes in the baseline environment are related to changes in disability. Experimental clinical trials will also provide evidence of whether the manipulation of various aspects of the environment influences disability.

The third and perhaps the most important challenge will be to implement complex analytical approaches in study designs. Disability theoretical frameworks posit that disability is the result of disease-specific person-level factors and the environment in which a person lives, that is, the interaction of the person within his or her environment. Studies to date have focused on assessment of the direct impact of the environment on disability and have not examined statistical interaction effects. Perhaps there is a certain threshold of functional limitation in combination with a certain type of restrictive environment that is conducive to greater disability. For example, people who are able to walk one or two blocks may be more strongly affected by restrictive communities than people who are able to walk several blocks. On the other hand, perhaps people with a combination of cognitive and physical impairments will be more adversely affected by restrictive environments than people with physical impairments alone. Large sample sizes and complex analytical strategies will be needed to assess interactive effects, and this could be imperative to understanding how the environment influences disability.

Lastly, the role of the environment on disability is likely to be quite complex, and important factors may need to be taken into consideration that are not clearly articulated in the current environment-disability literature. First, the role of behavioral factors in the person-environment interaction may be imperative. Do people adapt to barriers and remain active in their lives? Does one's ability to resolve the barriers and advocate for his or her needs mediate the relationship between restrictive environments and disability? Second, is disability the optimal outcome in the examination of person-environment interactions? Is the environment a determinant of disability, or does the environment influence other outcomes, such as satisfaction and quality of life, as some evidence suggests (Richards et al., 1999; Whiteneck et al., 2004a)?

REFERENCES

Badley EM, Rothman LM, et al. (1998). Modeling physical dependence in arthritis: the relative contribution of specific disabilities and environmental factors. *Arthritis Care and Research* 11(5):335–345.

Chaves ES, Boninger ML, et al. (2004). Assessing the influence of wheelchair technology on perception of participation in spinal cord injury. *Archives of Physical Medicine & Rehabilitation* 85(11):1854–1858.

Fange A and Iwarsson S (1999). Physical housing environment: development of a self-assessment instrument. *Canadian Journal of Occupational Therapy. Revue Canadienne d Ergotherapie* 66:250–260.

Fougeyrollas P (1995). Documenting environmental factors for preventing the handicap creation process: Quebec contributions relating to ICIDH and social participation of people with functional differences. *Disability and Rehabilitation* 17(3–4):145–153.

Fougeyrollas P, Bolduc M, et al. (1991). *Use of the Health and Activity Limitations Survey in Relation with Conceptual Framework of the ICIDH.* Ottawa, Ontario, Canada: Canadian Society of the ICIDH and Quebec Committee of the ICIDH.

Fougeyrollas P, Noreau L, et al. (1997). Measure of the quality of the environment. *ICIDH and Environmental Factors International Network* 9(1):32–39.

Freedman VA and Agree E (2005). Linking measures of assistive technology and disability. Workshop on Improving Survey Measures of Late-Life Disability. Sponsored by the Office of the Assistant Secretary for Planning and Evaluation, U.S. Department of Health and Human Services, Washington, DC.

Gandek B, Sinclair J, Jette A, Ware J. (In press). Development and initial testing of the participation measure for post-acute care (PM-PAC). *American Journal of Physical Medicine & Rehabilitation.*

Gray D, Gould M, et al. (2003). Environmental barriers and disability. *Journal of Architectural and Planning Research* 20(1):29–37.

Gray D, Hollingsworth H, et al. (2005). Participation and Environment Measurement System: PATS and FABS. Paper prepared for the American Public Health Association 133rd Annual Meeting, December 10-14, Philadelphia, PA.

IOM (Institute of Medicine) (1997). *Enabling America: Assessing the Role of Rehabilitation Science and Engineering.* Washington, DC: National Academy Press.

Iwarsson S (1997). *The Enabler. A Method of Analyzing Accessibility Problems in Housing.* Dalby/Lund, Sweden: Lund University.

Jette A, Keysor J, et al. (in press). Beyond function: predicting participation outcomes in a rehabilitation cohort. *Archives of Physical Medicine & Rehabilitation.*

Keysor J, Jette A, et al. (2005). Development of the home and community environment (HACE) instrument. *Journal of Rehabilitation Medicine* 37(1):37–44.

Keysor, J, Jette A, et al. (Submitted for publication). Does a prospective examination of the environment show a link with participation?

Letts L, Law M, et al. (1994). Person-environment assessments in occupational therapy. *American Journal of Occupational Therapy* 48(7):608–618.

Mann W, Ottenbacher K, et al. (1999). Effectiveness of assistive technology and environmental interventions in maintaining independence and reducing home care costs for the frail elderly: a randomized controlled trial. *Archives of Family Medicine* 8(3):210–217.

Meyers AR, Anderson JJ, et al. (2002). Barriers, facilitators, and access for wheelchair users: substantive and methodological lessons from a pilot study of environmental effects. *Social Science & Medicine* 55(8):1435–1446.

Noreau L, Fougeyrollas P, et al. (2002). The perceived influence of the environment on social participation among individuals with spinal cord injury. *Topics in Spinal Cord Injury* 7(3):56–72.

Richards JS, Bombardier CH, et al. (1999). Access to the environment and life satisfaction after spinal cord injury. *Archives of Physical Medicine & Rehabilitation.* 80(11):1501–1506.

Rochette A, Desrosiers J, et al. (2001). Association between personal and environmental factors and the occurrence of handicap situations following a stroke. *Disability & Rehabilitation* 23(13):559–569.

Sherbourne C & Stewart, A. (1991). The MOS Social Support Survey. *Social Science and Medicine* **32**:705–714.

Shumway-Cook A, Patla AE, et al. (2002). Environmental demands associated with community mobility in older adults with and without mobility disabilities. *Physical Therapy* 82(7):670–681.

Shumway-Cook A, Patla AE, et al. (2003). Environmental components of mobility disability in community-living older persons. *Journal of the American Geriatrics Society* 51(3):393–398.

Teel C, Dunn W, et al. (1997). The role of the environment in fostering independence: conceptual and methodological issues in developing an instrument. *Topics in Stroke Rehabilitation* 4:28–40.

Whiteneck G, Meade MA, et al. (2004a). Environmental factors and their role in participation and life satisfaction after spinal cord injury. *Archives of Physical Medicine & Rehabilitation* 85(11):1793–1803.

Whiteneck G, Gerhart KA, et al. (2004b). Identifying environmental factors that influence the outcomes of people with traumatic brain injury. *Journal of Head Trauma Rehabilitation* 19(3):191–204.

Whiteneck G, Harrison-Felix CL, et al. (2004c). Quantifying environmental factors: a measure of physical, attitudinal, service, productivity, and policy barriers. *Archives of Physical Medicine and Rehabilitation* 85:1324–1335.

WHO (World Health Organization). (2000). *International Classification of Functioning, Disability, and Health.* Geneva, Switzerland: World Health Organization.

E

Late-Life Disability Trends:
An Overview of Current Evidence

*Vicki A. Freedman**

A fundamental question in population aging research has been whether mortality declines in late life have been accompanied by a compression or an expansion of periods of morbidity and disability[1-3]. Gruenberg's theory[2] portends pandemic increases in chronic disease and disability, whereas Fries[1] suggested that as morbidity onset is postponed and more adults reach the limit to human life, aggregate declines will occur. Manton[3] proposed a third perspective, in which declines in mortality yield increases in the prevalence of chronic diseases whose rates of progression are slowed; hence, he predicts declines in the severity of disease and consequent disability even with increases in the prevalence of chronic disease. The competing theories have implications not only for the disability pathways at the end of life but also for trends in cross-sectional snapshots of the prevalence of disability among older Americans.

Numerous studies exploring late-life disability trends in the United States have been published over the last decade or so, sometimes with conflicting results[4,5]. Central to this debate are critical conceptual distinc-

*Vicki A. Freedman, Ph.D., Professor, Department of Health Systems and Policy, University of Medicine and Dentistry of the New Jersey, School of Public Health. This summary draws extensively upon collaborative efforts with Linda Martin of the Institute of Medicine and Robert Schoeni of the University of Michigan. Support for this paper was provided by National Institute on Aging Grant NIA R01AG021516. The analyses and views expressed are those of the author and do not necessarily represent those of the author's affiliation, the funding agency, or the Institute of Medicine Committee on Disability in America: A New Look.

tions and measurement issues. No studies thus far have tracked trends in late-life participation in society. Instead, most studies measure difficulty or the use of help with daily activities (related either to personal care or to living independently). Recent studies have also highlighted disparities in trends across demographic and socioeconomic groups[6–8].

Since these theories of population aging have been proposed, understanding of disability has evolved from a classic medical model, which attributes disability to underlying chronic conditions and impairments, to one that recognizes the fundamentally social and environmental components of disability[9,10]. As such, recent hypotheses as to the reasons for late-life disability trends have included the influence of chronic disease trends and related medical care; shifts in underlying physical, cognitive, and sensory functioning; changes to the environment, such as technological aids and rehabilitation technologies; and demographic shifts. This paper reviews the most recent evidence on trends in late-life disability in the United States, disparities therein, and current understanding of the reasons for those trends.

TRENDS IN LATE-LIFE DISABILITY

Studies of the 1960s and 1970s suggested that longer life implied worsening health, as measured by increases in self-reported disability and chronic disease[11,12]. Some have questioned whether these increases were due to changing social forces during the period that made reports of disability more acceptable[13].

The evidence for the 1980s and early 1990s was mixed, with Manton and colleagues reporting large declines in disability[14,15] and Crimmins and colleagues concluding that there was no clear ongoing trend[16]. At the request of the National Institute on Aging, the Committee on National Statistics of the National Research Council held a workshop to review the data and methods used to determine trends in disability at older ages[17]. The workshop report concluded that there had been modest declines in the proportion of older people with limitations in instrumental activities of daily living (IADLs) but inconsistencies across surveys in trends in activities of daily living (ADLs).

In the decade since that workshop more than a dozen studies have focused on late-life disability trends. A recent review[4] highlighted methodological considerations in the comparison of trends in prevalence across surveys and reported findings for a range of outcomes, including physical, cognitive, and sensory limitations as well as ADL and IADL disabilities. The authors found that of the 16 studies identified, 8 unique surveys were analyzed: for the purposes of trend analysis, 2 were rated as good, 4 were rated as fair, 1 was rated as poor, and 1 was rated as mixed (fair or poor,

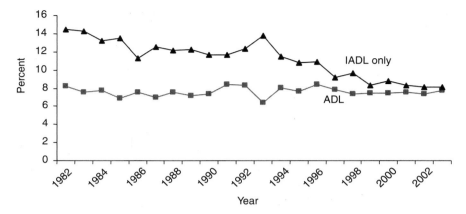

FIGURE E-1 Percentage of the community-based population ages 70 years and older reporting need for help with personal care or only routine care activities, 1982 to 2004. ADL=Needs help with personal care activities such as eating, bathing, dressing, or getting around the home. IADL only=Needs help only with routine needs, such as everyday household chores, doing necessary business, shopping, or getting around for other purposes.
SOURCE: Analysis of the 1982–2004 National Health Interview Survey.

depending on the outcome). Studies rated fair or good consistently showed substantial declines in IADL disability. For example, evidence from the National Health Interview Survey (NHIS) suggests that between 1982 and 2004 there has been a 6 percentage point decline in the population ages 70 years and older needing help with only routine care (but not personal care) activities such as shopping, preparing meals, and managing money, sometimes called IADLs (Figure E-1). Subsequent analysis of data from the National Long Term Care Survey (NLTCS) suggested that declines in three IADL activities—managing money, shopping for groceries, and doing laundry—were notably large from 1984 to 1999; however, among those reporting an ADL or an IADL disability, the severity of disability increased over time[18].

At the time that the review was published, there remained disagreement about whether or not there had been a decline in the proportion of older Americans with difficulty with self-care activities, such as bathing, dressing, toileting, and walking around inside, sometimes called ADLs. The answer was sorted out by a technical working group that analyzed five national surveys conducted from the early 1980s through 2001[19]. The 12-person panel prepared estimates using identical methodologies and investigated sources of the inconsistencies among the population ages 70 years and older. The panel found during the middle and late 1990s consistent declines on the order of 1 to 2.5 percent per year for two commonly used measures in the disability literature: difficulty with daily activities and help with daily activities. Mixed evidence was found for a third measure: use of help or equipment with daily activities. In comparing findings across surveys, the panel found that time period, definition of disability, treatment of the institutional population, and standardization of results by age were important considerations.

Trends in disability incidence have been much more difficult to characterize, in part because such estimates ideally involve equally spaced and relatively narrow time intervals[20]. Largely because of data constraints, only three studies to date have focused on trends in disability incidence rates in the United States[14,16,21]. Using different data and estimation strategies, all three studies show declines in the incidence of disabilities; two of the three suggest that rates of recovery have also declined[14,21].

DISPARITIES IN DISABILITY TRENDS

Although the literature on late-life health is relatively large and growing, relatively few studies have focused explicitly on disparities in trends for major demographic and socioeconomic groups. Comparisons across studies are complicated by several factors. First, with few exceptions[6–8] statistical tests of disparities in trends have been omitted. Second, in some cases conclusions are dependent on whether the disparity is measured in terms of differences in differences (e.g., Group 1 declined x percentage points more than Group 2) or in relative terms (e.g., the gap between Group 1 and Group 2 doubled from x percent to $2x$ percent). Third, demographic and socioeconomic groups and measures of disability and functioning vary widely across studies. A recent review[4] concluded that evidence on disparities in trends by race, education, sex, and age is limited and mixed, with no consensus yet emerging.

Racial disparities in late-life disability trends have received the most attention in the literature, with inconsistent results. For example, using data from the NLTCS, researchers found increasing racial disparities in the prevalence of chronic ADL or IADL disabilities during the 1980s and diminishing disparities during the 1990s[22,23]. Three studies of the NHIS (from 1982 to 1996 and from 1982 to 2002)[6–8] found no statistically significant changes in the relative gap between minorities and whites; however, there appears to have been a slight narrowing of the absolute size of the gap[7].

Reports of disparities in trends by education level have been more consistent. Declines in disability have been larger for those with more than a high school education[6–8,24]. For example, using data from the 1982 to 2002 NHIS, Schoeni and colleagues[6] found that older people with the least education (0 to 8 years) showed virtually no improvement in ADL or IADL disabilities, whereas those with 16 or more years of education experienced significant declines. Focusing on ADL disabilities, the authors found significant increases for the group with the least education and relatively flat trends for those with 16 or more years of education. Consequently, the socioeconomic gap in disability, which favored the more educated group in 1982, became much larger between 1982 and 2002 both in absolute terms and in relative terms[7]. However, findings for trends in cognitive functioning showed the reverse pattern with respect to education, with larger improvements among those with less than a high school education[25].

Conflicting evidence also exists with respect to disparities by other demographic characteristics. Sex differences in disability and functioning trends have been reported in one instance[24] but not in others [7,8,25,26]. With respect to age group, findings from the Survey of Income and Program Participation (SIPP) suggest that the largest absolute improvements in functioning between 1984 and 1993 occurred for the oldest old, but relative improvements were largest for those ages 50 to 64 years. In contrast, focusing on those ages 70 years and older in the NHIS, there appeared to be no statistically significant differences in disability trends by 10-year age groups from 1982 to 1996[8]. This finding appears to be sensitive to model specification, however. Further analysis of the NHIS data finds little change in the simple difference in the need for help with ADLs or IADLs across age groups, but the relative difference increased substantially, resulting in a widening relative gap[7]. That is, the rate in 1982 was roughly 200 percent higher for people ages 85 years and older than for people ages 70 to 74 years (a 32 percentage point gap), and this increased to nearly 400 percent by 2002.

Other important demographic factors have received little consideration in terms of whether gaps are widening or narrowing. For example, although nativity has been linked to mortality and health outcomes[27,28], late-life health trends have not been examined by place of birth. Furthermore, little evidence exists regarding disparities with respect to marital status, occupation, and wealth. Disparities by income quartiles have recently been investigated[7], with gaps for the first and fourth income quartiles following a pattern similar to that of education.

EVIDENCE ON WHY LATE-LIFE DISABILITY IS DECLINING

In part because of data limitations, thus far only limited research on possible explanations for these trends in late-life disability has been conducted. Four distinct realms have been explored to date: demographic and socioeconomic shifts; changes in chronic disease and related treatments; trends in underlying physical, cognitive, and sensory functioning; and environmental changes, particularly growth in the use of assistive devices. Research to date suggests that the decline is likely the result of a combination of factors and not any single underlying trend.

The improvement has been attributed in part to the shifting demographic and socioeconomic composition of the elderly population. Notably, the elderly as a group are much better educated today than they were in the mid-1980s; and such a change accounts for a substantial portion—but not all—of the decline in limitations[29]. The relationship between education and late-life functioning is complex and involves numerous indirect causal pathways. Education, along with other socioeconomic, demographic, and cultural factors, may, for example, influence the risk of disease, injury, and impairment by influencing access to health care throughout life, preventive care, occupational history, social standing (and the consequent stress and environmental exposures), and risk-taking behaviors. More educated people may have a greater ability to marshal resources to optimize their health outcomes and may more easily navigate the health care system, particularly in a managed care setting, in which referrals are needed for specialty care. Moreover, education may affect whether functional deficits result in disability through its influence on assistive device use and the environment. One analysis suggests that impending increases in education levels will continue to contribute to improvements in late-life functioning, albeit at a reduced rate[29].

Some evidence also suggests that the extent to which some chronic conditions are expressed in terms of disability may have been ameliorated in recent decades, in particular, for arthritis[26] and cardiovascular diseases[30], even as the prevalence of many of those conditions has increased in the older population[5,24,26]. It could be that earlier diagnosis and better management of such conditions has led to lower reported rates of disabilities; however, one investigation of the role of medication use in recent declines among the pre-retirement-age population did not demonstrate a link[31], and an investigation of medical procedures for cardiovascular disease provided only weak evidence [30].

A third area of focus has been on trends in underlying physical, cognitive, and sensory functioning. Physical functioning, most often measured with Nagi's functional limitations (difficulty with body movements such as reaching, bending, and lifting)[32], has shown consistently large declines[4]. For example, one of the only studies of its kind, a comparison of records from white Union Army veterans in 1910 with data for a sample of white men in the 1990s, suggested large declines in functional limitations (difficulty bending and walking)[33]. Analysis of data from SIPP[34] suggested substantial declines in the prevalence of difficulty with climbing stairs, lifting and carrying, and walking three blocks among older Americans between 1984 and 1993. Similar findings were evident from the 1984 and 1994–

1995 Supplements on Aging to the NHIS[26] and in additional analysis of the SIPP through 1999[35].

Evidence regarding trends in cognitive function among the elderly population is not as well developed, but one analysis of the Health and Retirement Study shows that from 1993 to 1998 the proportion of the population age 70 years and older who were severely cognitively impaired declined from 5.8 to 3.8 percent[25]. More recent analyses through 2000 suggest that some of this improvement may be due to methodological biases[36]; however, analyses based on the National Long Term Care Survey[37-39] also show declines in the prevalence of dementia among older Americans between 1982 and 1999.

The results with respect to sensory functioning are somewhat mixed. Analysis of Union Army records suggests that large declines in blindness and deafness have occurred over the century[33]. Analysis of SIPP data suggests substantial declines from 1984 to 1993 in the percentage of older Americans with difficulty seeing[34] and in the percentage with difficulty seeing or hearing through 1999[35]. Evidence from the Supplements on Aging to NHIS, however, shows that the rates of blindness, deafness, and hearing impairment remained constant between 1984 and 1995[40].

A final avenue of inquiry has focused on the role of assistive technology in disability trends. Assistive technologies are devices used to increase, maintain, or improve functional capabilities and include both portable aids, such as canes and walkers, and modifications to the environment, such as grab bars and ramps. As first reported a decade ago[41], shifts have been occurring in the forms of assistance provided to help people cope with disability in late life. In that study, between 1982 and 1989, equipment use without personal assistance increased among older people with mild chronic impairments and equipment use as a supplement to personal assistance increased among those with severe chronic impairments. During the same period, reliance on personal care without any supplemental equipment declined. The trend toward the use of equipment as a sole form of assistance with daily activities continued through the 1990s[18,19,42,43]. Estimates from six national surveys conducted over the period spanning 1999 to 2002 suggest that approximately 14 to 18 percent of the U.S. population age 65 or older uses assistive devices—most often, devices for mobility (canes, walkers) and bathing (grab bars, bath seats, railings)[44], although socioeconomic gaps that favor more advantaged groups persist [45]. A recent study decomposed the declines between 1992 and 2001 in the number of older people receiving help with ADLs into the contributions of demographic shifts, declines in underlying difficulty, and shifts toward the use of assistive technology. In that study, declines in underlying difficulty were most important, but shifts toward the use of assistive technology explained a substantial portion of the decline, helping to offset increases resulting from population growth and aging[43].

On a related note, some researchers have attributed declines in IADL disabilities to the increased availability of modern conveniences. For example, older Americans no longer have to go to the store to shop or to the bank to manage money, and many more have microwave ovens to facilitate cooking[18]. Moreover, many more seniors are living in supportive living environments that provide assistance with these tasks, such as continuing-care retirement communities, assisted living facilities, and other retirement communities.

SUMMARY AND FUTURE STEPS

In sum, much of the research performed thus far suggests that improvements in late-life functioning and disability have occurred over the past few decades. Declines have been concentrated in activities central to living independently: shopping, managing money, and doing laundry. Much smaller declines in difficulty with and the use of help with self-care activities have been observed. Despite these overall improvements, gaps by race have remained steady and gaps by socioeconomic status have widened.

The causes of these trends are not completely understood, although some results suggest that a combination of factors may be at work. Increases in educational attainment appear to be important, but these increases will not continue at the rates observed over the past two decades. A number of common chronic conditions appear to be less debilitating, and underlying physical functioning has improved. At least some of the declines in the use of help appear to be offset by increases in the use of assistive technologies. Still, there are a number of unanswered questions about the trends. For example, researchers have yet to sort out the role of medical care, the relative contributions of improvements in underlying functioning versus changes in the environment, the relative importance of late-life factors versus factors earlier in life, and changes in perceptions about the meaning of disability. More research in this area is clearly needed.

A number of data challenges will continue to complicate this area of inquiry. Much effort has gone into reconciling differences in trends across national surveys, which vary in their designs and the techniques that they use to measure late-life disability. Recently, attention has been given to ways to incorporate new measurement techniques into national surveys to enhance understanding of late-life trends[46]. The standardization of disability measures, for example, through the use of vignettes, may promote comparisons across surveys and across groups within surveys. The addition of measures of underlying functioning (assessed through performance measures), the environment (including assistive technologies), and participation or engagement may facilitate a more refined understanding of the shifts in population-level disability trends. Sorting out the roles of factors earlier in life may require panel surveys that start earlier in life. Inclusion of a standardized core set of disability measures that apply across all ages, as well as life course-specific measures, also may prove useful.

Looking forward, there is debate about the implications of these trends for public and private expenditures[18,47-49]. Some researchers are optimistic that the declines in rates of late-life disability will ultimately lead to (all else being equal) lower medical costs; others are dubious about whether declines will ultimately lead to savings. Whether declines in late-life disability will continue into the future is unclear, given, for example, the impending increases in rates of obesity[50] and related chronic conditions and the slowing increases in educational attainment[30].

Indeed, the impending growth of the older population suggests that it will be important to continue to achieve declines in rates of late-life disability. Projections of the size of the older population with disabilities, which depend upon assumptions about mortality and disability rates into the future, suggest that declines in disability rates will need to continue at the rates observed during the 1990s (on average, 1 to 2 percent per year) for this group to remain stable[51]. Projections that assume much lower rates of decline portend large increases in the number of older people with a disability, from 6 million today to 10 million in 2050[52]. How these population shifts will influence the composition of the population of people with disabilities is unclear and merits further study.

REFERENCES

1. Fries J. Aging, natural death, and the compression of morbidity. *New England Journal of Medicine* 1980;303(3):130–135.
2. Gruenberg EM. Failures of success. *Milbank Memorial Fund Quarterly* 1977;55(1):3–24.
3. Manton KG. Changing concepts of morbidity and mortality in the elderly population. *Milbank Memorial Fund Quarterly* 1982;60(2):183–244.
4. Freedman VA, Martin LG, Schoeni RF. Recent trends in disability and functioning among older adults in the United States: a systematic review. *Journal of the American Medical Association* 2002;288(24):3137–3146.
5. Crimmins E. Trends in the health of the elderly. *Annual Review of Public Health* 2004; 25(1):79.
6. Schoeni R, Freedman V, Martin L. Socioeconomic and demographic disparities in trends in old-age disability. University of Michigan Center for Demography of Aging Trends Network Working Paper Series 05-01. Ann Arbor: University of Michigan Center for Demography of Aging Trends Network; 2004.
7. Schoeni R, Martin L, Andreski P, Freedman V. Persistent and Growing Socioeconomic Disparities in Disability Among the Elderly: 1982-2002. *American Journal of Public Health,* 2005;95(11):2065-2070.

8. Schoeni RF, Freedman VA, Wallace RB. Persistent, consistent, widespread, and robust? Another look at recent trends in old-age disability. *Journals of Gerontology* 2001;56(4): S206–S218.

9. Pope AM, Tarlov AR, eds. *Disability in America: Toward a National Agenda for Prevention*. Washington, DC: National Academy Press; 1991.

10. Brandt EJ, Pope A, eds. *Enabling America: Assessing the Role of Rehabilitation Science and Engineering*. Washington, DC: National Academy Press; 1997.

11. Colvez A, Blanchet M. Disability trends in the United States population 1966–76: analysis of reported causes. *American Journal of Public Health* 1981;71(5):464–471.

12. Verbrugge LM. Longer life but worsening health? Trends in health and mortality of middle-aged and older persons. *Milbank Memorial Fund Quarterly* 1984;62(3):475–519.

13. Waidmann T, Bound J, Schoenbaum M. The illusion of failure: trends in the self-reported health of the U.S. elderly. *Milbank Quarterly* 1995;73(2):253–287.

14. Manton KG, Corder LS, Stallard E. Estimates of change in chronic disability and institutional incidence and prevalence rates in the U.S. elderly population from the 1982, 1984, and 1989 National Long Term Care Survey. *Journals of Gerontology* 1993;48(4): S153–S166.

15. Manton KG, Corder L, Stallard E. Chronic disability trends in elderly United States populations: 1982–1994. *Proceedings of the National Academy of Sciences USA* 1997;94(6):2593–2598.

16. Crimmins EM, Saito Y, Reynolds SL. Further evidence on recent trends in the prevalence and incidence of disability among older Americans from two sources: the LSOA and the NHIS. *Journals of Gerontology* 1997;52(2):S59–S71.

17. Freedman VA, Soldo BJ, eds. *Trends in Disability at Older Ages: Summary of a Workshop*. Washington, DC: National Academy Press; 1994.

18. Spillman BC. Changes in elderly disability rates and the implications for health care utilization and cost. *Milbank Quarterly* 2004;82(1):157–194.

19. Freedman VA, Crimmins E, Schoeni RF, Spillman BC, Aykan H, Kramarow E, et al. Resolving inconsistencies in trends in old-age disability: report from a technical working group. *Demography* 2004;41(3):417–441.

20. Wolf DA, Freedman VA, Marcotte JE, Ploutz-Snyder LL. Panel-data bias in estimates of demographic dynamics: disability dynamics at older ages. In: *Workshop on Incomplete Data in Event History Analysis*; December 7–8, 2000. Baltimore, MD: Johns Hopkins School of Hygiene and Public Health; 2000.

21. Wolf D, Mendes de Leon C, Glass T. Trends in rates of onset of and recovery from disability at older ages: 1982–1994. In: *International Conference on Health Policy Research*, October 17–19, 2003, Chicago, IL; 2003.

22. Clark DO. US trends in disability and institutionalization among older blacks and whites. *American Journal of Public Health* 1997;87(3):438–440.

23. Manton KG, Gu X. Changes in the prevalence of chronic disability in the United States black and nonblack population above age 65 from 1982 to 1999. *Proceedings of the National Academy of Sciences USA* 2001;98(11):6354–6359.

24. Crimmins E, Saito Y. Change in the prevalence of diseases among older Americans: 1984–1994. *Demographic Research* 2000;3 Available online. http://www.demographic-research.org/volumes/vol3/9/3-9.pdf. Last accessed: October 27, 2005.

25. Freedman VA, Aykan H, Martin LG. Aggregate changes in severe cognitive impairment among older Americans: 1993 and 1998. *Journals of Gerontology* 2001;56(2):S100–S111.

26. Freedman VA, Martin LG. Contribution of chronic conditions to aggregate changes in old-age functioning. *American Journal of Public Health* 2000;90(11):1755–1760.

27. Angel JL, Buckley CJ, Sakamoto A. Duration or disadvantage? Exploring nativity, ethnicity, and health in midlife. *Journal of Gerontology* 2000;56(5):S275-284.

28. Elo IT and Preston SH. 1997. Racial and ethnic differences in mortality at older ages. In LG Martin and BJ Soldo, eds. *Racial and Ethnic Differences in the Health of Older Americans*, Washington, D.C.: National Academy Press, pp. 10-42.

29. Freedman VA, Martin LG. The role of education in explaining and forecasting trends in functional limitations among older Americans. *Demography* 1999;36(4):461–473.

30. Cutler D. Intensive medical technology and the reduction in disability. In: Wise D, ed. *Analyses in the Economics of Aging*. Chicago, IL: University of Chicago Press; 2003.

31. Freedman VA, Aykan H. Trends in medication use and functioning before retirement age: are they linked? *Health Affairs* 2003;22(4):154–162.

32. Nagi SZ. Some conceptual issues in disability and rehabilitation. In: Sussman MB, ed. *Sociology and Rehabilitation*. Chicago, IL: American Sociological Association; 1966, pp. 100–113.

33. Costa DL. Changing chronic disease rates and long-term declines in functional limitation among older men. *Demography* 2002;39(1):119–137.

34. Freedman VA, Martin LG. Understanding trends in functional limitations among older Americans. *American Journal of Public Health* 1998;88(10):1457–1462.

35. Cutler DM. Declining disability among the elderly. *Health Affairs* 2001;20(6):11–27.

36. Rodgers WL, Ofstedal MB, Herzog AR. Trends in scores on tests of cognitive ability in the elderly U.S. population, 1993–2000. *Journals of Gerontology* 2003;58(6):S338–S346.

37. Manton KG, Stallard E, Corder L. Changes in morbidity and chronic disability in the U.S. elderly population: evidence from the 1982, 1984, and 1989 National Long Term Care Surveys. *Journals of Gerontology* 1995;50(4):S194–S204.

38. Manton KG, Stallard E, Corder LS. The dynamics of dimensions of age-related disability 1982 to 1994 in the U.S. elderly population. *Journals of Gerontology* 1998;53(1):B59–B70.

39. Manton K, Gu X, Ukraintseva S. Declining prevalence of dementia in the US elderly population. *Advances in Gerontology* 2005;16:30–37.

40. Desai M, Pratt LA, Lentzner H, Robinson KN. Trends in vision and hearing among older Americans. *Aging Trends* (National Center for Health Statistics) 2001;2:1–8.

41. Manton KG, Corder L, Stallard E. Changes in the use of personal assistance and special equipment from 1982 to 1989: results from the 1982 and 1989 NLTCS. *Gerontologist* 1993;33(2):168–176.

42. Russell JN, Hendershot GE, LeClere F, Howie LJ, Adler M. Trends and differential use of assistive technology devices: United States, 1994. *Advance Data* 1997(292):1–9.

43. Freedman V, Agree E, Martin L, Cornman J. Trends in the use of assistive technology and personal care for late-life disability, 1992–2001. *The Gerontologist*, in press.

44. Cornman JC, Freedman VA, Agree EM. Measurement of assistive device use: implications for estimates of device use and disability in late life. *The Gerontologist* 2005;45(3):347–358.

45. Freedman V, Martin L, Cornman J, Agree E, Schoeni R. Trends in assistance with daily activities: racial/ethnic and socioeconomic disparities persist in the U.S. older population. University of Michigan Center for Demography of Aging Trends Network Working Paper Series 05-02. Ann Arbor: University of Michigan Center for Demography of Aging Trends Network; 2004.

46. Freedman VA, Waidmann T. *Opportunities for Improving Survey Measures of Late-Life Disability: Workshop Overview*. Washington, D.C.: Office of the Assistant Secretary for Planning and Evaluation, U.S. Department of Health and Human Service; 2005.

47. Singer BH, Manton KG. The effects of health changes on projections of health service needs for the elderly population of the United States. *Proceedings of the National Academy of Sciences USA* 1998;95(26):15618–15622.
48. Cutler DM. The reduction in disability among the elderly. *Proceedings of the National Academy of Sciences USA* 2001;98(12):6546–6547.
49. Chernew, M.E., D.P. Goldman, F. Pan, and B. Shang. 2005. Disability and health care spending among Medicare beneficiaries. *Health Affairs* Web Exclusive W5:R42-R52.
50. Sturm R, Ringel JS, Andreyeva T. Increasing obesity rates and disability trends. *Health Affairs* 2004;23(2):199–205.
51. Waidmann TA, Liu K. Disability trends among elderly persons and implications for the future. *Journals of Gerontology* 2000;55(5):S298–S307.
52. Tilly J, Goldenson SM, Kasten J. Long-Term Care: *Consumers, Providers, and Financing: A Chart Book*. Washington, DC: Urban Institute; 2001.

F

Chronic Disease and Trends in Severe Disability in Working-Age Populations

*Jay Bhattacharya, Kavita Choudhry, and Darius Lakdawalla**

R ecent work has shown that rates of severe disability, measured by the inability to perform basic activities of daily living, have been rising in working-age populations. This paper examines the extent to which chronic disease trends can explain these disability trends. The primary findings are that for populations of 30- to 45-year-old individuals between 1984 and 1996, (1) the prevalence of disability fell dramatically among non-chronically ill individuals, (2) the rising prevalence of obesity explains about 40 percent of the rise in disability attributable to trends chronic illness, and (3) the rising prevalence of disability among chronically ill individuals explains about 60 percent of the rise in disability attributable to trends in chronic illness.

Over the past two decades, the rates of severe disability, as measured by limitations in instrumental activities of daily living (IADLs), such as the ability to prepare meals, shop, do housework, use the telephone, and take medications, have been declining in older populations. A consensus has

*Jay Bhattacharya, M.D., Ph.D., Assistant Professor of Medicine, Stanford University, Palo Alto, California, Kavita Choudhry, B.S., master's degree candidate at the Harvard John F. Kennedy School of Government, Boston, Massachusetts. Darius Lakdawalla, Ph.D., economist, RAND Corporation, Santa Monica, California. The authors are grateful for the financial assistance provided by the National Institute on Aging. The authors also thank Sara Laufer and Byung Kwang Yoo for helpful discussions. The analyses and views presented in this workshop paper are those of the authors and not necessarily those of the Institute of Medicine Committee on Disability in America: A New Look.

113

emerged that the health of the elderly population, at least on this measure, has been improving since the early 1980s and that this improvement in health is reflected in a declining rate of disability (see, e.g., Manton et al., 1997; Crimmins et al., 1997; Schoeni et al., 2001; Crimmins, 2004; Freedman et al., 2004). Much of this literature has pointed to improvements in medical and assistive technologies for the treatment of disabled individuals, as well as the improved prevention of disabling conditions among the elderly population, as the leading causes of these declines.

These declines in disability came as a surprise to researchers because they reversed the trends of increasing rates of disability seen among elderly people in the 1970s. Then, researchers argued that increases in longevity amounted to extensions of the time spent in disability by elderly people (see, e.g., Crimmins et al., 1989; Waidmann et al., 1995). Thus, they predicted, increases in longevity would inevitably be accompanied by growth in the incidence of disability (see, e.g., Gruenberg, 1977). This concern has been replaced with the happy prospect of a compression of morbidity into shorter periods at the end of longer lives.

On the other hand, the news has not been all good over the past 20 years. For both the elderly and the working-age populations, there have been increases in the prevalence of some important chronic conditions, such as obesity and asthma. Working-age populations in the United States are more likely to claim disability benefits now than they were in 1990 (Autor and Duggan, 2001; Bound and Waidmann, 2000). In addition to increases in the size of the work-limited population, severe activity of daily living (ADL)-style disabilities have also risen in the working-age population since 1980 (Lakdawalla et al., 2003a,b; 2004).

The difference in the rates of changes in disability between the elderly and the working-age populations over the past 20 years is puzzling. If the explanation is the use of medical technology and preventive medicine, then the question is why these have not benefited younger populations in the same way that they have benefited the elderly population. This explanation presumes that at the root there have been real changes in the health of the populations under consideration that have led to the observed changes in the prevalence of disabilities. However, is this root assumption correct? Over this period there has been real deterioration in some measures of health in working-age populations, such as the dramatic rise in obesity rates. It seems implausible that such changes would have had no effect on disability rates, but how much is the effect?

The main aim of this paper is to describe the existing evidence on disability and chronic health trends in the population under age 65 years and to present new estimates of a decomposition of disability trends among working-age populations into two parts: the part of the trend explained by changes in the prevalence of chronic disease and obesity and the part of the trend explained by changes in the prevalence of disability among people with chronic diseases. The main import of such a decomposition is that it may highlight preventable clinical conditions that are most likely to lead to disability. The optimal policies that need to be implemented to reduce disability will be quite different if disease prevalence is the primary cause than if disability prevalence among the chronically ill is the primary cause.

BACKGROUND

In this section, we make precise exactly what we mean when we say that someone has a disability. Perhaps not surprisingly, this turns out to be quite controversial and is the cause of much confusion when the results of papers that analyze disability are compared: they are quite frequently talking about different things. As we intimate in the introduction, the definition of disability that we adopt in this paper is closely related to ADL limitations. We then review the literature on trends in old-age disability. Next, we review the results on ADL disability among working-age populations obtained by some of the authors of the current paper. (To our knowledge, no other work has documented the trends in ADL disability in younger populations.) Finally, we summarize the large medical literature on chronic disease trends in working-age populations.

Defining Disability

Although everyone has some intuitive idea about what it means to be disabled, when it is examined closely, disability turns out to be a concept that is hard to define—and, hence, difficult to measure in population-based surveys. Disability is an elastic concept that changes both from one social environment to another at a single point in time and from one period to another over the life cycle (Berry and Hardman, 1998; Marshak et al., 1999). Definitions of disability thus vary widely and tend to be specific to a particular objective or agency (USDOL, 2005). These unique definitions serve the goals of, for example, removing discrimination through the Americans with Disabilities Act (P.L. 101-336), determining eligibility for special education services, and qualifying for Social Security disability benefits (USEEOC, 1995; Knoblauch and Soerenson, 1998; SSA, 2005).

Survey data on disabilities, which inform the policies established and practiced by the entities cited above, fall into two broad areas: activity limitations and work limitations. The former encompasses the most basic, mechanically oriented ADLs, such as dressing, eating, and bathing, as well as IADLs, which involve everyday behaviors that require a higher level of cognitive functioning than ADLs, such as grocery shopping, managing money, and preparing meals (Crimmins et al. 1997; Manton et al., 1997;

Stone, 1984). The latter definition, which is the one typically used in studies of disability in populations under age 65 years, measures whether individuals are restricted in their ability to work in the labor market as a result of disabling physical or mental conditions. Although both definitions of disability are potentially important for the optimal construction of different policies, the activity limitation definition that we focus on here has, perhaps, more direct clinical relevance.

Surveys that collect data on aging population niches—such as the National Long-Term Care Survey (NLTCS)—tend to gather activity limitation information, whereas nationally representative survey instruments, such as the Current Population Survey, emphasize work disability. Data from the 2000 census, however, include elements on long-lasting sensory impairments, ADLs and IADLs, cognitive ability, and work limitations; this recent change attests to an increasing need to understand what disability is, who is affected by disabilities and to what degree they are affected, and possible or likely trends in disability at all ages. There is also a growing movement to improve measures of current activity outcomes to better address ways in which overall quality of life and employment potential can be improved (see, e.g., Bierman, 2001).

The main data set that we rely on, those from the National Health Interview Surveys (NHISs), includes data on both work limitation-based measures of disability (which are the measures typically reported by analysts using the NHIS) and ADL limitation-based measures (which are the ones that we focus on in this paper).

Trends in Late-Life Disability

A broad set of the literature has looked at trends in disability in the American elderly population over the past two decades. Contributors to this literature have relied on different surveys and different definitions of disability but have consistently found declines—and sometimes sharp and accelerating declines—in disability among the elderly population.

Manton and colleagues (1997) use data from the 1982, 1984, 1989, and 1994 NLTCSs to investigate trends in the prevalence of disability in the elderly population. Defining disability as an inability to perform an ADL or IADL without aid for at least 90 days, they found that the age-adjusted prevalence of disability for 1994 decreased by 3.6 percent from that for 1982 (from 24.9 to 21.3 percent). The authors compare the size of the set of people with disabilities with that which would have occurred without the apparent declines in disability. There were 0.54 million and 1.2 million fewer disabled elderly people in 1989 and 1994, respectively, than there would have been had the 1982 rates stayed fixed (Manton et al., 1993, 1997). Manton and Gu (2001) updated these results using the latest wave of data from NLTCS. They confirmed a continuing decline in disability among the elderly population, especially among the oldest age groups.

Manton and colleagues also investigated the incidence of disability and the progression to increased forms of disability. They calculated the rates of being institutionalized from having one or two ADLs, three or four ADLs, five or six ADLs, or some number of IADLs exclusively in 1982 and 1984. The decline in the rate of disability accelerated from 0.27 percent per year from 1982 to 1989 to 0.34 percent from 1989 to 1994, with greater declines in older cohorts (Manton and Gu, 2001). The transition rates from 1982 to 1984 and from 1984 to 1989 were also improved (Manton et al., 1993). Manton (2003) and Pardes and colleagues (1999) attribute these recent improvements in the prevalence of disability among the elderly population to improvements in medical technology that enable seniors to delay both disability and death. They argue strongly that potential future medical breakthroughs (such as the treatment and prevention of senile dementia) hold the promise of further disability reductions for the elderly population.

Freedman and Martin (1998) used data from the 1984 and 1993 Surveys of Income and Program Participation (SIPP) to investigate trends in the prevalence of disability. Their definition of disability differs mildly from the one used by Manton and colleagues; they define it as difficulty seeing words in a newspaper, lifting and carrying 10 pounds, climbing stairs, or walking a quarter mile. The authors found that the prevalence of difficulty in each category declined over the study period. The prevalence ranged from 15.3 percent (difficulty seeing words in a newspaper) to 25.8 percent (walking three-quarters of a mile) in 1984 to 11.6 percent to 22.3 percent for the same categories, respectively, in 1993, a relative improvement of between 0.9 and 2.3 percent across functions.

Crimmins and colleagues (1997) confirmed net decreases in disability among the elderly population from 1982 to 1993, despite intermediate fluctuations. They used data from the Longitudinal Study of Aging (LSOA) (1984, 1986, 1988, and 1990) and NHIS (1982 to 1993) to track the prevalence of disability over time. They focused solely on the prevalence of disability in the population over 70 years of age. The overall prevalence of disability determined with data from NHIS (defined as an inability to perform personal or routine care) in 1982 was 21.1 percent, and in 1993 it was 19.5 percent. With data from LSOA they found that the proportions of individuals who were disabled (defined as an inability to perform an ADL without aid) in 1984, 1986, 1987, and 1990 were 18.8, 21.6, 21.3, and 20.5 percent, respectively. Although no visually striking trend exists in the plotted data sets, statistical analysis reveals a slight decrease in disability in the pooled population (controlling for age and sex). These decreases are more likely in the activities of IADLs (routine care) as opposed to ADLs (personal care). Hazard models applied to these data revealed that the rates of transition to disability and out of disability improved over time: the incidence of disability decreased 16 percent from the 1948 to 1986 period to the 1988 to 1990 period.

Using NHIS 1970, 1980, and 1990 data and a definition of disability that differs from the one that we rely on in this paper (any limitation in usual activity over the past 12 months), Crimmins and colleagues (1997) found fluctuations in the long-term prevalence of disability. Institutionalization rates have declined for most age groups but have stayed the same or increased for those older than age 80. Long-term disability increased for the population older than age 60 from 1970 to 1980 but decreased from 1980 to 1990. For example, males aged 65 to 69 in 1970, 1980, and 1990 had disability rates of 37.84, 43.68, and 39.39 percent, respectively; and for females the rates were 30, 36.2, and 30.56 percent, respectively. These prevalence figures are subject to assumptions made about the effects of question wording changes after 1982.

Crimmins and colleagues (1997) also investigated the relative contributions of disability-free and disabled years to life expectancy. They used the NHIS definition of years of active life expectancy: the "years when an individual's health does not affect ability to perform normal activities of life including both major and secondary activities" (p. S61). At age 65, total life expectancy increased from 1970 to 1990. (Mortality declines from 1980 to 1990 were one-third of the decline from 1970 to 1980 for females and three-quarters of that for males for that period.) However, the proportion of that increase that included disability-free years was small. From 1970 to 1980, disability-free life expectancy did not increase, but there was a slight increase from 1980 to 1990. McKinlay and colleagues (1989) also found that the disability-free life expectancy decreased for newborns and middle-aged women from 1964 to 1985. These findings do not entirely support the hypothesis of Fries (1980) that the active life span is increasing faster than the total life span.

Freedman and colleagues (2004) presented the most comprehensive work on documenting disability trends in the elderly population. That report presented the summary view of a large group of distinguished researchers on disability in the elderly population. The main goal of Freedman and colleagues was to explore comprehensively whether five different nationally representative data sets gave the same answer about the direction and extent of disability trends. They also looked at how different definitions of disability led to different trend estimates. They summarized their conclusions as follows:

> Although the evidence was mixed for the 1980s and it is difficult to pinpoint when in the 1990s the decline began, during the mid- and late 1990s, the panel found consistent declines on the order of 1 percent [to] 2.5 percent per year for two commonly used measures in the disability

literature: difficulty with daily activities and help with daily activities. Mixed evidence was found for a third measure: the use of help or equipment with daily activities (Freedman et al., 2004, pp. 434-435).

There has been one attempt to use statistical decompositions to measure the extent to which changes in chronic disease explain trends in elderly disability. Using NHIS data from 1984 and 1994, Freedman and Martin (2000) found that upper and lower body limitations declined over that decade. Using these same data, Freedman and Martin found that although the prevalence of many prominent chronic diseases rose over the same period, the prevalence of disability among those with chronic disease fell.[1]

Disability Trends in Working-Age Populations

Using data from the 1984 to 2000 NHISs, Lakdawalla and colleagues (2004) tracked changes in disability by age. They tracked two different measures of disability: personal care and routine needs disability. These are conceptually different from work limitation disabilities, which are also tracked by NHIS.[2]

Table F-1 shows how disability rates determined from the NHIS data changed between 1984 and 2000. The numbers in the personal care column in Table F-1 reflect the number of people per 10,000 population requiring assistance with personal care needs, whereas the numbers in the routine needs column reflect the number per 10,000 population requiring assistance with personal care needs or other routine needs.

From 1984 to 1996, Table F-1 shows that routine needs disability expanded significantly for individuals between the ages of 30 and 59 years. There were significant expansions in the more severe personal care limitation category for all individuals aged 18 to 39. For groups aged 30 to 59,

---

[1]Freedman and Martin (2000) rely on linear regression-based methods to decompose rates of disability growth. The validity of these methods depends strongly on the validity of the linearity assumption and on the low prevalence of jointly occurring chronic diseases.

[2]Specifically, NHIS respondents were asked: "Because of any impairment or health problem, does ___ need the help of other persons with personal care needs, such as eating, bathing, dressing, or getting around this home?" If they answered "no" to this question, they were then asked: "Because of any impairment or health problem, does ___ need the help of other persons in handling routine needs, such as everyday household chores, doing necessary business, shopping, or getting around for other purposes?" These questions allow respondents to be placed in one of three bins: (1) unable to perform personal care needs, (2) limited in performing other routine needs, or (3) not limited in personal care or routine needs. The NHIS questionnaire was redesigned in 1997, and the wording of the questions on disability were subtly altered, although it is still possible on the basis of the new questions to place individuals in the three bins. However, the NHIS designers discourage comparisons of data from before and after the redesign. Table F-1 consequently tracks trends separately between 1984 and 1996 and between 1997 and 2000.

TABLE F-1　Age-Specific Trends in the Proportion of People with Personal Care or Routine Care Needs Limitations per 10,000 Population, 1984 to 2000

| | Number of People per 10,000 Population in the Following Age Groups: | | | | | | | | | |
| | 18–29 | | 30–39 | | 40–49 | | 50–59 | | 60–69 | |
Year	Personal Care	Personal Care and Routine Needs	Personal Care	Personal Care and Routine Needs	Personal Care	Personal Care and Routine Needs	Personal Care	Personal Care and Routine Needs	Personal Care	Personal Care and Routine Needs
1984	23	82	30	118	63	212	111	400	256	765
1985–1986	25	75	37	125	53	200	108	423	212*	748
1987–1988	27	79	33	126	51	200	97	363	218*	701*
1989–1990	27	86	28	127	58	226	105	360	216*	674*
1991–1992	30*	101*	55*	173*	76	250*	130	449*	229	681*
1993–1994	26*	104*	48*	185*	71	272*	114	473*	231	763
1995–1996	31*	98	54*	181*	78	275*	126	464*	242	694*
Change 1984–1996	8	16	24	63	14	63	15	64	-14	-72
1997–1998	23	63	38	103	67	216	110	370	225	551
1999–2000	27	70	44	100	88	217	119	333	217	501
Change 1997–2000	4	7	5	-3	20	1	9	-37	-8	-50

NOTE: *Significantly different from base year (1984 or 1997–1998), according to two-tailed t test at the 95 percent level of confidence.
SOURCE: Lakdawalla et al. (2003a), based on NHIS data.

the absolute growth in personal plus routine needs disability was roughly 63 per 10,000 population. The largest percentage increase occurred for 30- to 39-year-olds, whose rate of disability rose by more than 50 percent over this period. According to either definition of disability, the population aged 60 to 69 actually became less disabled. This is consistent with the findings from previous research that the old are becoming less disabled.

Autor and Duggan (2001) gave a detailed analysis of the way in which changes in the incentives to claim eligibility for government disability insurance payments have affected reported rates of disability among working-age populations. Disability defined by eligibility for disability insurance should be kept conceptually distinct from notions of disability involving requirements for help with personal care or routine needs. Autor and Duggan's analysis, performed with the NHIS data, shows that over the period from 1970 to 1996, the overall rate of disability fell much more rapidly among those who are more educated. This difference in growth rates, however, does not appear when the data are analyzed within employment status groups. That is, among the employed and among those not in the labor force, disability is growing at the same rates across education groups. This suggests that growth in disability is coming from less educated people who are leaving the labor force at higher rates. Because incentives for disability insurance are also likely to be the strongest for this group (who tend to earn less than more educated individuals), this piece of evidence is consistent with an explanation that stresses the importance of disability insurance. This could be particularly important for those between the ages of 40 and 54 years. The per capita rate of disability awards was constant for this age group from 1984 to 1990, but it suddenly shot up between 1990 and 1992 as a result of increases in disability insurance payments.

The receipt of disability payment alone is unlikely to explain all of the trends in personal care and routine needs disability, because for other age groups the timing of disability award changes does not coincide with the timing of disability growth. The per capita award rate for those under age 40 years grew by 40 percent from 1984 to 1990, but it grew by only 14 percent from 1990 to 1996 (Autor and Duggan, 2001). In contrast, Lakdawalla and colleagues (2004) found that growth in disability among individuals over age 40 is concentrated entirely in the period from 1990 to 1996. Moreover, the per capita award rate grew by more than 20 percent for those between the ages of 55 and 64, whereas the reported disability rate actually declined for this age group (Autor and Duggan, 2001).

Chronic Disease in Working-Age Populations

In this section, we review trends in the prevalence of chronic health conditions in working-age populations (less than 65 years old) and the relation between these trends and trends in disability in the same population. Not surprisingly, trends in the prevalence of chronic health conditions vary by condition and by cohort; the evidence indicates that more recent cohorts are more likely to suffer from such chronic health conditions like asthma, diabetes (Mokdad et al., 2000), chronic bronchitis (ALA, 2002a), and obesity (Wolf and Colditz, 1998). They are less likely to suffer from heart disease, hypertension (Reynolds et al., 1999), or arthritis. However, the literature also indicates that the proportion of chronically ill people who have a disability is higher in younger cohorts, although the latter point has not been systematically investigated. The literature on disability in this population tends to focus mainly on disability that causes work limitations rather than on other ADL and IADL limitations, which renders much of the literature that we report on here incomparable with our own results reported below.

Respiratory diseases such as asthma and chronic bronchitis are increasing in prevalence among the nonelderly population. In 1982, 2.9 percent of 18- to 44-year-olds and 3.6 percent of 45- to 64-year-olds experienced an asthma attack; in 1996, these numbers increased to 5.7 and 4.9 percent, respectively (ALA, 2002b). Chronic bronchitis sufferers aged 18 to 44 years in 1982 comprised 2.5 percent of the population, whereas 4.4 percent of the 45- to 64-year-olds had chronic bronchitis. In 1996, these figures rose to 4.5 and 5.9 percent, respectively (ALA, 2002a). The prevalence of childhood disability due to asthma rose 232 percent from 1969 to 1995, whereas the prevalence of childhood disability due to all other chronic illnesses in childhood rose 113 percent—less than half as much—in the same time span (Newacheck and Halfon, 2000).

Both the prevalence and the incidence of self-reported diabetes increased from 1980 to 1994 (CDC, 1997). From 1990 to 1998, the prevalence rate for diabetes among 18- to 29-year-olds increased slightly, from 1.5 to 1.6 percent. However, much more striking increases are seen in other working-age groups: among 30- to 39-year-olds, the prevalence increased from 2.1 to 3.7 percent during the same period (a 69.9 percent rise); for 40- to 49-year-olds, the rate grew from 3.6 to 5.1 percent; in the group aged 50 to 59 years, the prevalence rose from 7.5 to 9.8 percent; and 60- to 69-year-olds saw an increase in diabetes prevalence from 10.9 to 12.8 percent over the period (Mokdad et al., 2000).

The prevalence of congestive heart failure was higher among people aged 40 to 65 years for the period 1988 to 1991 than among people in this age group from 1976 to 1980, with roughly twice as many people at each age experiencing this condition in the later time frame compared with the prevalence in the earlier period (NHLBI, 1996).

Although the recent rise in obesity has attracted considerable attention, growth in weight is not a recent or short-lived phenomenon. Costa and

Steckel (1997) documented large secular gains in average height-adjusted weight for men in different birth cohorts over the last century. Height-adjusted weight for people in their 40s, the age group with the highest labor force attachment, has increased by nearly 4 body mass index units (kilograms per square meter) over this period. To put this into perspective, an increase of this magnitude in the height-adjusted weight of a 6-foot-tall man would require a weight gain of approximately 30 pounds. Similar gains in weight are true for women and children (Bhattacharya and Currie, 2001).

Conversely, both the prevalence of arthritis and the prevalence of activity limitations caused by arthritis decreased for working-age people between 1989 to 1991 and 1997. In the earlier period, self-reported arthritis was noted by 6.6 percent of 25- to 34-year-olds, 12.7 percent of 35- to 44-year-olds, 22.6 percent of 45- to 54-year-olds, and 36.5 percent of 55- to 64-year-olds, whereas the proportions of individuals in these age groups limited in activity were 0.6, 1.5, 3.5, and 7.1 percent, respectively (CDC, 1994). In the later period, 5.5 percent of 25- to 34-year-olds had arthritis, whereas 10.5 percent of 35- to 44-year-olds, 19.4 percent of 45- to 54-year-olds, and 29.7 percent of 55- to 64-year-olds had the condition. Their activity limitation rates due to arthritis were 0.5, 1.3, 2.1, and 5.2 percent, respectively (CDC, 1997). Boult and colleagues (1996) note that a 1 percent biannual decrease in arthritis could result in 4 million person-years of increased activity limitations between the years 2001 and 2049.

The overall prevalence of disability (defined as an inability to work) among the working-age population aged 25 to 34 years decreased from 4.4 percent in 1988 to 3.6 percent in 1998, but during this period it increased from 5.9 to 7.0 percent for 35- to 44-year-olds, from 9.1 to 10.7 percent for 45- to 54-year-olds, and from 15.6 to 16.4 percent for 55- to 61-year-olds (McNeil, 2000). There is no published literature on disability trends in younger populations over this same time period when disability is defined in terms of an inability to perform ADLs or IADLs.

Chronic conditions have long been known to be an important cause of disability (see, e.g., Colvez and Blanchet, 1981). In 1972, the Social Security Administration Survey of Disabled and Nondisabled Adults indicated that 15 percent of the noninstitutionalized population aged 20 to 64 years reported being disabled because of a chronic condition, with women affected in larger proportions than men (Krute and Burdette, 1978). Twenty years later, in 1991–1992, SIPP data showed that 5.1 percent of 16- to 67-year-olds had a work disability that prevented them from working; in 1997, 5.6 percent of 16- to 64-year olds had a work disability that prevented them from working—an approximately 10 percent increase over the 6-year period (but note the 3-year difference in the upper ends of the reported age ranges) (McNeil, 1993, 2001).

Chronic conditions that were responsible for a great deal of work limitation in 1992 include heart disease, which accounted for 10.9 percent of people aged 18 to 69 years who had a work limitation in that year; arthritis, which was responsible for 8.3 percent of chronic conditions in this niche; respiratory diseases, which 5.6 percent of this group encountered; and diabetes, which caused work limitation in 3.3 percent of the segment (see the findings of Stoddard et al. [1998], based on 1992 NHIS data). There has been an upward trend in the proportion of diabetic working-age adults who report activity limitations. Among 20- to 44-year-olds with diabetes in 1964, 31.9 percent group indicated having activity limitations; this figure increased to 48.3 percent in 1989 for 18- to 44-year-olds. In the diabetic group aged 45 to 64 years, 46.4 percent had activity limitations in 1964, yet 54.7 percent of this same age group had similar limitations in 1989 (Songer, 1995).

Overall, there is much reason for concern over the fact that some important chronic diseases have become more prevalent in working-age populations. Although intuitively it seems plausible that these chronic disease trends can explain some of the rise in ADL-style disability that we reported above, it is not clear from the literature how much can be so explained. The purpose of the rest of the paper is to derive this figure.

DATA

The yearly NHISs provide a nationally representative set of individual-level data on demographics and health status that are designed to represent the noninstitutionalized population. Data have been collected every year since 1957. The stability of the NHIS design makes it particularly attractive for the analysis of long-term trends in disability. Although the survey was redesigned in 1982 and 1997, it is possible to construct quantitatively consistent estimates for the years from 1984 to 1996.

Before 1982, the NHIS disability data were based on an activity limitation variable. NHIS asked respondents whether their health limited their ability to perform work or housework. From their answers, they were then grouped into four categories: (1) unable to perform work or housework; (2) limited in the kind or the amount of work or housework; (3) limited in other activities, besides work or housework; or (4) not limited in any activities. After 1982, NHIS continued to ask the same question, but with one subtle difference. Retirees aged 45 years and older were asked different questions before and after 1982. Before that year, retirees were asked if their health would prevent them from working. Beginning in 1982, they were asked if their health interfered with their major activity, which need not be working. Not surprisingly, therefore, the reported rates of activity limitation among older individuals fell substantially in 1982 because elderly retirees are allowed to report a less strenuous major activity.

After 1982, however, NHIS asks a different question more appropriate for the analysis of disability. The survey began asking all respondents over age 60 years, as well as all of those aged 5 to 59 years who reported some activity limitation, if they need help with personal care.[3] This question is preferable to an activity limitation question, in which individuals are allowed to choose their major activity. Because more disabled individuals tend to report a less strenuous major activity, the activity limitation question tends to understate the absolute value of changes in disability. On the basis of a respondent's answer to the personal care question, he or she was placed in one of two categories: (1) unable to perform personal care needs or limited in performing other routine needs or (2) not limited in personal care or routine needs. Use of the responses to this question provides consistent measures of disability from 1984 to 1996.

NHIS also asks its respondents to answer a battery of questions regarding their medical histories. Among these questions are included probes about the presence of chronic disease. Most of these questions are asked in the form, "Has a doctor ever told you that you have [disease x]?" There is some legitimate concern that this method of asking about the prevalence of disease conditions might undersample people who are less likely to seek medical attention. If this is indeed the case, then the estimates that we present are underestimates of the true influence of chronic disease on disability.

Between 1984 and 1996, the NHIS questionnaire did not ask each of its respondents all the questions about disease prevalence. Instead, it separated the list of disease-related questions into six different condition lists and then randomly assigned each respondent to respond to one of the six condition lists. One consequence of this sampling strategy is that we cannot use data from NHIS to obtain information about whether, for example, a respondent has both hypertension and arthritis. Because these conditions are on different condition lists, the same respondent is never asked about both of these conditions. However, the condition lists were constructed so that diseases that frequently occur together in the population (such as hypertension and heart disease) were placed in the same condition list. Thus, we can use the data from NHIS to measure the covariance of commonly co-occurring conditions.

---

[3]More specifically, this question is asked of all people over age 60 years and all individuals aged 5 to 59 years who report being limited in their major activity. This procedure yields reliable estimates of disability, as long as every person under age 60 who needs help with personal care is also limited in his or her major activity.

METHODS

In this section, we briefly describe our decomposition of disability trends into two parts: disability attributable to changes in the prevalence of chronic disease and disability attributable to changes in the prevalence of disability among those with chronic diseases. A central challenge that we face is that there is no large national database of data from a survey that is repeatedly administered and that has samples large enough to state with any confidence how disability and chronic disease have changed within single-year age categories. To compensate for this fact, we combine information across age groups, using a well-specified smoothing technology. To learn about 60-year-olds, we take into account what happened to 59- and 61-year-olds with equal weight, 58- and 62-year-olds with less weight, and so on.[4] We elaborate on this basic strategy in Addendum A.

With this smoothing technology in hand, we describe our strategy for decomposing disability trends. Our aim is to determine the extent to which age-specific trends in disability can be explained by the observed trends in chronic health. Presumably, whatever is left over is explained by trends in other determinants of disability prevalence, such as public policy and (mechanically) by disability trends among those with no chronic illness.

Let D_t be a dummy variable indicating disability at time t, and let C_t be a dummy variable indicating chronic illness at time t. A basic law of probability allows us to decompose the probability (P) (or, equivalently, prevalence) of disability into one part attributable to the chronically ill population and another part attributable to the non-chronically ill population (pop.):

$$P[D_t] = P[D_t | C_t = 1] P[C_t = 1] +$$

(part attributable to non-chronically ill pop.)   (F-1)

Using Equation F-1, we can write the change in disability prevalence between $t-1$ and t, $\Delta P[D_t]$, as follows:

$$\Delta P[D_t] = \Delta P[D_t | C_t = 1] P[C_t = 1] + P[D_t | C_t = 1] \Delta P[C_t = 1] +$$

(change attributable to non-chronically ill pop.)   (F-2)

---

[4]All authors in the disability trends literature rely on some sort of smoothing; for example, many authors report changes in disability rates for people in different 5-year age categories.

Each term in Equation F-1 contributes two terms to Equation F-2: a term that reflects the change due to a change in the prevalence of chronic conditions and a term that reflects the change due to a change in the probability of disability among those with chronic conditions. We apply our smoothing technology to estimate how each of these terms has evolved over time in NHIS. In Addendum B, we extend this framework to account for changes in multiple chronic conditions.

The set of chronic diseases that we consider include all of the most common causes of severe ADL disability: arthritis, asthma, cancer, chronic obstructive pulmonary disease (COPD), diabetes, hypertension, heart disease, stroke, and obesity.[5] The set of jointly occurring conditions that we consider include heart disease and hypertension, diabetes and hypertension, hypertension and stroke; heart disease and stroke, and all conditions interacted with obesity. The last set of interactions is possible because NHIS does not ask about body height or body weight within one of the six randomly assigned condition lists; rather, it asks about these variables in a part of the questionnaire that asks questions of all respondents.

RESULTS

In this section, we present our decomposition of the trends in disability prevalence between 1984 and 1996, as measured by the inability to perform personal care tasks. Recall Table F-1, which shows an increasing prevalence of disability among populations under age 60 years over that time period. We focus on trends between 1984 and 1996 because Table F-1 shows either small or mixed changes in the prevalence of disability between 1997 and 2000. We do not analyze routine needs disability trends here because the results are similar to the personal care disability trends that we do present here.

Table F-2 presents an overview of our results. It shows, in aggregate, the extent to which changes in smoothed disability prevalence between 1984 and 1996 can be attributed to chronic disease trends. Given our discussion to this point, it should not be surprising that the top row of Table F-2 shows increases in total disability prevalence over this period for 30- and 45-year-olds (by 20 and 46 cases per 10,000 population, respectively) and decreases for 60-year-olds (by 89 cases per 10,000).

The next rows of Table F-2 show that chronic illness plays a critical role in explaining these changes in disability prevalence. Among 30-year-

---

[5]We calculated obesity by using NHIS respondents' self-reported body height and body weight and constructing a body mass index (BMI), which equals height (in meters) divided by weight (in kilograms) squared. A person is defined as obese if his or her BMI is over 30.

TABLE F-2   A Decomposition of Changes in the Prevalence of Disability Due to Chronic Disease, 1984 to 1996

Parameter	Age 30	Age 45	Age 60
Total change in disability	20	46	–89
Change attributable to chronically ill population	61	100	–27
• Change attributable to prevalence of chronic illness	24	43	38
• Change attributable to disability prevalence among chronically ill	37	57	–66
Change attributable to non–chronically ill population	–41	–53	–62

NOTE: Prevalence rates are measured as the number of cases per 10,000 population. This table is based on the authors' calculations performed with NHIS data.

olds with chronic disease, disability rates rose by 61 cases per 10,000 population. About 24 of these cases can be attributed to changes in the prevalence of chronic illness, and 37 of these cases can be attributed to changes in the prevalence of disability among the chronically ill population. Among 45-year-olds with chronic disease, the prevalence of disability rose by 100 cases per 10,000. About 43 of those cases are attributable to changes in the prevalence of chronic disease, and 57 are attributable to changes in the prevalence of disability among the chronically ill population. Among 60-year-olds with chronic disease, disability rates actually fell by 27 cases per 10,000. Changes in the prevalence of chronic disease alone would have caused an increase in the prevalence of disability by 38 cases per 10,000. However, the prevalence of disability among the chronically ill population decreased dramatically, causing a decline in the attributable disability prevalence by 66 cases per 10,000.

The bottom row of Table F-2 shows how much of these changes in disability prevalence are attributable to non-chronically ill populations. The results are striking: there were large declines in the prevalence of disability in these populations for all age groups. In other words, if chronic disease prevalence and disability prevalence among the chronically ill population had remained constant between 1984 and 1996, there would have been declines in overall disability prevalence by 41, 53, and 62 cases per 10,000 population for 30-, 45-, and 60-year-olds, respectively.

Tables F-3, F-4, and F-5 present, in some detail, the results of our decomposition for 30-, 45-, and 60-year-olds, respectively. The data in these tables were estimated by using smoothed versions of the probabilities

TABLE F-3   A Decomposition of Changes in the Prevalence of Disability for 30-Year-Olds Due to Chronic Disease, 1984 to 1996

Chronic Disease	Change in Disability Due to Change in Prevalence	Change in Disability Due to Change in $P[D_t \mid C_t]$	Total Contribution to Change in Disability Rate	Percent Contribution to Change in Disability Rate
Arthritis	−1.0	0.7	−0.3	−1
Asthma	1.7	6.1	7.8	13
COPD	1.0	2.6	3.5	6
Diabetes	−0.2	3.2	3.0	5
Heart disease	−0.6	12.0	11.3	19
Hypertension	−2.7	7.7	5.0	8
Cancer	0.0	0.0	0.0	0
Obesity	20.3	−3.4	16.9	28
Stroke	−1.6	−5.2	−6.8	−11
Obesity and heart disease	0.0	21.1	21.1	35
Obesity and hypertension	−0.8	−7.0	−7.7	−13
Total	24.2	36.8	61.0	100
Total change in disability, 1984 to 1996			19.9	33
Remainder attributable to change among people without chronic conditions			−41.0	−67

NOTE: Prevalence rates are measured as the number of cases per 10,000 population. This table is based upon the authors' calculations performed with data from NHIS. Because of space constraints, we include an abridged version of the complete table. Rows with combinations of chronic diseases that contribute less than 10 percent to column totals are excluded. These include stroke and hypertension; obesity and diabetes; obesity and arthritis; heart disease and stroke; heart disease and hypertension; heart disease, hypertension, and stroke; and asthma and COPD. A complete version of the table is available upon request from the lead author.

listed in Equation F-2 for each chronic condition evaluated at the age indicated. The first data column in each table shows how much of the total change in disability prevalence is due to the change in the prevalence of chronic disease *j* between 1984 and 1996. The second data column shows how much of the total change in disability prevalence is due to the change in disability rates among those who have condition *j* in absolute terms. The last two data columns show the sum of those smoothed probabilities in absolute terms and as a percentage of the total change attributable to chronic disease. These last two columns represent the total contribution of changes in condition *j* on changes in disability prevalence.

Table F-3 shows the decomposition for 30-year-olds. The single largest

TABLE F-4   A Decomposition of Changes in Disability Prevalence for
45-Year-Olds Due to Chronic Disease, 1984 to 1996

Chronic Disease	Change in Disability Due to Change in Prevalence	Change in Disability Due to Change in $P[\,D_t \mid C_t\,]$	Total Contribution to Change in Disability Rate	Percent Contribution to Change in Disability Rate
Arthritis	−3.6	3.6	−0.1	0
Asthma	4.4	8.5	12.9	13
COPD	3.1	21.3	24.4	24
Diabetes	0.2	5.9	6.0	6
Heart disease	−0.8	−6.9	−7.7	−8
Hypertension	−9.4	24.2	14.8	15
Cancer	0.0	0.0	0.0	0
Obesity	30.0	−1.5	28.6	29
Stroke	−3.9	−8.9	−12.8	−13
Asthma and COPD	−3.7	−10.4	−14.0	−14
Obesity and arthritis	14.6	7.3	21.9	22
Obesity and diabetes	1.7	14.0	15.7	16
Stroke and hypertension	11.8	−6.2	5.6	6
Total	43.4	56.6	100.0	100
Total change in disability, 1984 to 1996			46.7	47
Remainder attributable to change among people without chronic conditions			−53.3	−53

NOTE: Prevalence rates are measured as the number of cases per 10,000 population. This table is based on the authors' calculations performed with data from NHIS. Because of space constraints, we include an abridged version of the complete table. Rows with combinations of chronic diseases that contribute less than 10 percent to column totals are excluded. These include obesity and hypertension; obesity and heart disease; heart disease and stroke; heart disease and hypertension; and heart disease, hypertension, and stroke. A complete version of the table is available upon request from the lead author.

source of increased chronic disease prevalence resulting in disability among 30-year-olds is an increase in obesity. If the prevalence of all other chronic diseases had stayed the same while obesity rates increased, as they actually did, our decomposition suggests that the disability rates in this age group would have risen by 20 cases per 10,000 population. This calculation ignores the increase in the prevalence of obese individuals with other chronic diseases. Thus, the increasing prevalence of obesity by itself explains a third of the rise in disability in this group.

TABLE F-5 A Decomposition of Changes in Disability Prevalence for 60-Year-Olds Due to Chronic Disease, 1984 to 1996

Chronic Disease	Change in Disability Due to Change in Prevalence	Change in Disability Due to Change in $P[\,D_t\,|\,C_t\,]$	Total Contribution to Change in Disability Rate	Percent Contribution to Change in Disability Rate
Arthritis	−9.1	2.8	−6.4	−23
Asthma	12.1	−7.8	4.3	16
COPD	−4.4	21.6	17.2	62
Diabetes	0.6	−32.1	−31.5	−114
Heart disease	−14.9	−17.5	−32.3	−117
Hypertension	−21.5	−24.7	−46.1	−167
Cancer	−6.2	0.0	−6.2	−22
Obesity	55.3	−21.2	34.1	123
Stroke	13.5	−13.6	−0.1	0
Asthma and COPD	16.9	2.4	19.3	70
Heart disease, hypertension, and stroke	−3.0	1.4	−1.5	−6
Heart disease and hypertension	−18.7	14.0	−4.7	−17
Heart disease and stroke	−23.6	−19.1	−42.8	−155
Obesity and arthritis	40.6	−0.4	40.2	145
Obesity and diabetes	−8.4	−22.9	−31.3	−113
Obesity and heart disease	3.8	−6.2	−2.4	−8
Obesity and hypertension	2.4	61.9	64.3	232
Stroke and hypertension	2.9	−4.7	−1.8	−7
Total	38.4	−66.1	−27.7	−100

Total change in disability, 1984 to 1996	−89.9	−325
Remainder attributable to change among people without chronic conditions	−62.3	−225

NOTE: Prevalence rates are measured as the number of cases per 10,000 population. This table is based on the authors' calculations performed with data from NHIS. Because of space constraints, we include an abridged version of the complete table. Rows with combinations of chronic diseases that contribute less than 10 percent to column totals are excluded. These include obesity and hypertension; obesity and heart disease; heart disease and stroke; heart disease and hypertension; and heart disease, hypertension, and stroke. A complete version of the table is available upon request from the lead author.

Table F-3 also shows that increases in the probability of disability among the chronically ill population are an important source of the overall rise in disability. Increases in disability rates among heart disease patients explain 20 percent of the overall rise attributable to chronic disease, whereas increases in disability rates among obese heart disease patients explain a further 35 percent of the overall rise. Heart attack survival rates increased substantially over this period. Our evidence suggests that improvements in therapy kept people alive but increasingly in a disabled state, at least for 30-year-olds. Increases in disability rates among asthma and hypertension patients also explain 10 and 13 percent of the rise, respectively. Stroke patients were more likely to be disabled in 1996 than they were in 1999, providing evidence of improvements in care for stroke patients.

Table F-4 shows the results of our decomposition for 45-year-olds. As was the case for 30-year-olds, Table F-3 shows that obesity is a major source of the increase in disability in this group, explaining 30 percent of the overall increase in disability. The increase in the prevalence of obese individuals with arthritis, diabetes, or hypertension together explains a further 20 percent of the overall rise. The increase in the prevalence of individuals with stroke and hypertension explains 12 percent of the overall rise.

Table F-4 also shows that (by holding disease prevalence fixed) increases in the prevalence of disability among individuals with COPD (21 percent of the overall increase), hypertension (24 percent), and asthma (9 percent) are also important sources of rising rates of disability in this group. Obese individuals with diabetes in this age group are also increasingly likely to be disabled. Increasing disability in the latter group explains a further 14 percent of the overall increase in disability attributable to the chronically ill. As was the case for 30-year-olds, there is evidence of improvements in disability rates among some subsets of the chronically ill population. For example, 45-year-old stroke patients and patients with both asthma and COPD were less likely to be disabled in 1996 than they were in 1984. In contrast to the findings for the 30-year-olds, 45-year-old nonobese heart disease patients with no history of hypertension were also less likely to be disabled in 1996 than they were in 1984.

Table F-5 shows our decomposition for 60-year-olds. For 60-year-olds with chronic disease, obesity is again the largest single source of increasing chronic disease prevalence that results in increasing disability, although asthma and stroke are also important sources. The declining prevalences of hypertension and heart disease, on the other hand, play important roles in the overall decline in the prevalence of disability for this age group. Table F-5 shows, with few exceptions, that the disability rates among the chronically ill population declined substantially. In particular, disability among patients with asthma, diabetes, heart disease, hypertension, stroke, and obesity declined by 8, 32, 18, 25, 14, and 21 cases per 10,000 population, respectively. However, disability among patients with both heart disease and hypertension rose by 14 cases per 10,000; among obese individuals with hypertension, disability rose by 62 cases per 10,000. Similarly, disability rose among patients with arthritis (3 cases per 10,000) and with COPD (22 cases per 10,000).

Although the results that we present here may seem to tell a complicated story, they can be summarized simply. With the exception of an increasing prevalence of obesity, changes in chronic disease prevalence cannot account for the increasing prevalence of disability in the population under age 60 years. Within chronically ill populations, however, people were more likely to be disabled in 1996 than they were in 1984. Thus, the two main sources of increasing disability among those under age 60 years are increases in the numbers of obese individuals and an increasingly disabled chronically ill population.

DISCUSSION AND CONCLUSIONS

Although previous literature has established rising disability rates in younger populations and falling disability rates in older populations (results that we confirm), the decomposition estimated in this paper is a starting point in understanding why the prevalence of disability has moved as it has. Our main results are as follows:

• Between 1984 and 1996, the rising prevalence of obesity has been an important source of the rise in the prevalence of disability for all age groups that we examined.
• Among populations in age groups under age 60 years, changes in the prevalence of other chronic diseases (including heart disease, hypertension, diabetes, and cancer) have had a mixed or small impact on overall disability rates.
• Among populations in age groups under age 60 years, chronically ill populations were substantially more likely to be disabled in 1996 than they were in 1984, whereas non-chronically ill populations were substantially less likely to be disabled in 1996 than in 1984.
• Among populations in age groups ages 60 years and older, both chronically ill and non-chronically ill populations were less likely to be disabled in 1996 than they were in 1984.

One important limitation in our work is that we do not explicitly measure the effect on disability rates of trends in some conditions that afflict working-age populations, including traumatic brain injuries, multiple sclerosis, mental retardation/developmental disability, blindness, and depression. In our methodology, individuals with these conditions for whom measurements were not obtained are treated as if they were not chronically ill. This limitation suggests a reinterpretation of our finding that non-chronically ill populations have become substantially less disabled over time. What this finding really means is that non-chronically ill populations, alongside populations of individuals with conditions that we did not measure, have become substantially less disabled over time.

Even if an increase in disability prevalence meant nothing more than an increase in the set of people unable to perform basic activities like dressing themselves, such increases would be a source of considerable concern, at least to newly disabled individuals and their caretakers. The well-established link between disability prevalence and medical care expenditures by the elderly population heightens the importance of this phenomenon: disability is closely linked to public expenditures on health insurance. In the remainder of this section, we consider some of the consequences of our findings for future Medicare expenditures.

The well-documented decline in disability among older populations over the past 25 years has led some authors to forecast projections of future Medicare expenditures substantially more optimistic than those that would be predicted if disability trends were ignored (see, e.g., Pardes et al., 1999; Manton and Gu, 2001). Such optimistic forecasts have been criticized because disability rates have been increasing among younger populations (Lakdawalla et al., 2003a, 2004). As these younger populations age into eligibility for Medicare and if they remain increasingly disabled, then future cohorts of elderly individuals may not enjoy further declines in disability. Accounting for both the rising rates of disability among younger populations and the falling rates of disability among older populations results in considerably less optimistic forecasts of future spending on Medicare. A key issue related to the accuracy of these alternate forecasts relates to the permanence of disability. If the development of disability at younger ages augurs disability at older ages, then the less optimistic forecasts are correct. On the other hand, if the disability that develops at younger ages is transitory, then the original optimistic forecasts are more likely true.

The decomposition of disability trends reported in this paper is directly germane to the permanence of disability in younger populations. We emphasize two different sources of the changes in disability: (1) changes in the prevalence of chronic disease and (2) changes in the probability of disability among chronically ill populations. If chronic disease prevalence is a major source of the rise in the prevalence of disability, then the rise in disability is more likely to be permanent. Because most chronic illnesses are permanent, unless these diseases cause younger populations to die at substantial rates before the age of 65 years (although given rising life expectancies and improved medical technologies, this is not likely to be the case), the rising disability rates caused by an increasing prevalence of chronic disease implies permanent increases in disability. With the exception of a rising prevalence of obesity, we find that the rising prevalence of chronic disease does not, on net, explain the rise in disability among populations between 18 and 59 years old; hence, we do not find empirical support for this particular argument that the changes in disability are permanent.

We do, however, find that the increasing prevalence of obesity is an important source of the rise in disability among younger populations. Of course, an individual who becomes obese does not necessarily remain so forever; that is, weight loss is possible, although it is difficult. However, a case can be made that once an obese individual has a disability, it can be hard to recover, so this result buttresses the argument that the changes in disability are permanent. In the case of obesity, though, this argument is further complicated by the fact that the health effects of increased body weight are different for the younger and the older populations. In older populations, increased body weight can sometimes be protective against conditions that commonly lead to disability (for example, the increased bone density that accompanies increased weight leads to fewer hip fractures).

Alternatively, if rising rates of disability among chronically ill populations (as opposed to rising chronic disease prevalence) are a major source of the rise in the prevalence of disability, then the overall rise in the prevalence of disability may or may not be permanent, depending on why the chronically ill are more likely to be disabled. A rising prevalence of disability due to this source suggests strongly that a chronically ill population is sicker now than it was before, but this fact does not establish the cause and may be due to a number of reasons. For example, the rising prevalence of disability among the chronically ill population may be due to improved medical care; that is, chronically ill people who otherwise would have died when they were treated with the old technology are kept alive with the new technology but are in a disabled state. On the other hand, perhaps the chronically ill population is sicker for reasons that have little to do with technological changes. For example, an increasingly obese populace might produce both more diabetics and a more severely ill diabetic population. Whether these changes in the chronically ill population result in permanent increases in the prevalence of disability and what effect these changes will have on the disability rates of future elderly cohorts are empirical issues that require further research. In any case, it should be clear that accurate forecasts of future Medicare expenditures cannot be constructed by ignoring the increasing prevalence of disability among younger populations.

ADDENDUM A:
ESTIMATING CHANGES IN AGE-PREVALENCE CURVES

To describe the method that we use to produce smooth age-specific prevalence functions—the overlap polynomial method[6]—it is helpful to introduce some notations. Let N represent the number of observations in the data set. Each observation i taken in $year_i$ consists of information about i's self-reports regarding disability limitations (d_i) and age (age_i).[7] Given these data, we estimate the following logit model of disability prevalence using each year of data available:

$$P[d_i | age_i, year_i] = \frac{1}{1 - \exp\left[g_1(age_i)\beta_1 + g_2(year_i)\beta_2 + g_1 * g_2\beta_3\right]}$$

(F-A-1)

where β_1, β_2, and β_3 are parameters to be estimated, g_1 is the overlap polynomial in age, and g_2 is the overlap polynomial in year.

In effect, we calculate the prevalence of disability at each age and year in the context of a logistic distribution. The g functions allow the presence of disability to vary flexibly with the year of observation and the age cohort of the respondent. Age and year enter the model through the g functions, which are specified by using an overlap polynomial.

The age polynomials are defined as

$$g_1(age_i) = \sum_{j=0}^{K}\left[\Phi\left(\frac{age_i - k_{j+1}}{\sigma_1}\right) - \Phi\left(\frac{age_i - k_j}{\sigma_1}\right)\right]p_j(age_i; \beta_{1j})$$

(F-A-2)

where $p_j(age_i; \beta_{1j})$ $j = 0, \ldots, K + 1$ are all nth-order polynomials in age_i.[8] The terms $k_0 \ldots k_{K+1}$ are called "knots," and σ_1 is a smoothing parameter; all of these are fixed before estimation. With this smoothing technique, the knots define the age intervals. When the value of the smoothing parameter approaches 0, the age profile over each interval simply equals the average disability level within that interval. In this case, the age profile reduces to a step function, in which each interval constitutes a separate step. As the smoothing parameter increases, the estimator uses increasingly more information from outside each interval. In the extreme, as the smoothing param-

---

[6]See Garber and MaCurdy (1993) for a description of the overlap polynomial methodology.

[7]It is possible to adapt this method to use with other covariates.

[8]We use first-degree polynomials. Although we experimented with higher-order polynomials, we find that they add to the costs of computation with no change in the final results.

eter approaches infinity, there is no meaningful distinction between any two intervals. The allowance of nonzero values for the smoothing parameters eliminates the sharp discontinuity of the growth rates at the knots. One advantage of the use of overlapping polynomials over the use of traditional splines is that the function and all its derivatives are automatically continuous at the knots, without the imposition of any parameter restrictions.

The overlap polynomial for year g_2 and its interaction with g_1 allow flexible changes in the age-prevalence relationship over time. It is defined as

$$g_2\left(year_i\right) = \sum_{j=0}^{M} \left(\left[\Phi\left(\frac{year_i - m_{j+1}}{\sigma_2}\right) - \Phi\left(\frac{year_i - m_j}{\sigma_2}\right)\right]\right) q_j\left(year_i; \beta_{2j}\right)$$

(F-A-3)

As before, the m terms represent the knots, while the σ term represents the smoothing parameter.

The object of the maximum-likelihood logit estimation is to obtain consistent estimates for β_1, β_2 and β_3. By using these estimates, it is straightforward to generate age-prevalence profiles representative for any particular year. Let $\rho_{t,a}$ be the disability prevalence among a-year-olds in year t. Then,

$$\rho_{t,a} = \frac{1}{N} \sum_i P\left[d_i = 1 \middle| age_i - a, year_i = t; \hat{\beta}_1, \hat{\beta}_2, \hat{\beta}_3\right]$$

(F-A-4)

APPENDIX B: DECOMPOSING CAUSES OF CHANGES IN AGE-SPECIFIC DISABILITY

The aim here is to determine the extent to which age-specific trends in disability can be explained by observed trends in chronic health. Presumably, whatever is left over is explained by trends in other determinants of the prevalence of disability, such as public policy and (mechanically) by disability trends among those with no chronic illness.

For each person i (suppressed for clarity), let D_t be a dummy indicating self-reported disability at time t and let $C_t = \{C_{1t}, C_{2t},...,C_{Kt}\}$ be a vector of dummy variables, each of which indicates whether a particular chronic condition is present and observed (by the econometrician) at time t. For illustration, consider just the first chronic condition, C_1t. The probability of disability can be written as follows:

$$P\left[D_t\right] = P\left[D_t \middle| C_{1t} = 1\right] P\left[C_{1t} = 1\right] + P\left[D_t \middle| C_{1t} = 0\right] P\left[C_{1t} = 0\right]$$

(F-A-5)

The proportion of the people with disabilities that is attributable to people with $C_1 t$ is simply the first of two terms in the previous equation, whereas the second term is the proportion of the people with disabilities that is attributable to people without $C_1 t$ (although these people may have other chronic conditions or may report being disabled because of public policy, accidents, or other health trends). Using Equation F-A-5, we can decompose the change in disability prevalence between $t-1$ and t, $\Delta P[D_t]$, as follows:

$$\Delta P[D_t] = \Delta P[D_t | C_{1t} = 1] P[C_{1t} = 1] + P[D_t | C_{1t} = 1] \Delta P[C_{1t} = 1]$$
$$+ \Delta P[D_t | C_{1t} = 0] P[C_{1t} = 0] + \Delta P[D_t | C_{1t} = 0] P[C_{1t} = 0]$$

$$(F\text{-}A\text{-}6)$$

Each term in Equation F-A-5 contributes two terms to Equation F-A-6: a term that reflects the change due to a change in the prevalence of the condition and a term that reflects the change due to a change in the probability of disability among those with the condition.

Now, let E_t be the portion of disability prevalence that can be explained by the chronic conditions in C_t when they are observed singly. Define E_t as a generalization of the first term in Equation F-A-5:

$$E_t = \sum_{k=1}^{K} P[D_t | C_{kt} = 1] P[C_{kt} = 1] \qquad (F\text{-}A\text{-}7)$$

Let ΔE_t be the portion of the change in disability prevalence between $t-1$ and t that can be explained by the chronic conditions in C_t:

$$\Delta E_t = \Delta P[D_t | C_{1t} = 1] P[C_{1t} = 1] + P[D_t | C_{1t} = 1] \Delta P[C_{1t} = 1]$$
$$+ \Delta P[D_t | C_{2t} = 1] P[C_{2t} = 1] + P[D_t | C_{2t} = 1] \Delta P[C_{2t} = 1] \qquad (F\text{-}A\text{-}8)$$
$$+ \Delta P[D_t | C_{Kt} = 1] P[C_{Kt} = 1] + P[D_t | C_{Kt} = 1] \Delta P[C_{Kt} = 1]$$

To show how E_t and $P[D_t]$ are related, consider the case in which the presence of only two chronic conditions are observed (i.e., $K = 2$). In that case, the proportion of disability attributable to each of the conditions can be decomposed as follows:

$$P\left[D_t\middle|C_{1t} = 1\right]P\left[C_{1t} = 1\right] = P\left[D_t\middle|C_{1t} = 1, C_{2t} = 1\right]P\left[C_{2t} = 1\middle|C_{1t} = 1\right]P\left[C_{1t} = 1\right]$$
$$+ P\left[D_t\middle|C_{1t} = 1, C_{2t} = 0\right]P\left[C_{2t} = 0\middle|C_{1t} = 1\right]P\left[C_{1t} = 1\right]$$
$$P\left[D_t\middle|C_{2t} = 1\right]P\left[C_{2t} = 1\right] = P\left[D_t\middle|C_{1t} = 1, C_{2t} = 1\right]P\left[C_{1t} = 1\middle|C_{2t} = 1\right]P\left[C_{2t} = 1\right]$$
$$+ P\left[D_t\middle|C_{1t} = 0, C_{2t} = 1\right]P\left[C_{1t} = 0\middle|C_{2t} = 1\right]P\left[C_{2t} = 1\right]$$

$$(\text{F-A-9})$$

Notice that the first terms of both decompositions in Equation F-A-9 are identical and represent the contribution of people who have both chronic conditions to the prevalence of disability. For this case of $K = 2$, note that $E_t = P\left[D_t\middle|C_{1t} = 1\right]P\left[C_{1t} = 1\right] + P\left[D_t\middle|C_{2t} = 1\right]P\left[C_{2t} = 1\right]$. Thus,

$$E_t = P\left[D_t\middle|C_{1t} = 1, C_{2t} = 0\right]P\left[C_{1t} = 1, C_{2t} = 0\right]$$
$$+ P\left[D_t\middle|C_{1t} = 0, C_{2t} = 1\right]P\left[C_{1t} = 0, C_{2t} = 1\right] \qquad (\text{F-A-10})$$
$$+ 2P\left[D_t\middle|C_{1t} = 1, C_{2t} = 1\right]P\left[C_{1t} = 1, C_{2t} = 1\right]$$

On the other hand, the true probability of disability attributable to the two conditions, $P\left[D_t\middle|C_{1t} + C_{2t} \geq 1\right]$, can be decomposed as follows:

$$P\left[D_t\middle|C_{1t} + C_{2t} \geq 1\right] = P\left[D_t\middle|C_{1t} = 1, C_{2t} = 0\right]P\left[C_{1t} = 1, C_{2t} = 0\right]$$
$$+ P\left[D_t\middle|C_{1t} = 0, C_{2t} = 1\right]P\left[C_{1t} = 0, C_{2t} = 1\right]$$
$$+ P\left[D_t\middle|C_{1t} = 1, C_{2t} = 1\right]P\left[C_{1t} = 1, C_{2t} = 1\right]$$

$$(\text{F-A-11})$$

By comparing Equations F-A-10 and F-A-11, it is evident that E_t overestimates the portion of disability attributable to chronic conditions by the joint prevalence term, $P\left[D_t\middle|C_{1t} = 1, C_{2t} = 1\right]P\left[C_{1t} = 1, C_{2t} = 1\right]$. That is, by taking each of the observed chronic conditions singly, E_t produces an upper bound on how much disability prevalence can be explained by chronic health conditions. It is easy to generalize this argument to more than two conditions, although the proof requires the introduction of some cumbersome notation, so it is omitted here. The principle is the same, though: E_t

overcounts disability compared with that counted by $P\left[D_t \left| \sum_{k=1}^{K} C_{kt} \geq 1\right.\right]$
because it includes too many joint prevalence terms. Thus, in Equation F-A-8, ΔE_t measures how an upper bound (to the contribution of observed trends in chronic conditions to disability) changes over time.

Although it would be attractive to use Equation F-A-11 to evaluate exactly how the trends in chronic health conditions explain trends in disability, for practical reasons it is not possible to do so. In particular, implementation of our strategy by use of Equation F-A-11 would require large amounts of data for people with every conceivable set of multiple conditions. In practice, this is impossible because there are many combinations of conditions that are rare in the population. Also, as we note above, NHIS does not ask all people about all chronic conditions; rather, it randomly assigns each respondent to respond to one of six condition lists.

On the other hand, we can implement the main insight of Equation F-A-11 by expanding the condition set that we consider to include all common combinations of conditions. For example, because diabetes in combination with heart disease is common, we include three conditions in our calculations from this set: diabetes with heart disease, diabetes alone, and heart disease alone. By doing this we limit the error due to overcounting for all the common disease combinations.

REFERENCES

ALA (American Lung Association, Epidemiology and Statistics Unit). (2002a) Trends in Chronic Bronchitis and Emphysema: Morbidity and Mortality. Online. (The link is no longer available. For the most recent data, go to http://www.lungusa.org/atf/cf/{7A8D42C2-FCCA-4604-8ADE-7F5D5E762256}/COPD1.pdf. Last accessed September 23, 2005.)

ALA. (2002b) Trends in Asthma Morbidity and Mortality January 2001. Online. (The link is no longer available. For the most recent data, go to http://www.lungusa.org/atf/cf/{7A8D42C2-FCCA-4604-8ADE-7F5D5E762256}/ASTHMA1.PDF. Last accessed September 23, 2005).

Autor D, Duggan M. (2001). The Rise in Disability Recipiency and the Decline in Unemployment. Working Paper 8336. Cambridge, MA: National Bureau of Economic Research.

Berry J, Hardman M. (1998) Lifespan Perspectives on the Family and Disability. Needham Heights, MA: Allyn & Bacon.

Bhattacharya J, Currie J. (2001) Youths and nutritional risk: malnourished or misnourished? In Risky Behavior among Youths. Gruber J (ed.). Chicago, IL: University of Chicago Press.

Bierman A. (2001) Activity status: the sixth vital sign. Journal of General Internal Medicine (16):785–786.

Boult C, Altmann M, Gilbertson D, Yu C, Kane R. (1996) Decreasing disability in the 21st century: the future effects of controlling six fatal and nonfatal conditions. American Journal of Public Health 86(10):1388–1393.

Bound J, Waidmann T. (2000) Accounting for Recent Declines in Employment Rates among the Working-Aged Disabled. Working Paper 7975. Cambridge, MA: National Bureau of Economic Research.

CDC (Centers for Disease Control and Prevention). (1994) Arthritis prevalence and activity limitations—United States, 1990. *Morbidity and Mortality Weekly Report* 43(24):433–438.

CDC. (1997) Trends in the prevalence and incidence of self-reported diabetes mellitus—United States, 1980–1994. *Morbidity and Mortality Weekly Report* 46(43):1014–1018.

Colvez A, Blanchet M. (1981) Disability trends in the United States population 1966–76: analysis of reported causes. *American Journal of Public Health* 71(5):464–471.

Costa DL, Steckel RH. (1997) Long-term trends in health, welfare, and economic growth in the United States. In *Health and Welfare during Industrialization*. Floud R, Steckel RH (eds.). Chicago, IL: University of Chicago Press, pp. 47–89.

Crimmins EM. (2004) Trends in the health of the elderly. *Annual Review of Public Health* 25:79–98.

Crimmins EM, Saito Y, Ingegneri D. (1989) Changes in life expectancy and disability-free life expectancy in the United States. *Population and Development Review* 15(2):235–267.

Crimmins, EM, Saito Y, Reynolds SL. (1997) Further evidence on recent trends in the prevalence and incidence of disability among older Americans from two sources: the LSOA and the NHIS. *Journal of Gerontology* 52B(2):S59–S71.

Freedman VA, Martin LG. (1998) Understanding trends in activity limitations among older Americans. *American Journal of Public Health* (88):1457–1462.

Freedman VA, Martin LG. (2000) Contribution of chronic conditions to aggregate changes in old age functioning. *American Journal of Public Health* 90(11):1755–1760.

Freedman VA, Crimmins E, Schoeni RF, Spillman BC, Aykan H, Kramarow E, Land K, Lubitz J, Manton K, Martin LG, Shinberg D, Waidmann T. (2004) Resolving inconsistencies in trends in old-age disability: report from a technical working group. *Demography* 41(3): 417–441.

Fries JF. (1980) Aging, natural death, and the compression of morbidity. *New England Journal of Medicine* (303):130–135.

Garber A and MaCurdy T. (1993) Nursing home discharges and the exhaustion of Medicare benefits. *Journal of the American Statistical Association* (88):727–736.

Gruenberg EM. (1977) The failures of success. *Milbank Memorial Fund Quarterly* 55(1):3–34.

Knoblauch B, Sorenson B. (1998) IDEA's Definition of Disabilities. ERIC Digest E560. Online. · http://www.ed.gov/databases/ERIC_Digests/ed429396.html. Last accessed September 29, 2002.

Krute A, Burdette ME. (1978) 1972 Survey of disabled and nondisabled adults: chronic disease, injury, and work disability. *Social Security Bulletin* 41(4):3–17.

Lakdawalla D, Goldman D, Bhattacharya J, Hurd M, Joyce G, Panis C. (2003a) Forecasting the nursing home population. *Medical Care* 41(1):8–20.

Lakdawalla D, Goldman D, Bhattacharya J, Hurd M, Joyce G, Panis C. (2003b) A response to the points by Manton and Williamson on forecasting the nursing home population. *Medical Care* 41(1):28–31.

Lakdawalla D, Bhattacharya J, Goldman D. (2004) Are the young becoming more disabled? *Health Affairs* 23(1):168–176.

Manton KG. (2003) Forecasting the nursing home population. *Medical Care* 41(1):21–24.

Manton, KG, Gu X. (2001) Changes in the prevalence of chronic disability in the United States black and nonblack population above age 65 from 1982 to 1999. *Proceedings of the National Academy of Sciences USA* 98(11):6354–6359.

Manton KG, Corder L, Stallard E. (1993). Estimates of change in chronic disability and institutional incidence and prevalence rates in the U.S. elderly population from the 1982, 1984, and 1989 national long term care survey. *Journal of Gerontology: Social Sciences* 48(4):S153–S166.

Manton KG, Corder L, Stallard E. (1997) Chronic disability trends in elderly United States populations: 1982–1994. *Proceedings of the National Academy of Sciences USA* (94):2593–2598.

Marshak LE, Seligman M, Prezant F. (1999) *Disability and the Family Life Cycle: Recognizing and Treating Developmental Challenges.* New York: Basic Books.

McKinlay JB, McKinlay SM, Beaglehole R. (1989) A review of the evidence concerning the impact of medical measures on recent mortality and morbidity in the United States. *International Journal of Health Services* 19(2):181–208.

McNeil JM. (1993) Americans with Disabilities: 1991–92. Current Population Reports, P79-33, U.S. Bureau of the Census. Online. http://www.bls.census.gov/sipp/p70-33.pdf. Last accessed September 23, 2005.

McNeil JM. (2000) Employment, Earnings, and Disability. Paper prepared for the 75th Annual Conference of the Western Economic Association International, Vancouver, British Columbia, Canada, June 29–July 3.

McNeil JM. (2001) Americans with Disabilities: 1997. Current Population Reports, P79-33, U.S. Bureau of the Census. Online. http://www.bls.census.gov/sipp/p70s/p70-73.pdf. Last accessed September 23, 2005.

Mokdad AH, Ford ES, Bowman BA, Nelson DE, Engelgau MM, Vinicor F, Marks JS. (2000) Diabetes trends in the U.S.: 1990–1998. *Diabetes Care* 23(9):1278–1283.

Newacheck, PW, Halfon N. (2000) Prevalence, impact, and trends in childhood disability due to asthma. *Archives of Pediatrics and Adolescent Medicine* 154(3):287–293.

NHLBI (National Heart, Lung, and Blood Institute). (1996) Data Fact Sheet: Congestive Heart Failure in the United States: A New Epidemic. Bethesda, MD: U.S. Department of Health and Human Services.

Pardes H, Manton KG, Lander ES, Tolley HD, Ullian AD, Palmer H. (1999) Effects of medical research on health care and the economy. *Science* 283:36–37.

Reynolds SL, Crimmins EM, Saito Y. (1999) Cohort differences in disability and disease presence. *The Gerontologist* 38(5):578–590.

SSA (U.S. Social Security Administration). (2005) Social Security Disability Planner. Online. http://www.ssa.gov/dibplan/dqualify4.htm. Last accessed September 23, 2005.

Schoeni RF, Freedman VA, Wallace RB. (2001) Persistent, consistent, widespread, and robust? Another look at recent trends in old-age disability. *Journal of Gerontology* 56(4):S206–S218.

Songer TJ. (1995) Disability in diabetes. In *Diabetes in America*, 2nd ed. National Diabetes Data Group. Washington, DC: U.S. Government Printing Office.

Stoddard, S., L. Jans, J. Ripple, L. Kraus. (1998) *Chartbook on Work and Disability in the United States, 1998.* Washington, DC: U.S. National Institute on Disability and Rehabilitation Research.

Stone, DA. (1984) *The Disabled State.* Philadelphia, PA: Temple University Press.

USDOL (U.S. Department of Labor, Office of Disability Employment Policy). (2005) How Does the Federal Government Define 'Disability'? Online. http://www.dol.gov/odep/faqs/federal.htm. Last accessed September 23, 2005.

USEEOC (U.S. Equal Employment Opportunity Commission). (1995) Executive Summary: Compliance Manual Section 902, Definition of the Term Disability. Online. http://www.eeoc.gov/policy/docs/902sum.html. Last accessed September 23, 2005.

Waidmann T, Bound J, Schoenbaum M. (1995) The illusion of failure: trends in the self-reported health of the U.S. elderly. *Milbank Quarterly* 73(2):253–287.

Wolf A, Colditz G. (1998) Current estimates of the economic cost of obesity in the United States. *Obesity Research* 6(2):97–106.

G

Trends in Disability in Early Life

*Ruth E. K. Stein**

This paper provides an overview of the trends in disability in early life and has five main sections. The first section identifies key demographics that may be important to the Institute of Medicine (IOM) Committee on Disability in America: A New Look. The second section reviews traditional measures of childhood disability in use over the past several decades and the trends that they show. The third section highlights newer approaches to the assessment of disability among children and youth and what is known about trends determined by the use of these newer techniques. The fourth provides some examples of changes in disability patterns, and the last section provides conclusions with some implications for the committee.

DEMOGRAPHICS

Children younger than 18 years of age constitute 25 percent of the population in the United States. Over the past half-century there has been an increase in the number of children in the population, from 44 million in 1950 to 73 million in 2003, and this number is expected to rise to 80 million by 2020.[1] There has also been a dramatic change in the composi-

---

*Ruth E. K. Stein, M.D., Professor of Pediatrics, Albert Einstein College of Medicine, Children's Hospital at Montefiore, New York City. The analyses and views presented in this workshop paper are those of the author and not necessarily those of the Institute of Medicine Committee on Disability in America: A New Look.

tion of the child population. While white non-Hispanic children represented 75 percent of the nation's children in 1980, by the year 2020 they are expected to be a little over 50 percent of the child population.[2] In contrast, the proportion of minority children is increasing and the Hispanic child population is growing at the fastest rate and will exceed one in five children within the next few years.[3]

These data are important for a number of reasons, especially because of the strong association between membership in a minority group and poverty. Poverty is a major correlate of poor child health and has been shown to have important long-term health consequences, such that morbidity and mortality are strongly associated with income. The proportion of children in poverty has remained relatively stable at about 16 percent, but most recently, in 2003 (the last year for which statistics are available) that proportion was 18 percent.[4] Moreover, 29 percent of children live below 150 percent of the federal poverty level (FPL) and 39 percent live below 200 percent of the FPL.[4]

Although the absolute numbers and the recent suggestion that the percentage may be increasing are of concern, the more important point is that children are the one age group in U.S. society whose financial status has not improved over time.[5] In fact, in the 1960s, before the institution of Medicare, elderly people were considered the most financially disadvantaged age group. However, over the ensuing years the rate of poverty among the elderly population has fallen by almost two-thirds, but the proportion of children who are poor today is about the same as it was in the 1960s. At that time, children were less likely to be poor than the elderly, but today, the rate of poverty among children exceeds that among elderly people, so that about two-thirds more children than elderly people are poor.[5] Among minority children in 2003, 29 to 34 percent of black and Hispanic children were poor, whereas 9 percent of white non-Hispanic children were poor.[5]

A recent paper also suggests a growing intergenerational inequity in public spending.[6] Between 1965 and 2000, per capita public spending grew more rapidly for elders than for children, so children today are getting a smaller share of the pie.

Children in poverty are much more likely to be rated as having poorer health than other children.[7] Among the children in families with incomes below the FPL, 71 percent of the children are rated to be in excellent or very good health, whereas 89 percent of the children in families whose incomes are above 200 percent of the FPL are rated to be in excellent or very good health.[4]

DISABILITY

Although the rates of disability among the young are considerably lower than those among people in older age groups, disability is nevertheless of great importance in the child population. Among the reasons for this importance is that those with disabling health conditions have long-term survival, with the overwhelming majority now surviving well into adulthood. Thus, disabilities in children result in extremely large cumulative costs to society, their family units, and the individual members of their families. Moreover, the health of children as a group is critical to society because of the key role that children play as perhaps the single most precious of society's natural resources. Undoubtedly, therefore, the health of children is integrally linked to the health of the nation's and society's future.

In addition, as was recently highlighted in a report of the Board of Children, Youth, and Families, *Children's Health, the Nation's Wealth: Assessing and Improving Child Health,*[8] a child's health has been demonstrated to have effects that may reach far into adulthood. It is becoming increasingly evident that many, if not most, of the most important causes of adult disability have their origins during childhood, even though they may not be causing any obvious health problem or disabilities during childhood. This is a key point, and its implications will be discussed below.

The predominant notion of disability in the United States is derived from two central concepts based on the effects of injury and illness for adults: (1) the effects of having a condition on one's ability to work to support oneself and (2) self-care as reflected in independence in activities of daily living (ADLs). Other concepts of disability, such as the International Classification of Functioning, are relatively new.[9] This creates a problem when early life and disability are being discussed, because neither the concept of work nor the concept of independence in ADLs is an adequate way of defining disability among children. Independence in ADLs is not the norm, especially in younger children, who are fully dependent, and only a few of the very most severely impaired older children actually qualify as being disabled by virtue of limitations of ADLs. In 1987 the Office of Technology Assessment of the U.S. Congress attempted to estimate the number of children with dependence on technology for bodily function and ADLs. Its estimates varied up to 40-fold, depending on the level of technology dependence and the criteria used.[10]

Moreover, the functioning of children is always a moving target, as children mature at different rates, live in different cultures with different expectations of independence and self-sufficiency, and grow up in environments that vary markedly in the demands that they place on the performance of activities by children. All these factors make it hard to conclude whether a child's function is or is not within the normal range by the use of a short set of questions or some other relatively efficient modality.[11]

These difficulties with the assessment of functioning in children leave only traditional measures of assessment that are built on the notion of work. For children, substitutes for work have customarily been activity limitations in schoolwork for those over age 5 years and play for those under age 5 years. I would submit that there are very few even very impaired children who cannot play. So this leaves a rather significant paradox, in which very few children under age 5 appear to be disabled, even though many of these children are considered disabled as they age without experiencing changes in their health status or level of impairment. This suggests that current techniques for the identification of the level of disability in children are not optimal. Another reason for the rise in the rate of the disability with age is that additional children become disabled later as a result of either disease progression or the onset of new conditions or injuries.

Nevertheless, questions about functional limitations affecting participation in school and play have been used and are very similar to the types of questions used for adults that Jay Bhattacharya and colleagues reviewed in Appendix F. Such questions have been used rather frequently in national surveys over time. As mentioned in other appendixes in this volume, inconsistencies in the wording of the questions for children and adults have occurred across data sets and over time, but questionnaires have been a major means of tracking disabilities in children. Wording changes have been tracked in a number of studies[12,13] and are not reviewed here, but it should be noted that they may contribute to some of the changes in trends over time. It should also be emphasized, however, that the trends have continued even during periods in which the wording and administration of data collection have been stable. In a 1998 paper, Newacheck and Halfon[14] showed that in the 1960s the rate of functional or activity limitations in children was a little below 2 percent; in the early 1980s this rate went up to about 3.5 percent. These rates continued to increase to the present rate of about 7 percent.[13]

Another study that examined the differences between white and black non-Hispanic children showed differences in the raw percentages of functional or activity limitations in children. It appeared that higher proportions of black children and youth than white children and youth are affected, but poverty accounted for all of these patterns. When the data were controlled for poverty, the differences completely disappeared.[13] The bottom line is that over a 40-year period, the proportion of children reported to have major limitations in their activities related to play and school has gone from less than 2 percent to close to 7 percent. Within the population, all studies show higher rates of major activity limitations among older children than younger children and higher rates among males than females. At present, children over the age of 5 years are consistently reported to have rates of major activity limitations over 8 percent.[4]

The overwhelming majority of limitations in major activities is related to school participation and the need for special education. The higher level of special education for males is responsible for most of the difference by gender. Relatively few children are reported to be limited in major activities in any other way.[4] Additionally, broader definitions such as the one adopted by Child Trends Data Bank report that as many as 18 percent of 5- to 17-year-olds have at least one limitation of activity.[15]

Another way of looking at the traditional measures of disability is examination of the rate of Supplemental Security Income (SSI) enrollment among children. These data provide only a rough notion of the rates of disability among children because they are limited to poorer children, a consequence of the program's income restrictions that make children in middle-class homes ineligible for this benefit. In addition, the eligibility criteria for SSI require the child to have a significant impairment or a fatal condition. Nevertheless, according to those statistics, a rather significant rise in the number of children reported to have disabilities could be seen in the 1990s. In the early 1990s about 290,000 children[16] were receiving SSI, but by the end of the decade that number rose to 960,000.[17] However, that increase is due in large part to two concurrent changes: the U.S. Supreme Court decision in *Sullivan v. Zebley*, which broadened the criteria for eligibility,[18] and a revision of the medical standards for assessing health mental impairment, which increased the number of qualifying conditions from 4 to 11.[19]

NEWER APPROACHES

Although the methods described above are the traditional ways in which disability has been measured in children and youth, there are real problems with these work-related measures. First, there is a lack of a baseline against which functioning in children can be measured. Children are involved with the acquisition of function; except in instances of later onset of illness or injury, it is not possible to assess what the child would have been able to do if he or she did not have the condition that caused the disability. That is, children are involved in habilitation, not *re*-habilitation. To complicate matters more, wide variations in cultural norms and expectations exist across society, and these influence how children are assessed. Wide variations in what is accepted as normal development also exist.[11,20] The standard that children must meet before they are considered to have a disability is actually pretty low (and one that most healthy children pretty easily exceed). In real instances children and youth are not considered disabled because they have previously functioned above normal, and when their functioning is impaired to the level that meets the minimum baseline expectations, they continue to be classified as being free of a disability.

A recent example is an adolescent who had won an athletic scholarship to a university and who had been recruited for a professional baseball team. He then developed a condition that impaired his arm so that he could not play baseball. This adolescent is going to lose both his educational opportunity and a very major activity in his life, but he would probably not be counted as disabled by the standards that are now used.

However, the real problem with the use of school or play as the work analog for children and youth is that the real work of childhood is maturation and development of the child's potential—the acquisition of new capacities and skills—not going to school and playing. This notion of child health was recently endorsed by the Board of Children, Youth, and Families (Institute of Medicine and National Research Council) report on the health of children. It defines children's health as "the extent to which individual children or groups of children are able or enabled to develop and realize their potential; satisfy their needs; and develop the capacities that will allow them to interact successfully with their biological, physical and social environments"[8] (page 33). In the assessment of disabilities in children, individuals who are unable to develop and realize their potential, satisfy their needs, or interact with their environments—rather than those who cannot play or participate in school—should be counted. That is quite different from the current standard.

An important consideration in the search for alternative ways of measuring disabilities in children is the measurement of chronic conditions that lead to disability over time in childhood as well as those that may portend disabilities in later life. This is critical, because it is known that many chronic conditions lead to disability, especially if they are inadequately treated. From a prevention focus, the time to identify and catch chronic conditions and minimize the chance that they will produce a long-term disability is early in the child's life. This is important to avoid the extra burdens of disability over a lifetime.

In comparison to disabilities in adults, which tend to result from a cluster of relatively frequent conditions that account for a large portion of the burden of disability, the range of chronic conditions that produce disabilities among children is extremely diverse; and a far larger proportion of the burden of disabling conditions in childhood results from very rare conditions. The percentage of children with chronic conditions has been estimated by the use of a variety of tools and a large number of national surveys over the years and has varied from a low in the single digits to a high in the low 30s.[21,22] In the Child Health Supplement of the 1988 National Health Interview Survey, conducted by the National Center for Health Statistics, the estimate was 31 percent.[23] It should be noted that these percentages are based on counts of conditions, not of children.

A series of concerns surrounded these estimates, especially because a child, once he or she is labeled as having a condition, was counted forever after. Additionally, it seemed important to distinguish those who carried a label from those who were actually experiencing a consequence of having a condition. Furthermore, the condition lists used to identify children in such surveys were long and cumbersome and inevitably were unable to list all conditions, so that those with serious and disabling but rarer conditions were likely being missed. These factors, combined with the growing evidence that raising a child with a wide variety of health conditions posed similar challenges and required similar assistance from service systems, led to the endorsement of what has been called the "noncategorical" or "generic" approach to the identification of children with chronic conditions. It is based on continuing concern that the large number of individual conditions cannot be inventoried, that there have been negative effects of providing services and advocacy for each condition separately, and that there are inherent inequities in doing so.[24,25,26,27]

In 1993, my colleagues and I at the Albert Einstein College of Medicine proposed that children with chronic conditions could be identified by the consequences of their conditions.[27] Three major types of consequences were identified: whether the conditions imposed functional limitations compared to the functioning of their age-mates, whether they produced dependence on compensatory mechanisms or assistance, or whether they required more than the usual level of services. Others have since published similar definitions[28] and endorsed similar concepts,[29] and a variety of noncategorical or generic approaches have been used. One advantage of this approach is that it counts children, not conditions, and it has been estimated that between one-third and one-half of children have more than one condition.

A number of tools have been developed to operationalize these concepts, and three of these employ survey techniques: the Questionnaire for Identifying Children with Chronic Conditions (QuICCC), which has 39 items[30]; the Questionnaire for Identifying Children with Chronic Conditions—Revised (QuICCC–R), which has 16 items[31]; and the Children with Special Health Care Needs (CSHCN) screener, which is the shortest (and which some have called the "quickest"), with 5 items.[32] Only the first of these instruments was specifically designed for epidemiological purposes. However, the brevity of the CSHCN screener, which was originally designed for the purposes of quality assessment in health insurance plans, and its ability to identify so many children with disabilities quickly has made it an appealing instrument for many other purposes, including estimation of the prevalence of disabilities within populations. It has now been incorporated into many large-scale surveys on a national basis, such as the National Survey of Children with Special Health Care Needs (2000, 2005), the National Survey of Child Health, the National Health Interview Survey, and the Medical Expenditure Panel Survey.

The most comprehensive of these instruments, QuICCC, was almost entirely incorporated into the National Health Interview Survey on Disability (NHIS-D; 1994–1995) and produced estimates of rates of disability in children between 14.8 and 18 percent from the NHIS-D by the use of different analytic algorithms.[33,34] As in the case of the estimates obtained by using traditional measures of activity limitations, the numbers increased with the ages of the children, were higher for males, and were considerably higher among those whose family incomes were at or near the poverty level and whose parents had low levels of education.[34]

More recently, the CSHCN screener has been used in the State and Local Area Immunization Telephone Survey Children on Special Health Care Needs, funded by the Maternal and Child Health Bureau, and produced an estimate of disability among children of 12.9 percent.[35] Later national estimates of the rates of disability among children based on the CSHCN screener from the Medical Expenditure Survey suggest a rate of 17.6 percent. It is unclear whether this represents a true increase in prevalence or is related to differences in the methodologies related to the implementation of the CSHCN screener. The 2005 National Survey of Children with Special Health Care Needs is in the field and is again using the CSHCN screener.

Before leaving discussion of this approach to identification, it is worth noting that significant numbers of children have conditions that cause considerable consequences and are not identified by the functional limitations questions, even in the longest instrument. In fact, only 49 to 66 percent of the children identified as having disabilities by QuICCC are identified by 16 functional limitations items alone.[30,33,36] Most importantly, among the more than 50 diagnoses inventoried in the validation study, children with the same diagnoses were found to have different types of consequences as a result of their disabling conditions. Except for the fact that children with more types of consequences were more likely to have multiple diagnoses than those with only one type of consequence, the type of consequence was not useful in identifying classes of children with disabilities.[36] For example, a child with asthma might have only functional limitations or, when he or she was properly treated, might have been identified only by dependence on medication or might have intermittent inadequately treated asthma and experience only increased service use. This underscores the deficits that occur from the use of only functional limitations for the identification of children with disabilites.[36]

TRENDS IN DISABILITY

To evaluate trends in disability, it might be useful to look at a few examples for which data on trends in childhood disability are available. These trends have gone in different directions and make it hard to provide a single message about what is happening with childhood disability.

Blood Lead Levels

From 1976 to 1980, 88.2 percent of children 1 to 5 years of age had blood lead levels that were more than 10 micrograms of lead per deciliter. By 1988 to 1991, that figure had fallen to only 8.6 percent of children in that age group. It continued to fall so that in 2003 only 1.6 percent of children ages 1 to 5 years had blood lead levels of 10 micrograms of lead per deciliter.[37] This is a result of major changes in the environment, especially as a result of the elimination of the use of lead paint and lead-containing gasoline.[8]

Although this particular threshold of the blood lead level is not associated with measurable disability, it is a good marker for the level of population exposure to environmental lead, which at high levels of body burden is associated with significant cognitive as well as behavioral effects in children. High blood lead levels cause significant disability and even at low levels cause some impairment of the intellectual quotient.

Spina Bifida

Failure of the neural tube to fuse during fetal development is a cause of major childhood disability, regardless of the measure used. Another example of a success in lowering disability among children has resulted from the unraveling of the complicated interaction of genetics and environmental folic acid deficiency during pregnancy in a vulnerable subset of the population.[8] The inclusion of folic acid supplements to women of childbearing age has led to marked declines in the rates of both spina bifida and anencephaly. The Neural Tube Defect Ascertainment Project reported a 31 percent decline in the rate of spina bifida after fortification of the mother's diet with folic acid and a 19 percent decline in the rate of anencephaly.[38] Thus, the rate of the two conditions combined decreased from 7.6 to 5.4 per 10,000 births in a 3-year period (1997 through 1999).

Asthma

Asthma presents a very different pattern, one of increasing disability among children. There has been a steady increase in the proportion of U.S. children with asthma. A dramatic rise in the prevalence of asthma has been seen since the 1980s, with the rate almost doubling from the 1980s to the present.[39] Although many cases are mild and do not cause the significant disability seen in children with neural tube defects, the prevalence is much higher. More than 5 percent of children have asthma, which makes the prevalence of asthma 100 times greater than that of spina bifida, so that even if only a small percentage of children experience disability because of asthma, the increase in their numbers significantly overshadows the decline in the numbers of children with spina bifida.

Low Birth Weight

One of the successes of modern medicine has been the survival of low-birth-weight infants. As the rate of mortality has declined and the rates of low birth weight and preterm birth have increased somewhat, more children in the low-birth-weight population are surviving.[40] Although most low-birth-weight children do well, these survivors still experience far higher rates of morbidity and more significant rates of disabilities than children born at term with higher birth weights.[41] Another concern is that the infant mortality rate is not decreasing at the same rate among all the racial and ethnic groups. As a result, there are real disparities in the rate of infant mortality by race and ethnicity. The trends in low birth weight are also not evenly distributed, so that the rate of low birth weight among blacks is higher than that among the rest of the population.[42] A rapid rise in multiple births is also being seen, which is another reason for the increases in the rates of low birth weight and disabilities associated with low birth weight.[41]

Obesity

Members of the IOM committee have probably seen information from the Centers for Disease Control and Prevention depicting the rise in the proportion of the adult population experiencing obesity from less than 10 percent in most states to more than 25 percent in many states. This is an issue that has not been limited to adults.

In the 1960s the rates of obesity among children were 4 to 5 percent. Now the rates of obesity, considered a body mass index (BMI) more than 2 standard deviations above the mean for age and gender, are consistently close to 15 percent among adolescents and late-school-age children. This is an epidemic with great consequences for the future. Again, people in minority groups are the most affected. The rates among black and Mexican-American children have been increasing over time, and the rates of obesity are increasing among males as well as females. Among older Hispanic children, one in four meets or exceeds the criterion for being overweight.[43]

Although many people do not consider obesity per se to be a disability, this dramatic rise in the rate of obesity among children has major implications for the rates of disability for the children now and later in their lives. Excess BMI is associated with a variety of the conditions that cause disability, including cardiovascular problems, type II diabetes mellitus, hypertension, and hypercholesterolemia. The incidence of type II diabetes among children and adolescents has increased dramatically over time and at the Children's Hospital at Montefiore, the incidence equals that of type I diabetes, something that was previously unheard of.[44]

IMPORTANT OMISSIONS

Finally, two major omissions in this summary are noteworthy. First, the presenters were asked to exclude from discussion children who are institutionalized, who are not surveyed in any of the household-based surveys, and mental health morbidity, which is a major growing cause of disability among children and youth. Nevertheless, it would be inappropriate not to mention that institutionalized children are among those with the most severe disabilities. In addition, mental health conditions are among the leading causes of disability among children and youth and have extremely important implications for long-term well-being and functioning.

IMPLICATIONS

So what does the information presented here mean for the IOM committee? Current approaches to childhood disability that focus only on the severely disabled show low rates compared with those of adults, with a modest but consistent upward trend among children and youth. These disabilities have major implications for the young people who experience them, for their families, and for society as a whole. However, if the purpose of disability policies is to minimize impairment and lifetime disability, then I believe that the current emphasis on those with the most severe childhood disability is misguided.

I think that a broader conceptualization for the assessment of milder disabilities and conditions among the young is needed so that the precursors of disability that would allow the minimization of future impairment and disability can be tracked. Furthermore, this mismatch of agendas, in which the focus is on those who already are experiencing severe impairment, is going to increase dramatically as the genomic revolution allows children who are at biologic risk to be identified much earlier. This has real implications for the specialized preventive services that those children are going to need to prevent or postpone the onset of their disabilities.

There is an urgent need to address these issues and to redefine how society identifies and thinks about disability among the young, both for the children themselves and their current health and for their future health and their ability to be productive members of society in the long run.

REFERENCES

1. U.S. Census Bureau Population Estimates and Projections. http://childstats.gov/ americaschildren/pop1/asp. Accessed July 21, 2005.
2. U.S. Census Bureau Population Estimates and Projections. http://childstats.gov/ americaschildren/pop3/asp. Accessed July 21, 2005.
3. U.S. Census Bureau Population Estimates and Projections. http://childstats.gov/ americaschildren/pop3/asp. Accessed July 21, 2005.
4. Federal Interagency Forum on Child and Family Statistics. *America's Children: Key Indicators of Well-Being*. Washington, DC: U.S. Government Printing Office, 2005.
5. National Center for Health Statistics. *Health, United States, 2004, with Chartbook on Trends in the Health of Americans*. Hyattsville, MD: National Center for Health Statistics, 2004.
6. Newacheck PW and Benjamin AE. Intergenerational equity and public spending. *Health Affairs* 23:142–146, 2004.
7. U.S. Census Bureau Population Estimates and Projections. http://childstats.gov/ americaschildren/hea1/asp. Accessed July 21, 2005.
8. National Research Council and Institute of Medicine. *Children's Health, the Nation's Wealth: Assessing and Improving Child Health*. Committee on the Evaluation of Children's Health. Board of Children, Youth, and Families, Division of Behavioral and Social Sciences and Education. Washington, DC: National Academies Press, 2004.
9. Chatterji S, Ustun B, Sadana R, Salamon JA, Mathers CD, and Murray CJL. The conceptual basis for measuring and reporting on health. Global Programme on Evidence for Health Policy Discussion Paper 45. Geneva, Switzerland: World Health Organization, 2002.
10. U.S. Congress, Office of Technology Assessment. *Technology-Dependent Children: Hospital v. Home Care: A Technical Memorandum*. OTA-TM-H-38. Washington, DC: U.S. Government Printing Office, May 1987.
11. Stein REK and Jessop DJ. Functional status II(R): a measure of child health status. *Medical Care* 28:1041–1055, 1990.
12. Newacheck PW, Budetti PP, and Halfon N. Trends in activity-limiting chronic conditions among children. *American Journal of Public Health* 76:178–184, 1986.
13. Newacheck PN, Stein REK, Bauman LJ, et al. Disparities in the prevalence of disability between black and white children. *Archives of Pediatrics and Adolescent Medicine* 157:244–248, 2003.
14. Newacheck PW and Halfon N. Prevalence and impact of disabling chronic conditions in childhood. *American Journal of Public Health* 88:610–617, 1998.
15. Child Trends Data Bank. www.childtrendsdatabank.org. Accessed July 21, 2005.
16. Perrin JM and Stein REK: Reinterpreting disability: changes in SSI for children. *Pediatrics* 88:1047–1051, 1992.
17. Social Security Administration, Office of Policy, Office of Research, Evaluation and Statistics. *Children Receiving SSI, December 2003*. SSA Publication 13-11830. Washington, DC: U.S. Government Printing Office, 2005.
18. *Sullivan v. Zebley*, 88–1377. U.S. Supreme Court, February 20, 1990.
19. Perrin JM, Kuhlthau K, McLaughlin TJ, Etner SL, and Gortmaker SL. Changing patterns of conditions among children receiving Supplemental Security Income disability benefits. *Archives of Pediatric and Adolescent Medicine* 153:80–84, 1999.
20. Stein REK. Measurement of children's health. *Ambulatory Pediatrics* 4:365–370, 2004.
21. Gortmaker S and Sappenfield W. Chronic childhood disorders: prevalence and impact. *Pediatric Clinics of North America* 31:3–18, 1984.

22. Jessop DJ and Stein REK. Consistent but not the same: effects of method on chronic conditions rates. *Archives of Pediatrics and Adolescent Medicine* 149:1105–1110, 1995.

23. Newacheck PW and Taylor WR. Childhood chronic illness: prevalence, severity, and impact. *American Journal of Public Health* 82:364–371, 1992.

24. Pless IB and Pinkerton P. *Chronic Childhood Disorder: Promoting Patterns of Adjustment.* Chicago, IL: Year Book Medical Publishers, 1975.

25. Hobbs N and Perrin JM. *Issues in the Care of Children with Chronic Illness: A Sourcebook on Problems, Services, and Policies.* San Francisco, CA: Jossey-Bass, 1985.

26. Stein REK and Jessop DJ. What diagnosis does not tell? The case for a noncategorical approach to chronic illness in childhood. *Social Science and Medicine* 29:769–778, 1989.

27. Stein REK, Bauman LJ, Westbrook LE, Coupey SM, and Ireys HT. Framework for identifying children who have chronic conditions: the case for a new definition. *The Journal of Pediatrics* 122:342–347, 1993.

28. McPherson M, Arango P, Fox H, et al. A new definition of children with special health care needs. *Pediatrics* 102:137–140, 1998.

29. Perrin EC, Newacheck P, Pless IB, Drotar D, Gortmaker SL, Leventhal J, Perrin JM, Stein REK, Walker DK, and Weitzman M. Issues involved in the definition and classification of chronic health conditions. *Pediatrics* 91:787–793, 1993.

30. Stein REK, Westbrook LE, and Bauman LJ. The questionnaire for identifying children with chronic conditions (QuICCC): a measure based on a noncategorical approach. *Pediatrics* 99:513–521, 1997.

31. Stein REK, Silver EJ, and Bauman LJ. Shortening the questionnaire for identifying children with chronic conditions (QuICCC): what is the consequence? *Pediatrics* 107(4):pe61, 2001.

32. Bethell C, Read D, Stein REK, Blumberg SJ, Wells N, and Newacheck PW. Identifying children with special health care needs: development and evaluation of a short screening instrument. *Ambulatory Pediatrics* 2:38–48, 2002.

33. Stein REK and Silver EJ. Operationalizing a conceptually-based noncategorical definition: a first look at US children with chronic conditions. *Archives of Pediatrics and Adolescent Medicine* 153:68–74, 1999.

34. Stein REK and Silver EJ. Comparing different definitions of children with chronic conditions in a national data set. *Ambulatory Pediatrics* 2:63–70, 2002.

35. van Dyck PC, Kogan MD, McPherson MG, Weissman GR, and Newacheck PW. Prevalence and characteristics of children with special health care needs. *Archives of Pediatrics and Adolescent Medicine* 158(9):88:4–90, 2004.

36. Westbrook LE, Silver EJ, and Stein REK. Implications for estimates of disability in children: a comparison of definitional components. *Pediatrics* 101:1025–1030, 1998.

37. Centers for Disease Control and Prevention, National Center for Environmental Health. Lead research, as quoted by Trends Data Bank. www.childtrendsdatabank.org. Accessed July 21, 2005.

38. March of Dimes, personal communication. Data from National Birth Defects Prevention Network-Centers for Disease Prevention and Control.

39. Centers for Disease Control and Prevention. Childhood asthma prevalence before and after the 1997 redesign of the National Health Interview Survey—United States. *Morbidity and Mortality Weekly Report* 49:908–911, 2000.

40. Martin JA, Kochanek K, Strobino DM, Guyer B, and MacDorman MF. Annual summary of vital statistics—2003 *Pediatrics* 115:619–634, 2005.

41. Hack M, Taylor HG, Drotar D, Schluchter M, Cartar L, Andreias L, Wilson-Costello D, and Klein N. Chronic conditions, functional limitations, and special health care needs of school-age children born extremely low birth weight in the 1990s. *Journal of the American Medical Association* 294:318-325, 2005.

42. U.S. Census Bureau Population Estimates and Projections. http://childstats.gov/americaschildren/hea5/asp. Accessed July 21, 2005.

43. U.S. Census Bureau Population Estimates and Projections. http://childstats.gov/americaschildren/hea3/asp. Accessed July 21, 2005.

44. Hannon TS, Rao G, and Arslanian SA. Childhood obesity and type 2 diabetes mellitus. *Pediatrics* 16:473–480, 2005.

H

Aspects of Disability
Across the Life Span:
Risk Factors for Disability in Late Life

Jack M. Guralnik[*]

I have been working on the epidemiology of disability and risk factors for disability for 20 years. Until the Institute of Medicine (IOM) report *Disability in America* was published nearly 15 years ago (IOM, 1991), we were in a kind of wilderness in some respects. The IOM report, in elaborating on Nagi's model of disability (Nagi, 1991), gave us a framework for our work. I trust that this workshop and the larger study of which it is a part will make a similar contribution to disability research in the future. It is particularly important that the study report focus on operational concepts that epidemiologists (like me) who undertake large population studies can use to measure disability and the steps from disease to disability in a valid, reliable manner.

This paper describes classic epidemiologic research on risk factors for disability and points out some of the challenges in trying to sort out the main causes of disability in the older population. I will note how aspects of this research relate to some of the mechanisms and pathways in the Nagi-IOM model.

In the early 1980s, the National Institute on Aging initiated a set of four large population-based studies called the Established Populations for Epidemiologic Studies of the Elderly (EPESE). The basic approach was to

---

[*]Jack Guralnik, M.D., Ph.D. Acting Chief, Laboratory of Epidemiology, Demography and Biometry, National Institute on Aging, Bethesda, Maryland. The analyses and views presented in this workshop paper are those of the author and not necessarily those of the Institute of Medicine Committee on Disability in America: A New Look.

study risk factors for the onset of disability in a population or subpopulation that was free of disability and then examine the development of incident cases of disability and the risk factors that predicted its onset. The condition that I will discuss is mobility disability, defined here as an inability to walk a quarter mile and an inability to climb a set of stairs.

When my colleagues and I started our study, 72 percent of the cohort of 10,000 individuals was free of mobility problems at the baseline (Guralnik et al., 1993). Over a period that included four annual follow-ups, 53 percent of this group maintained mobility, 35 percent lost mobility, and a small percentage died without any evidence of mobility loss. At the baseline, we collected data on a number of chronic conditions that we hypothesized might predict mobility loss. We found the odds ratio for the loss of mobility to be in the range of about 1.2 to 1.5 for people with baseline reports of heart attack, stroke, diabetes, dyspnea, or exertional leg pain compared with the risk for people free of these conditions.

A considerable amount of cross-sectional and longitudinal research, including some studies documented in these appendixes, has investigated a variety of potential risk factors for disability. A range of physical and behavioral risk factors have been shown to be associated with disability. These factors include low levels of physical activity, smoking, high and low body mass index, weight loss, heavy and no alcohol consumption, high levels of medication use, poor self-rated health, and reduced social contacts. Andreas Stuck did a very nice job of summarizing this body of research in a 1999 paper (Stuck, 1999).

Among the chronic conditions that have been shown in epidemiologic studies to be associated with disability are heart disease and stroke, osteoarthritis, hip fracture, diabetes, peripheral artery disease, chronic obstructive pulmonary disease, cancer, visual impairment, depression, and cognitive impairment. This list of conditions is in no particular order, and people frequently ask what conditions are the primary causes of disability. This is actually a much more complicated question than it initially appears to be.

Some of the issues involved in assessments of the overall impact of a chronic condition on disability include the strength of the association between the condition (risk factor) and a particular disability; the prevalence of the risk factor; and—putting these together—something called an "attributable risk," which has been assessed for some conditions. Also, it is important to consider the disability outcome of interest, as Alan Jette has done (Jette, 1994). For example, are you assessing the difficulty of performing a certain activity or, more narrowly, the human assistance required to perform the task?

Another important issue is population characteristics, such as age and gender. The main causes of disability may be different in men and women. For example, Ettinger and colleagues found arthritis-musculoskeletal dis-

TABLE H-1   Most Common Diseases Reported to Cause Difficulty with Specific Tasks

Activity	Men		Women	
	Disease	Percent	Disease	Percent
Walking ½ mile	Arthritis	33	Arthritis	43
	Heart disease	13	Heart disease	12
	Injury	9	Lung disease	9
Doing heavy housework	Heart disease	26	Arthritis	45
	Arthritis	24	Heart disease	15
	Lung disease	11	Old age	8
Bathing	Stroke	25	Arthritis	57
	Arthritis	21	Injury	11

SOURCE: Adapted from Ettinger et al. (1994).

ease and injury to be more important causes of disability for women than for men, whereas men are more likely to experience disability in association with heart disease, lung disease, and stroke (Ettinger et al., 1994). For both women and men, arthritis and musculoskeletal disease led as causes of disability by a considerable margin (reported by 50 percent of women and 30 percent of men), with heart disease being the next most often reported (reported by 13 percent of women and 16 percent of men).

When the investigators looked not only at overall disability but also at specific conditions, they again found different results for men and women and found different results depending on the type of disability. As shown in Table H-1, for limitations related to the ability to walk one-half mile, do heavy housework, or bathe, women reported arthritis as the main cause for each of these limitations. For men, arthritis was the top reported cause for limitations in walking one-half mile; but for heavy housework, heart disease is slightly more important as a cause, and for limitations in bathing, stroke has a slightly greater role than arthritis.

As mentioned earlier, the way in which disability is assessed affects what is found. For example, Suzanne Leveille has been interested in pain and its effect on functioning and disability. She and her colleagues have found consistent results in a number of different studies that show a significant association between pain and difficulties in climbing stairs and lifting as well as difficulties with activities of daily living (ADLs) (Leveille et al., 1999). However, if the measure is whether someone is not able to perform an activity at all, there is some increase related to levels of pain, but the relationship (the odds ratio) is not significant.

Another study by Leveille and colleagues shows similar results (Leville et al., 2001). For the categories of mild pain (at least one site), moderate pain (at least two sites), and widespread pain (at least three sites and both upper and lower body sites), people with pain report more difficulty with ADLs than people without pain; but people with pain are not more likely to be unable to perform ADLs or to need help from another person.

In addition to individual chronic conditions, the co-occurrence of multiple conditions or comorbidities is very important in the older population. EPESE data show that as the number of chronic conditions increases, the risk of developing a new disability goes up rather dramatically for both men and women (Guralnik et al., 1993). Those who are not disabled at the baseline but who have four or more chronic conditions at that time are almost three times as likely to report mobility loss at follow-up.

Some research suggests that synergistic or multiplicative effects on disability levels may exist for specific combinations of chronic conditions. This is difficult research to do, even with fairly large sample sizes. It is still not clear that a greater effect results from such combinations of conditions than would be expected simply from the additive effects of each condition.

In addition to identifying relationships, colleagues and I have also tried to identify mechanisms by which risk factors operate in contributing to disability. Two examples of this work involve diabetes and low socioeconomic status as risk factors for disability.

For diabetes, we first looked at the association between diabetes and several different functional or disability outcomes: mobility problems, ADL disability, and severe walking limitation (i.e., an inability to walk or walking less than 0.4 meters per second). We also included an additional objective measure of lower-extremity performance, the Short Physical Performance Battery (SPPB). Next we added into our statistical models several specific conditions and impairments (e.g., peripheral neuropathy, hypertension, and visual impairment) that are associated with diabetes. We then looked at the attenuation of the diabetes-function association, as measured by the odds ratio (for discrete outcomes) or the beta coefficient (for continuous outcomes).

For each outcome, we found that each of the diabetes-related conditions reduced the initial association between diabetes and the functional outcomes (Volpato et al., 2002). No condition predominates, but when taken together, the conditions explain about 80 percent of the statistical association between diabetes and, especially, mobility and ADL outcomes. In addition, most of the conditions appear to be clinically plausible as explanatory factors.

In other studies, we have looked at socioeconomic status (specifically, educational level) as a risk factor related to both total life expectancy and disability-free life expectancy. From the EPESE cohort from North Caro-

---

Nagi-IOM model of disabling process (simplified):

Disease → Impairment → Functional limitation → Disability

ICF model (simplified):

Disease → Body functions and structure → Activity → Participation

---

FIGURE H-1   Models of the pathway from disease to disability.

lina, we found that for both white and African-American men and women, higher education is associated with longer life expectancy and longer disability-free life expectancy at age 65 years (Guralnik et al., 1993).

Many other studies likewise show a relationship between socioeconomic status and disability outcomes. What might be the mechanisms here? Some findings from the InChianti Study (so named because it was undertaken in the Chianti region of Italy) are interesting. The focus was different physiologic subsystems that affect walking. These include the central and peripheral nervous systems, the muscular system, bones and joints, sensory systems, and the energy delivery system. Antonia Coppin, who is in my research group, looked at a variety of different impairments in these subsystems and how they mediate the relationship between low levels of education and both lower-extremity functioning and gait speed (Coppin et al., in press). She found two conditions that have a particularly high impact: trail making (a test of executive functioning that is related to educational status) and leg power. When all the factors are added into the analysis, they explain a very large proportion of the difference in lower-extremity function between people with lower and higher levels of education.

Beyond this research, we have also attempted to do empirical research using the IOM model (Figure H-1). This has worked quite well. I present here examples that look at disease and impairment and subsequent functional limitations and then functional limitations and subsequent disability. We are trying to sort out just how our work will relate to the new *International Classification of Functioning, Disability and Health* (ICF) model (WHO, 2001), but so far we have based a lot of our research on the Nagi-IOM model. In operationalizing this model, the work of Lois Verbrugge and Alan Jette (1994) has been very valuable.

One way that we have measured functional limitations uses the SPPB mentioned earlier, an approach first used in the EPESE study (Guralnik et al., 1994; Guralnik et al., 2000). This battery has three components: standing balance, timed 4-meter walk, and the time required to rise from a chair five times. Each component is scored categorically from 0 to 4, and these scores contribute to a summary performance score that ranges from 0 to 12.

In the Women's Health and Aging Study, colleagues and I looked at individuals every 6 months. We analyzed data for people who had documented acute medical events—hip fracture, stroke, myocardial infarction (MI), and congestive heart failure (CHF). Women with none of these conditions clearly had the least decline in performance; those with hip fracture fared the worst (Ostir et al., 2002). (Changes in summary scores were –0.29 for no condition, –1.48 for CHF, –2.30 for MI, –2.63 for stroke, and –3.09 for hip fracture over the 6 month period when these events occurred.)

Another study looked at depression as a risk factor for declines in the same objective performance measure (Penninx et al., 1998). That study found that people with greater numbers of symptoms of depression had greater declines in the SPPB.

We have also studied the transition from functional limitation to disability. In one part of the EPESE study, we found that the higher (better) that the performance was on the SPPB, the less likely it was that an individual who was nondisabled at the start of the study would have an ADL or mobility limitation 4 years later (Guralnik et al., 1995). Using the results of this study in a clinical trial of exercise to prevent disability, we are employing the SPPB to target people without disabilities who have functional limitations and who are therefore at high risk of progressing to disability (Rejeski et al., 2005).

The pace and the course of disability in the older population are also of interest. Colleagues and I have evaluated, using annual interviews over a 6-year period, what we call severe catastrophic and severe progressive disability, defined as follows:

• Severe disability: the individual needs help with three or more of six ADLs (eating, dressing, bathing, transferring, using the toilet, and walking across a small room)

• Catastrophic severe disability: an individual with severe disability in whom no ADL disability was identified in the preceding two interviews

• Progressive severe disability: an individual with severe disability in whom one or two ADLs were identified in the preceding interview

We found that catastrophic disability is more common in the young old. Progressive disability is most common in those ages 85 years and older, a pattern consistent with what we think of the frailty of old age (Ferrucci et al., 1996).

Although I have not considered them here, environmental and personal

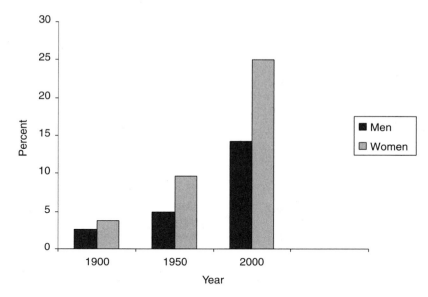

FIGURE H-2 Percentage of American men and women age 50 years or older projected to survive to age 90 years and older. Compiled from U.S. life tables, National Center for Health Statistics.

factors should not be forgotten, as they may affect the progression of potentially disabling conditions. The disabling potential of many of the conditions that I have discussed is affected by the physical environment, access to assistive technologies, and other environmental conditions.

Let me close by recalling the demographic context for this discussion. Figure H-2 shows data that I developed from U.S. life tables starting in 1900. It shows the proportion of 50-year-old people expected to live to age 90 years or older. That proportion was tiny in 1900, but in 2000 more than 25 percent of 50-year-old women were projected to live to be 90 years old and older.

Figure H-3 shows data that I compiled from EPESE data, specifically, data on disability in the year before death. For people in their 90s, the rate of disability in the years before death is extremely high. So, although the age-adjusted or age-specific rates of disability are declining in the United States, the overall numbers of older people with disabilities and the societal impact of disability will grow because so many more people will be in the very old age groups. Thus, identification of the causes of disability and interventions that can mitigate these causes or their effects will be increasingly important.

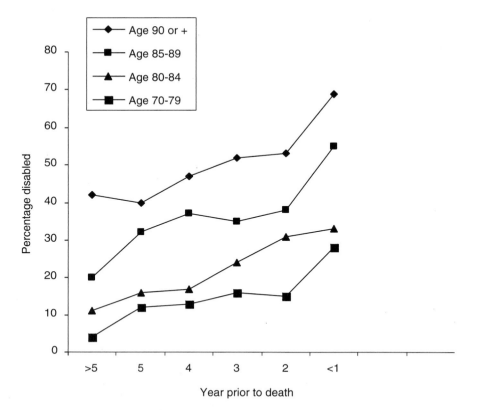

FIGURE H-3 Percentage of individuals age 70 years or older defined as disabled by year before death.

REFERENCES

Coppin AK, Ferrucci L, Lauretani F, Phillips C, Chang M, Bandinelli S, Guralnik JM. Low socioeconomic status and disability in old age: evidence from the InChianti Study for the mediating role of physiological impairments. *The Journals of Gerontology. Series A, Biological Sciences and Medical Sciences*, in press.

Ettinger WH Jr, Fried LP, Harris T, Shemanski L, Schulz R, Robbins J. Self-reported causes of physical disability in older people: the Cardiovascular Health Study. CHS Collaborative Research Group. *Journal of the American Geriatric Society* 1994 Oct;42(10):1035–1044.

Ferrucci L, Guralnik JM, Simonsick E, Salive ME, Corti MC, Langlois J. Progressive versus catastrophic disability: A longitudinal view of the disablement process. *The Journals of Gerontology. Series A, Biological Sciences and Medical Sciences* 1996;51:M123-M130.

Guralnik JM, LaCroix AZ, Abbott RD, et al. Maintaining mobility in late life. I. Demographic characteristics and chronic conditions. *American Journal of Epidemiology* 1993;137:845–857.

Guralnik JM, Simonsick EM, Ferrucci L, Glynn RJ, Berkman LF, Blazer DG, Scherr PA, Wallace RB. A short physical performance battery assessing lower extremity function: Association with self-reported disability and prediction of mortality and nursing home admission. *The Journals of Gerontology. Series A, Biological Sciences and Medical Sciences* 1994;49:M85-M94.

Guralnik JM, Ferrucci L, Simonsick EM, Salive ME, Wallace RB. Lower-extremity function in persons over the age of 70 years as a predictor of subsequent disability. *New England Journal of Medicine* 1995; Mar 2;332(9):556–561.

Guralnik JM, Ferrucci F, Pieper CF, Leveille SG, Markides KS, Ostir GV, Studenski S, Berkman LF, Wallace RB. Lower extremity function and subsequent disability: Consistency across studies, predictive models, and value of gait speed alone compared to the short physical performance battery. *The Journals of Gerontology. Series A, Biological Sciences and Medical Sciences* 2000;55:M221-231.

IOM (Institute of Medicine). *Disability in America*. Washington, DC: National Academy Press, 1991.

Jette, AM. How measurement techniques influence estimates of disability in older populations. *Social Science Medicine* 1994; 38:937–942.

Leveille SG, Guralnik JM, Hochberg M, Hirsch R, Ferrucci L, Langlois J, Rantanen T, Ling S. Low back pain and disability in older women: independent association with difficulty but not inability to perform daily activities. *The Journals of Gerontology. Series A, Biological Sciences and Medical Sciences* 1999; Oct;54(10):M487–M493.

Leveille SG, Ling S, Hochberg MC, Resnick HE, Bandeen-Roche KJ, Won A, Guralnik JM. Widespread musculoskeletal pain and the progression of disability in older disabled women. *Annals of Internal Medicine* 2001; Dec 18;135(12):1038–1046.

Nagi, S. Disability Concepts revisited: implications for prevention, pp. 309–327. In *Disability in America*. Institute of Medicine. Washington, DC: National Academy Press; 1991.

Ostir GV, Volpato S, Fried LP, Chaves P, Guralnik JM. Women's Health and Aging Study. Reliability and sensitivity to change assessed for a summary measure of lower body function: results from the Women's Health and Aging Study. *Journal of Clinical Epidemiology* 2002; Sep;55(9):916–921.

Penninx BW, Guralnik JM, Ferrucci L, Simonsick EM, Deeg DJ, Wallace RB. Depressive symptoms and physical decline in community-dwelling older persons. *Journal of the American Medical Association* 1998; Jun 3;279(21):1720–1726.

Rejeski WJ, Fielding RA, Blair SN, Guralnik JM, Gill TM, Hadley EC, King AC, Kritchevsky SB, Miller ME, Newman AB, Pahor M. The Lifestyle Interventions and Independence for Elders (LIFE) pilot study: Design and methods. *Contemporary Clinical Trials* 2005;26:141-54.

Stuck AE, Walthert JM, Nikolaus T, Bula CJ, Hohmann C, Beck JC. Risk factors for functional status decline in community-living elderly people: a systematic literature review. *Social Science Medicine* 1999; Feb;48(4):445–469.

Verbrugge LM, Jette AM. The disablement process. *Social Science Medicine* 1994; Jan;38(1):1–14.

Volpato S, Blaum C, Resnick H, Ferrucci L, Fried LP, Guralnik JM. Women's Health and Aging Study. Comorbidities and impairments explaining the association between diabetes and lower extremity disability: The Women's Health and Aging Study. *Diabetes Care* 2002; Apr;25(4):678–683.

WHO (World Health Organization). *International Classification of Functioning, Disability, and Health*. Geneva, Switzerland: World Health Organization; 2001.

I

Health Care Transition of Adolescents and Young Adults with Disabilities and Special Health Care Needs: New Perspectives

John Reiss and Robert Gibson[*]

In the United States, almost 9.4 million children and youth have special health care needs (Centers for Disease Control and Prevention, National Center for Health Statistics, 2000), and approximately 500,000 turn 18 years old annually (Newacheck and Taylor, 1992). The large and growing number of young adults with special health care needs and disabilities is a result of medical advances that have been made over the past 25 years. Today, many children who once would have died from severe congenital disorders and other serious medical conditions survive into adulthood (Blum, 1995; Gortmaker et al., 1993).

More than 15 years ago, in anticipation of the challenges that these young people might face in accessing health care and the demands they would place on the pediatric and adult health care systems, Surgeon General C. Everett Koop convened a conference entitled Growing Up and Getting Medical Care: Youth with Special Health Care Needs (Magrab and Miller, 1989). The conference drew much needed attention to this emerging issue and created a national agenda for developing a seamless health care system that would allow youth to easily move from child-centered (pediatric) to adult-oriented health care (Blum, 2002; Reiss, 1999). Because the

---

[*]John Reiss, Ph.D. Associate Professor of Pediatrics and, Institute for Child Health Policy, University of Florida, Gainesville. Robert Gibson, Ph.D., MSOTR/L, Research Associate, Institute for Child Health Policy, University of Florida, Gainesville. The analyses and views presented in this workshop paper are those of the author and not necessarily those of the Institute of Medicine Committee on Disability in America: A New Look.

transition to adulthood represents a critical turning point in the life course, suboptimal transition experiences may affect the ability of people with childhood onset chronic conditions to participate in society and live fulfilling lives as adults (Halfon and Hochstein, 2002).

The last decade and a half has seen an ever-expanding number of policy and consensus statements, practice guidelines, position papers, conference reports, calls to action, editorials, program descriptions, and small research studies that address various aspects of health care transitions for young people (Reiss and Gibson, 2002). In 2002, the American Academy of Pediatrics (AAP), the American Academy of Family Physicians (AAFP), and the American College of Physicians-American Society of Internal Medicine (ACP-ASIM) released a consensus statement (American Academy of Pediatrics et al., 2002) that sets out six steps to ensure that all young people with special health care needs are provided with the support that they need to transition to adult-oriented medical care. (See Box I-1 below). To implement these and other similar recommendations will require changes in professional education, clinical practice, organizational procedures and structures, public policies, and research priorities (Scal, 2002; Blum, 2002; Reiss and Gibson, 2002; Reiss et al., 2005; Lotstein et al., 2005).

For the purposes of this paper, *health care transfer* refers to the point in time when an individual changes from one primary or specialty care provider to another. This paper focuses on one important example, the transfer from pediatric to adult care. *Health care transition* refers to a planned process that for youth includes the preparation for transfer from pediatric to adult-oriented health care, the transfer itself, and the establishment of the young adult in the adult health care system. *Child-centered care* and *pediatric care* refer to primary and specialty health care that is provided to individuals under the age of 18 years by pediatricians, family physicians, pediatric nurse practitioners, and other child health care professionals. Such care is characterized by attention to processes of physical, mental, and emotional development that continue from infancy through adolescence and includes involvement by parents, who oversee and provide much care to children in the home. During this period, parents have the legal responsibility for decisions about a child's care, although young people generally become more involved in decision making as they mature. *Adult-oriented health care* refers to health care that is provided to individuals over the age of 18 and that places greater emphasis on personal responsibility and patient autonomy.

HEALTH CARE TRANSITION VIEWED
AS A DEVELOPMENTAL PROCESS

As noted by Rosen (2004), health care transition occurs "contemporaneously with the dramatic physical, cognitive, psychological and social development of adolescence" (p. 126) and within the broader context of the developmental tasks associated with the transition from adolescence to adulthood (i.e., increased independence, legal responsibility, work, financial self-sufficiency, and the formation of adult partnerships and new families). For young adults with disabilities or special health care needs, health care transition is a "dynamic lifelong process that seeks to meet their individual needs as they move from childhood to adulthood. The goal is to maximize lifelong functioning and potential through the provision of high-quality, developmentally appropriate health care services that continue uninterrupted as the individual moves from adolescence to adulthood" (American Academy of Pediatrics et al., 2002, p.1304). Furthermore, transition involves a "reorientation of clinical relations to mirror the young person's increasing maturity and emerging adulthood" (American Academy of Pediatrics et al., 2002, pp.1304-5).

Our research on the real-life experience of health care transitions revealed that for the youth and families that were most successful in transition, the shift occurred as a developmental process that progressed through three stages. These stages are: envisioning a future, age of responsibility, and age of transition (Reiss et al., 2005).

The first stage, envisioning a future, starts at the time of diagnosis and focuses on the establishment of a future-oriented perspective. Questions about future education, employment options, independent living in the community, and health care needs should help to prompt families and providers to formulate long-term goals and initiate activities that promote the child's future independence.

The second stage, the age of responsibility (ages 6 to 14 years), centers on the young person mastering and independently carrying out developmentally appropriate and age-appropriate tasks. These tasks include such routine activities as learning to dress oneself and managing personal hygiene, as well as specific health care tasks, such as taking medications independently, learning about one's illness or disability and communicating with health care providers.

The first two stages lay the foundation for the broad range of the transition-specific activities that occur during the final stage, the age of transition. This stage is divided into two periods, adolescence (ages 15 to 17 years) and young adulthood (ages 18 to 25 years), the dividing point being the legal age of adulthood (age 18 years in the United States). It is during the stage of transition that the young person develops and refines the knowledge and skills needed to interact with the adult-oriented health care system independently and take the lead role in medical decision making. New adult-oriented providers are identified and selected and the challenge of maintaining health insurance coverage is addressed.

PROVIDER POLICIES AND PRACTICES

In the United States, children receive child-oriented health care from pediatricians, family physicians, pediatric nurse practitioners, or other child health care professionals. Transfers from pediatric to adult-oriented care typically appear to be based on a young person's age rather than his or her readiness or ability to negotiate the adult health care system (Reiss et al., 2005). Many pediatric physicians, especially those who provide primary care, have a policy to discharge their patients when they finish college or reach a certain age, which is typically by the age of 21 years (American Academy of Pediatrics, Council on Child Health, 1972; see also commentary by Litt, 1998. The 1972 statement remains current AAP policy [personal communication, Stephanie Mucha Skipper, M.P.H., Manager, Council on Children with Disabilities, AAP]). In addition, some professional medical associations have guidelines on age as part of licensing or specific accreditations. For example, the national professional guidelines for pediatric nurse practitioners restrict their practice to individuals aged 21 years and under, except under certain circumstances (National Association of Pediatric Nurse Practitioners, 2004).

Children's health services and agencies may have maximum age policies defined in their charters, by-laws, or other corporate operating procedures. Examples include the 18-21 upper age limit for State Title V CHSCN Programs (Reiss and Lamar, 2003) and the 18 year old age limit for Shriners Hospitals (Ben Ali Shriners, 2005). Hospitals that serve both children and adults typically have policies that require inpatients over a certain age (for example, age 18 years) to be cared for on floors for adults rather than in the pediatric section of the hospital (Personal communication, Terrance Flotte, MD, Chairman Department of Pediatrics, University of Florida, November 8, 2005). These inpatient policies appear to be related to a number of factors, including staff training and expertise, the availability of size- and age-appropriate medical equipment and technology, the perceived appropriateness of the care environment, and tradition.

An abrupt transfer out of pediatric care can also be prompted by an adolescent's display of adult behaviors. More generally, pediatric providers may hesitate to treat adolescents and young adults who are sexually active, pregnant, abusing illegal substances, acting out or challenging authority, or adjudicated to the juvenile justice system (Reiss et al. 2005, Rosen, 2004).

The primary concern about using a young person's age or behavior as a criterion for transfer to adult care is that transfers may be implemented without a process for determining whether the individual is prepared for the world of adult-oriented medicine.

BENEFITS AND CHALLENGES OF THE TRANSFER FROM
PEDIATRIC TO ADULT CARE

How young people move from pediatric to adult-oriented health care is not well documented or understood. For many healthy young people, a typical sequence appears to be (1) a period during which a young person stops seeing child-oriented providers, (2) a period during which the individual is not well connected to the health care system, and (3) a time in middle age when emerging acute and chronic health care problems such hypertension prompt the reestablishment of a relationship with one or more health care professionals. This pattern may be most characteristic of healthy young men, who may only occasionally need treatment for an injury or acute illness. Young adult women with needs for gynecological and obstetric care have more motivation to establish a relationship with a health care professional. Although data from the National Health Interview Survey show a sharp drop after age 18 for both males and females in the proportion of people who have a usual place to go for health care, the drop is much greater for males than females—from approximately 95 percent for both groups in the under-18-age group to approximately 65 percent for males and 80 percent for females aged 18 to 24 (Centers for Disease Control and Prevention, 2004).

Overall, our sense is that for many young people the move from pediatric to adult-oriented care is less a transition (a planned purposeful process) than a series of discontinuous events. Although such an unplanned process is not ideal, it may not substantially interfere with the progress that most young adults make in addressing the tasks of young adulthood, such as completing education and training, getting a job, moving toward financial self-sufficiency, living independently, starting a family of their own, and establishing their place in adult society (Havighurst, 1972; Elliot and Feldman, 1990; Carnegie Council on Adolescent Development, 1995).

In contrast, young adults with disabilities and special health care needs do not have the option of dropping out of the health care system for an extended period of time. Doing so can have serious, even life-threatening health consequences. Furthermore, for many of these young people, progress toward adult roles and responsibilities depends, in part, on access the health care that helps them to be as healthy and as functional as possible (Viner, 1999).

The move from pediatric to adult-oriented health care presents both potential benefits and challenges or risks for young adults with disabilities or special health care needs. The potential benefits include

• receipt of age-appropriate preventive and primary care that supports adult roles and functioning and that includes screening for and treatment of common adult health problems, for example, cholesterol and hypertension screening and counseling about exercise and weight;

• increased attention to sexuality, fertility, and reproductive health issues;

• promotion of a more active role for the young adult in learning about, managing, and making decisions about their health and health care; and

• improved access to adult inpatient services and to subspecialists trained to treat adults.

Potential challenges associated with the transition of young adults to adult-oriented providers also exist. They include

• difficulty finding primary and specialty care providers who have experience with and current knowledge of certain pediatric-onset conditions and who are interested in treating young adults with these conditions;

• loss of access to pediatric professionals and providers who have unique knowledge about the pediatric onset conditions, the history of a disabling condition for a particular young person, and the personal and family circumstances of that individual, including the medical care and other support provided by family members;

• changes in a therapeutic regimen that may, if not carefully presented and monitored, cause confusion and compromise a young adult's adherence to the regimen; and

• limited preparation of young adults to assume, as appropriate, the adult patient role in making decisions and independently carrying out self-care and other medical tasks and responsibilities.

The transfer to adult care has potential psychosocial as well as health consequences. Potential psychosocial benefits include the promotion of age-appropriate social and emotional development, greater self-reliance, a positive self-image, and an increased sense of competence. The transfer may also broaden the young person's system of interpersonal and social supports beyond those developed in childhood and adolescence.

At the same time, a transfer to adult care may present psychosocial challenges, including the loss of familiar formal and informal social supports provided by the pediatric health system. Young people may also be overwhelmed by their new adult responsibilities of medical decision making, self-care, and self-advocacy and the challenge of navigating the unfamiliar adult health care system. Some young people, especially those for whom transfer is abrupt, may experience the transfer to adult-oriented care as a punishment or rejection. For people with disabilities that are associated with shortened life expectancy, the transfer to adult care may bring an increased awareness of mortality and increased anxiety, including anxiety about age-related exacerbations and complications of their condition.

Not only patients but also health care professionals may experience challenges with the transfer of older pediatric patients. These challenges include having to terminate long-term, emotionally significant relationships with young adults and their families (Sawyer et al., 1997). Some pediatricians do not trust that their young adult patients will receive the necessary care and guidance in the adult health care system that they have received from the pediatric health care system (Schidlow and Fiel, 1990; Reiss et al., 2005). Sometimes, pediatricians may be dismayed to find prior pediatric patients returning to see them as adults whose health has deteriorated after they have unsuccessfully sought care from the adult-oriented health care system (Reiss et al., 2005). For clinical researchers involved in long-term research on pediatric onset conditions, continued follow up can become even more difficult when their patients move from pediatric to adult care.

For adult care providers, the timely transfer of key medical information can be a challenge (Coleman and Boult, 2003; Rubin, 2003), not unique to this transition but nonetheless a significant concern. Some young adults with complex conditions come to their new adult providers with little or no written information about their history or current course of treatment. Others come with multiple volumes of documentation that may date back to the patient's initial stay in a neonatal care unit. In either case, this presents the new providers with very time-consuming tasks of collecting or assessing information, tasks for which there is little or no specific reimbursement by health plans.

FORCES AND FACTORS THAT AFFECT TRANSFERS AND TRANSITIONS

In addition to the challenges for patients, families, and providers that are associated with the transfer to adult-oriented health care, a number of systems-level forces and factors impede the smooth transfer from pediatric to adult care systems. Two—health care funding and professional education—are discussed here. The policies and procedures of health care professionals and facilities were described earlier.

Funding of Health Care Services

Two aspects of health care funding may complicate smooth transfers from pediatric to adult providers. The first of these involves the lower rates of insurance for young adults with special health care needs compared to other young adults. Young adults with disabilities and chronic conditions have a relatively higher rate of being uninsured than younger or older individuals (Callahan and Cooper, 2004; Collins et al., 2004; Fishman, 2001; White, 2002). Employment-based family health insurance plans have age limits (generally between the ages of 19 and 23 years), after which coverage for children is no longer offered (Collins et al., 2004). Young adults with special health care needs who are insured are less likely than their insured peers to have employment-based insurance because the unemployment and underemployment rates for that population are so high (White, 2002; Fishman, 2001). They are more likely than their peers to be insured through state Medicaid programs (McManus et al., 1991). Medicaid typically provides a significantly lower rate of payment to providers than employment-based coverage or Medicare, which may discourage physicians from accepting Medicaid patients (Kaiser, 2002; Yudowsky et al., 2000). Because the SSI disability criteria for children (age 0 to 17) are less restrictive than the criteria for adults, youth who are insured through Medicaid because they qualify as disabled under the Supplemental Security Income (SSI) Program may lose both SSI and Medicaid when they turn 18 (Reiss, Wallace and McPherson, 2002; Loprest and Wittenberg, 2005).

The second funding issue involves the differences in the scope of health plan coverage for children and adolescents compared to that for adults, especially in public programs. Medicaid, the State Children's Health Insurance Program, and the state Title V Children with Special Health Care Needs Screener Program offer benefits to children that are not equally available to adults in need. For example, Medicaid's Early and Periodic Screening, Diagnostic, and Treatment (EPSDT) program, which covers recipients under the age of 21, requires that specified services be provided to children even if a state's Medicaid program does not cover the service for other beneficiaries (Centers for Medicare and Medicaid Services, 2005). The EPSDT program also requires state programs to provide information to families and to help them use available services appropriately. Unfortunately, the scope of this coverage as written is not matched by the actual delivery of services. The U.S. General Accounting Office has reported that Medicaid-eligible children often do not receive critical EPSDT services (General Accounting Office, 2001). Notwithstanding this shortfall, many children with special health care needs will experience a loss of financial access to certain services when they become adults, even if they continue to be covered by Medicaid. This can complicate the transition to adult care and frustrate patients, families, and providers.

Education of Pediatric and Adult Health Care Professionals

Some studies suggested that factors that affect the transition from pediatric to adult-oriented care are associated with the differences between the training of pediatricians and adult physicians (Rosen, 1995, 2004; Watson,

2005; McDonagh, 2005). Most general and specialty medical care physicians receive the majority of their clinical training in residencies and fellowships that address the diseases and health care needs either of children (those under age 21 years) or of adults, but rarely both.

One exception to this pattern of age segregation is Med-Peds, in which physicians receive 2 years of residency training in pediatrics and 2 years of residency training in internal medicine (Lannon et al., 1999; American Academy of Pediatrics, undated). Another exception is adolescent medicine, in which physicians trained in pediatrics or internal medicine receive additional training in the care of adolescents and young adults (American Board of Internal Medicine, 2005; American Board of Pediatrics, 2005). However, these two specialty areas of training are relatively new, and the number of physicians who have completed Med-Peds or adolescent medicine programs is small and geographic distribution is uneven (Lannon et al., 1999). Family physicians are prepared to provide primary care from birth through old age. Nonetheless, they receive very limited training in the complex pediatric onset conditions for the growing number of patients with these conditions who in earlier times would not have reached adulthood or middle age (Blum, 1995).

Beyond the initial training of physicians, medical journals, professional organizations, research, and conferences tend to be organized into distinct age-related realms. This separation limits the formal and informal connections between pediatric and adult-oriented primary and specialty care providers and also reinforces the suggestion that pediatric and adult-oriented medicine constitute two separate subcultures of biomedicine (Cassell, 2004; Good, 1994; Rosen, 1995; Reiss et al., 2005). As noted by Dr. Christine Cassell (President, American Board of Internal Medicine), "as health professionals, we do not often think of culture as affecting our actions and attitudes . . . Culture is a term we apply freely to explain the behavior and attitudes of people who think and act differently from ourselves" (Cassell, 2004, p. xv). Although empirical data regarding cultural differences between pediatrics and adult-oriented medicine are limited, we believe it is important to recognize the power of medical cultures and their relevance to health care transitions involving the move of children with special health care needs from one medical subculture (pediatrics) to another (adult-oriented medicine).

IMPROVING THE TRANSFER PROCESS

As noted earlier, the AAP, AAFP, and ACP-ASIM have developed a consensus statement on the health care transitions for children with special health care needs. An excerpt from that statement appears in Box I-1. It recognizes that much remains to be done to improve health care transitions and outcomes for young adults with special health care needs.

The consensus statement recommends the creation of an up-to-date detailed written transition plan for children with special health care needs by the time they reach 14 years of age. At a minimum, this plan should include what services need to be provided, who will provide them, and how they will be financed. The importance of developing a transition plan in early adolescence is also reflected in the Individuals with Disabilities Education Act (2004, PL 108-446), which mandates the development of a transition plan for all students who receive special education services by age 16 years.

A variety of instruments for transition planning currently exist (see National Center of Medical Home Initiative for CSHCN, 2005 for a listing). These instruments have both strengths and weaknesses. A review of these transition planning instruments as part of the development of a comprehensive transition planning tool for youth and their families (Reiss and Gibson, 2005) suggest that transition plans should address the following eight areas: (1) the youth's long-term goals; (2) the youth's knowledge about his or her condition or disability; (3) the youth's health behaviors; (4) tasks related to taking medication, conducting clinical tests, and using equipment; (5) the youth's behaviors related to health care visits; (6) tasks related to transfer to adult providers (e.g., locating and selecting adult providers and transferring medical information); (7) tasks related to other aspects of adulthood (e.g., education, work, and independent living); and (8) skills for accessing care through the adult-oriented health care system (e.g. making appointments, maintaining and using health insurance, and providing informed consent).

A strategy that is similar in many respects to that outlined in the consensus statement has been suggested by Forbes and colleagues (2001) in a report for the National Coordinating Centre for National Health Service of Great Britain on continuity of care during the transfer from pediatric to adult medicine. The authors of the report reviewed more than 120 publications that addressed continuity of care for youth with disabilities and special health care needs, identified practices that address continuity, and assessed the relative merits evidence for those practices.

The report proposed that strategies can be classified into general approaches or models. We have simplified and relabeled these, for the purposes of this review, as: 1) youth and family education and preparation; 2) practitioner-focused clinical education and training; and 3) systems development.

Youth and Family Education and Preparation

As discussed by Forbes and colleagues, youth- and family-focused interventions address the logistical, developmental, and emotional challenges of the transfer to adult-oriented care. These interventions are designed to

---

**Box I-1
Health Care Transitions for Young Adults with
Special Health Care Needs**

This policy statement represents a consensus on the critical first steps that the medical profession needs to take to realize the vision of a family-centered, continuous, comprehensive, coordinated, compassionate, and culturally competent health care system that is as developmentally appropriate as it is technically sophisticated. The goal of transition in health care for young adults with special health care needs is to maximize lifelong functioning and potential through the provision of high-quality, developmentally appropriate health care services that continue uninterrupted as the individual moves from adolescence to adulthood. . . . The goals of this policy statement are to ensure that by the year 2010 all physicians who provide primary or subspecialty care to young people with special health care needs 1) understand the rationale for transition from child-oriented to adult-oriented health care; 2) have the knowledge and skills to facilitate that process; and 3) know if, how, and when transfer of care is indicated.

1. Ensure that all young people with special health care needs have an identified health care professional who attends to the unique challenges of transition and assumes responsibility for current health care, care coordination, and future health care planning. This responsibility is executed in partnership with other child and adult health care professionals, the young person, and his or her family. It is intended to ensure that as transitions occur, all young people have uninterrupted, comprehensive, and accessible care within their community.
2. Identify the core knowledge and skills required to provide developmentally appropriate health care transition services to young people with special health care needs and make them part of training and certification requirements for primary care residents and physicians in practice.

---

help youth acquire the knowledge and skills that they need to interact independently and effectively with the adult health care system and to support families through this process. Activities associated with this type of intervention include individualized needs assessment; the use of checklists and health care transition planning materials and support; individualized or group training on self-care, communication, medical decision making, and life skills; peer support; and the education of parents to promote their child's independence.

Practitioner-Focused Clinical Education and Training Interventions

Practitioner-focused interventions are designed to ensure that the clinical expertise regarding childhood-onset disabilities and special health care needs found in the pediatric system continues to be available to the young

3. Prepare and maintain an up-to-date medical summary that is portable and accessible. This information is critical for successful health care transition and provides the common knowledge base for collaboration among health care professionals.

4. Create a written health care transition plan by age 14 together with the young person and family. At a minimum, this plan should include what services need to be provided, who will provide them, and how they will be financed. This plan should be reviewed and updated annually and whenever there is a transfer of care.

5. Apply the same guidelines for primary and preventive care for all adolescents and young adults, including those with special health care needs, recognizing that young people with special health care needs may require more resources and services than do other young people to optimize their health. Examples of such guidelines include the American Medical Association's *Guidelines for Adolescent Preventive Services (GAPS)*, the National Center for Education in Maternal and Child Health's *Bright Futures: Guidelines for Health Supervision of Infants, Children, and Adolescents*, and the US Public Health Service's *Guidelines to Clinical Preventive Services*.

6. Ensure affordable, continuous health insurance coverage for all young people with special health care needs throughout adolescence and adulthood. This insurance should cover appropriate compensation for 1) health care transition planning for all young people with special health care needs, and 2) care coordination for those who have complex medical conditions.

SOURCE: American Academy of Pediatrics et al., 2002. See also, American Medical Association, 2000; Green and Palfrey, 2000; and U.S. Preventive Services Task Force, 1996. Permission to use requested from *Pediatrics*.

adult once he or she transfers to adult providers. These interventions include the provision of clinical training to adult primary and specialty care providers who may not have experience in treating childhood-onset conditions. They also include the availability of pediatric providers to provide ongoing consultation and technical assistance to adult providers and the implementation of shared clinics. In shared clinics, pediatric and adult providers work together over a period of time to manage the care of patients and learn from each other regarding the development and implementation of developmentally appropriate health care for young adults.

Systems Development

Systems-level actions focus on the organizational issues that arise because pediatrics and adult-oriented medicine tend to function as separate and distinct health care delivery systems. Actions include the promotion of good communication; the sharing of patient-specific information across pediatric and adult programs and services; and the modification of standard practices, procedures, and staffing patterns to better meet the changing needs of youth as they move through the transition process. Changes of these sorts also involve the linking of the health care system with the educational system and the other institutions and organizations that have served a child with special needs. Strategies for improving communication and information exchange include regular meetings among pediatric and adult staff to share patient-specific information before the transfer of care, the development of a model medical summary form, and care coordination (which ensures that appointments with adult providers are scheduled and kept). Modifications to standard practices include implementation of transition clinics; the provision of more flexible services (such as longer medical visits, visits after traditional office hours, and the provision of services in schools and other nontraditional settings); and the addition of staff whose time is dedicated to providing training or developmentally appropriate care and psychosocial support.

On the basis of their review, Forbes and colleagues concluded that the quantity and the quality of the empirical evidence do not allow determination of the absolute or the relative impact that the various family-focused, professional-focused, and organization-focused health care transition interventions and related activities have on the transfer of care. This lack of evidence on impact is related to a number of methodological problems, including small sample sizes, the lack of control groups, and measurement problems. Additionally, most of the real-world health care transition programs that have been studied have included activities that fall under two or three of the intervention categories discussed above (Betz, 2004). This blending of intervention methods, along with the confounding of patient-family factors, such as disease severity, health status, cognitive ability, family functioning, and psychosocial status, contribute to the difficulty of determining what health care transition interventions are helpful to whom, when, and under what circumstances.

There is general agreement about the needs and directions for health care transition in the Consensus Statement, the work of Forbes and colleagues (2001), and the suggestions of Rosen, (2004). As Rosen (2004) states, although the empirical evidence is not conclusive, the body of published work on health care transition does provide practical guidance and that there are now "some fundamental principles of transition that have achieved nearly universal endorsement . . . [which] provide a framework" (p. 126) for the further development and study of health care transition services for young people with special health care needs. These principles and promising approaches include the following: (1) transition should occur within a developmental context; (2) the timing of the transfer from pediatric to adult-oriented health care should be flexible; (3) self-care is a critical competency for youth with special needs; (4) the adequate exchange of information between the pediatric and the adult physicians is a critical component of the transition process; (5) successful transition requires coordination; (6) transition should include joint visits; (7) transition planning should include the family; (8) young adults require adult-oriented primary and preventive care; and (9) adequate infrastructure is necessary to support transition (Rosen, 2004).

Further research is clearly necessary to assess what practices best prepare young people and their families for transition. Research can also help guide changes in medical education, policies and procedures and improvements in health systems and community infrastructure that will better assist young adults with disabilities and special health care needs to work and live independently in their communities.

DIRECTIONS FOR FUTURE RESEARCH

Based on our work and the work of others cited in this appendix, we see several areas for transition research. The lists of research topics below follow the categories set out by Forbes and colleagues (2001).

First are research questions that are relevant to the needs of youth and family members in transition. These include

- What information, training, and other support are most effective in helping families to anticipate and prepare for health care transition?
- At what age should transition preparation begin and what age or age range constitutes the best target date for transfer to adult-oriented medical systems?
- What characteristics of youth and families predict successful transition outcomes?
- What are the social and psychological impacts on the young person of transfer to adult-oriented care?

A second category of research needs focuses on the preparation of health care providers to facilitate and promote transition. Questions include

- What research and professional activities will best alert the adult-oriented medical community of the growing need of providers for young adults with disabilities and special health care needs?
- What knowledge and skills are necessary to address the continuing developmental as well as medical needs of young adults with disabilities and special health care needs? What are the best methods for getting ad-

equate numbers of adult-oriented providers acquainted with this knowledge and these skills?

• What supports such as a standardized transition notes or joint medical visits are most effective in getting transition information conveyed among health care providers?

• What else can be done to establish better communication between pediatric and adult-oriented providers to support the transition process?

A third area for research involves knowledge to guide system changes that will support successful health care transitions. Questions include

• What characteristics of health care systems predict successful transition outcomes?

• What are the medical and health care experiences of healthy adolescents and young adults (ages 16 to 26) as well as those with disabilities as they transition to adult-oriented providers? What type of care do they access, from whom do they receive their care and how is this care paid for?

• What are the costs and the benefits of health care transition services and support (including long-term costs)?

• What models and strategies are used by professionals, providers, and others to transition youth with disabilities and special health care needs to the adult health care system? How do they affect outcomes?

• What are the short-term and the long-term health consequences of aging out of the pediatric health care system?

Some of these suggestions will require new information sources and research strategies. They will require long-term studies to track health behaviors and encounters through adolescence into adulthood.

CONCLUSION

About 9.4 million children and youth in the United States have special health care needs, and more than 90 percent of these children and youth will live to see their 21st birthday. As young adults, these individuals need age-appropriate medical care that will help them be healthy, active, contributing members of society. However, these young adults face a broad range of challenges as they graduate from the pediatric system and turn to the adult-oriented system for the health care. These challenges are the product of a variety of forces and factors, both individual and systemic. Although the available evidence does not provide us with a surefire fix for these problems, it does point out steps that can be taken to make progress. These steps involve the implementation of promising health care transition practices and principles more broadly, the evaluation of the effectiveness of demonstration projects in a more systematic fashion, and the provision of the resources needed to finance quality health care services and support for young adults with disabilities and special health care needs.

REFERENCES

American Academy of Pediatrics. Medicaid: Empowering Beneficiaries on the Road to Reform. Testimony for the Record of the Hearing before the Committee on Energy and Commerce, U.S. House of Representatives, September 8, 2005. Available online at http://www.house.gov/commerce_democrats/medicaidblockgrant/109-stmt-aap-090805.pdf.

American Academy of Pediatrics, American Academy of Family Physicians, and American College of Physicians-American Society of Internal Medicine. A consensus statement on health care transition for young adults with special health care needs. *Pediatrics* 2002;110:1304–1306.

American Academy of Pediatrics, Council on Child Health. Age limits of pediatrics. *Pediatrics* 1972;49:463.

American Academy of Pediatrics, Section on Internal Medicine-Pediatrics. *Internal Medicine-Pediatrics 101.* Undated. Available online at http://www.aap.org/sections/med-peds/101.htm.

American Board of Internal Medicine. Policies for added qualifications in adolescent medicine. 2005. Available online at http://www.abim.org/cert/policies_aqadol.shtm.

American Board of Pediatrics. Certification in the pediatric subspecialties. 2005. Available online at http://www.abp.org/certinfo/subspec/ssproc.htm.

American College of Physicians. ACPOnline: Selected medical curricula. A guide to expanding educational objectives in internal medicine residency. Available online at http://www.acponline.org/srf/smc.htm#adolescentmedcine. Accessed February 8, 2005.

American Medical Association, Department of Adolescent Health. *Guidelines for Adolescent Preventive Services (GAPS): Clinical Evaluation and Management Handbook.* Chicago, IL: American Medical Association, 2000.

Ben Ali Shriners. Hospital Eligibility, 2005. Available online at http://www.ben-ali-shriners.org/HospElig.htm.

Betz C. Transition of adolescents with special health care needs: Review and analysis of the literature. *Issues in Comprehensive Pediatric Nursing* 2004;27:179–241.

Blum R. Transition to adult health care: setting the stage. *Journal of Adolescent Health* 1995;17:3–5.

Blum R. Introduction. *Pediatrics* 2002;110:1301–1303.

Callahan ST, Cooper WO. Gender and uninsurance among young adults in the United States. *Pediatrics* 2004;113:291–297.

Carnegie Council on Adolescent Development. *Great Transitions: Preparing Adolescents for a New Century.* New York: Carnegie Corporation of New York, 1995.

Cassell C. Forward. In *The Cultures of Caregiving, Conflict and Common Ground among Families, Health Professionals and Policy Makers.* Levine C and Murray T (eds.) Baltimore, MD: The Johns Hopkins University Press, 2004.

Centers for Disease Control and Prevention, National Center for Health Statistics. Figure 2.2, Early release of selected estimates based on data from the 2003 National Health Interview Survey. Released June 30, 2004. Available online at http://www.cdc.gov/nchs/data/nhis/earlyrelease/200406_02.pdf.).

Centers for Medicare and Medicaid Services. State Medicaid manual. Baltimore, MD: Centers for Medicare and Medicaid Services, 2005. Available online at http://www.cms.hhs.gov/manuals/45_smm/pub45toc.asp.

Coleman E, Boult C. Improving the quality of transitional care for persons with complex care needs. Position Statement of the American Geriatrics Society Health Care Systems Committee. Journal of the American Geriatrics Society 2003;51:556–557.

Collins S, Schoen C, Tenney K, Doty M, Ho A. *Rite of Passage? Why Young Adults Become Uninsured and How New Policies Can Help.* Commonwealth Fund Issue Brief May, 2004. Available online at__http://www.cmwf.org/programs/insurance/collins_riteofpassage_ib_649.pdf

Committee on Children with Disabilities, American Academy of Pediatrics. Continued Importance of Supplemental Security Income (SSI) for Children and Adolescents With Disabilities. *Pediatrics* 2001;107:790–793.

Elliott G, Feldman S. *At The Threshold, The Developing Adolescent.* Cambridge, MA: Harvard University Press, 1990.

Fishman E. Aging out of coverage: young adults with special health care needs. *Health Affairs* 2001;20:254–266.

Forbes A, While A, Ullman R, Lewis S, Mathes L, Griffiths P. A *Multi-Method Review to Identify Components of Practice Which May Promote Continuity in the Transition from Child to Adult Care for Young People with Chronic Illness or Disability.* National Co-ordination Centre for National Health Service, Service Delivery and Organization R & D. London, March 2001. Available online at http://www.sdo.lshtm.ac.uk/pdf/coc_transition_forbes.pdf

General Accounting Office (now Governmental Accountability Office). *Medicaid: Stronger Efforts Needed to Ensure Children's Access to Health Screening Services.* GAO-01-749. Washington, DC: GAO, 2001. Available online at http://www.gao.gov/new.items/d01749.pdf.

Gesensway D. Internists wanted for complex adolescent care. *ACP Observer* 2004;24(10): 1,14–15.

Good B. *Medicine, Rationality and Experience: An Anthropological Perspective.* Cambridge, England: Cambridge University Press, 1994.

Gortmaker SL, Perrin JM, Weitzman M, et al. An unexpected success story: transition to adulthood in youth with chronic physical health conditions. *Journal of Research on Adolescence* 1993;3:317–336.

Green M, Palfrey JS, eds. *Bright Futures: Guidelines for Health Supervision of Infants, Children, and Adolescents.* 2nd ed. Arlington, VA: National Center for Education in Maternal and Child Health, 2000.

Halfon N, Hochstein M. Life course health development: an integrated framework for developing health, policy, and research. *Milbank Quarterly* 2002;80:433–479.

Havighurst RJ. *Developmental Tasks and Education.* New York: McKay, 1972.

Health Services and Resources Administration, U.S. Department of Health and Human Services. The National Survey of Children with Special Health Care Needs Chartbook, 2001. Available online at http://mchb.hrsa.gov/chscn/ <http://mchb.hrsa.gov/chscn/>.

Individuals with Disabilities Education Act (2004). PL 108-446. Available online at http://thomas.loc.gov/.

Kaiser Family Foundation. National Survey of Physicians Part IV: Doctor, Payers and Low Income Patients. Publication #3223. Menlo Park, CA, 2002.

Lannon C, Oliver T, Guerin R, Day S, Tunnessen W. Internal medicine-pediatrics combined residency graduates. *Archives of Pediatric and Adolescent Medicine* 1999;153: 823–828.

Levine C, Murray T (eds.). *The Cultures of Caregiving*. Baltimore, MD: The Johns Hopkins University Press, 2004.

Litt I. Commentary on "Age Limits of Pediatrics". *Pediatrics* 1998 (July supplement);102 (Supplement No. 1):249–250. Available online at http://pediatrics. aappublications.org/cgi/content/full/102/1/S1/249.

Loprest P, Wittenburg D. *Choices, Challenges, and Options: Child SSI recipients Preparing for the Transition to Adult Life*. Washington, DC: The Urban Institute, May 2005. Available online at http://www.urban.org/Template.cfm?NavMenuID=24&template=/TaggedContent/ViewPublication.cfm&PublicationID=9277

Lotstein D, McPherson M, Strickland B, Newacheck P. Transition planning for youth with special health care needs: results from the National Survey of Children with Special Health Care Needs. *Pediatrics* 2005;115:1562–1568.

Magrab P, Millar HEC. *Surgeon General's Conference: Growing Up and Getting Medical Care*. Washington, DC: Georgetown University Child Development Center, 1989.

McDonagh JE. Growing up and moving on: transition from pediatric to adult care. *Pediatric Transplantation* 2005;9(3):364–372.

McManus M, Flint S, Kelly R. Adequacy of physician reimbursement for pediatric care under Medicaid. *Pediatrics* 1991;87(6):909–920.

National Association of Pediatric Nurse Practitioners. *Scope and Standards of Practice*. Cherry Hill, NJ: National Association of Pediatric Nurse Practitioners, 2004.

National Center of Medial Home Initiative for CSHCN. Transition Publications. Available online at www.medicalhomeinfo.org/publications/transitions.

Newacheck PW, Taylor WR. Childhood chronic illness: prevalence, severity, and impact. *American Journal of Public Health* 1992;82:364–371.

Reiss J. Executive summary. *Transition Revolution: You Can Make It Happen in Health Care Conference*. Gainesville: Institute for Child Health Policy, University of Florida, 1999.

Reiss J, Gibson R. Health care transition: destinations unknown. *Pediatrics* 2002;110:1307–1314.

Reiss J, Gibson R. *Health Care Transition Workbooks Series*. Gainesville: Institute for Child Health Policy, University of Florida, 2005.

Reiss J, Gibson R, Walker L. Health care transition: youth family and providers perspectives. *Pediatrics* 2005;115:112–120.

Reiss J, Lamar D. Directory of State Title V CSHCN Programs: Eligibility criteria and scope of services, 2003. Available online at: http://cshcnleaders.ufl.edu./TitleVDirectory

Reiss J, Wallace H, McPherson M. Supplemental Security Income Program for Children in H Wallace, G Gordon, K Jaros et al, (eds.). *Health and Welfare for Families in the 21st Century* (2ed). Sudbery, MA: Jones and Bartlett, 2002.

Rosen D. Between two worlds: bridging the cultures of child health and adult medicine. *Journal of Adolescent Health* 1995;17:10–16.

Rosen D. Transition of young people with respiratory diseases to adult health care. *Pediatric Respiratory Reviews* 2004;5:124–131.

Rubin K. Transitioning the pediatric patient with Turner's syndrome from pediatric to adult care. *Journal of Pediatric Endocrinology & Metabolism* 2003;16:651–659.

Sawyer S, Blair S, Bowes G. Chronic illness in adolescents: transfer or transition to adult services. *Journal of Pediatric and Child Health* 1997;33:88–90.

Scal P. Transition for youth with chronic conditions: primary care physicians' approaches. *Pediatrics* 2002;110:1315–1321.

Schidlow D, Fiel S. Life beyond pediatrics: Transitions of chronically ill adolescents from pediatric to adult health care systems. *Medical Clinics of North America* 1990;74(5):1113–1120.

U.S. Preventive Services Task Force, Public Health Service. *Guidelines to Clinical Preventive Services*. 2nd ed. Washington, DC: US Public Health Service, 1996.

Viner R. Transition from pediatric to adult care. Bridging the gaps or passing the buck? *Archives of Disease in Childhood* 1999;81(3):271–275.

Watson AR. Problems and pitfalls of transition from pediatric to adult renal care. *Pediatric Nephrology* 2005;20(2):113–117.

White P. Access to health care: health insurance considerations for young adults with special health care needs/disabilities. *Pediatrics* 2002;110:1328–1335.

Yudkowsky BK, Tang SS, Siston AM. *Pediatrician Participation in Medicaid and SCHIP: Results of a Survey*. Chicago: American Academy of Pediatrics, October, 2000. Available online at http://www.aap.org/statelegislation/med-schip/Introduction.PDF.

J

Secondary Conditions and Disability

*Margaret A. Turk**

rofessionals disagree about the definition of the term *secondary condition.* Definitions vary (to the extent that they are explicit), and
concepts are often confused or misunderstood. The term itself is
relatively new. It came on the scene in 1986 through the work of Michael
Marge of the National Council on Disability.

Although the term itself was new, the concept that people with disabilities experienced ongoing health problems that were somehow associated
with their primary disabling conditions was not new either to them or to
the clinicians who treated them. This paper reviews the evolution of the
concept of a secondary condition, describes its components, discusses areas
of disagreement regarding the definition, and places secondary conditions
within the taxonomies of disabilities used in rehabilitation science and
clinical practice.

HISTORY

As Heidegger posited (Heidegger, 1964), to name something is to call it
into being. After Michael Marge named it, the concept of the "secondary
condition" was identified and highlighted in the Institute of Medicine's

*Margaret A. Turk, M.D., Professor of Physical Medicine and Rehabilitation, State Uni-
versity of New York Upstate Medical University at Syracuse, Syracuse, New York. The analyses and views presented in this workshop paper are those of the author and not necessarily
those of the Institute of Medicine Committee on Disability in America: A New Look.

(IOM's) 1991 report *Disability in America* (Pope and Tarlov, 1991) and its 1997 report *Enabling America* (Brandt and Pope, 1997). Both reports defined secondary conditions specifically in terms of physical or mental health problems.

The new concept was embraced, especially by the federal funding agencies, such as the National Center for Medical Rehabilitation Research (NCMRR), the National Institute for Disability Related Research (NIDRR), and the Centers for Disease Control and Prevention (CDC). These agencies initially funded research to identify and define secondary conditions and then supported further studies to evaluate interventions that can be used to prevent or modify such conditions. The concept also became a part of the strategic planning cores within the agencies.

Recognizing the potential to improve the prevention of secondary conditions, CDC organized national conferences highlighting their epidemiology as well as preventive and modifying strategies. The conferences promoted discussions that enriched the understanding of secondary conditions. Individuals with disabilities were active participants in the discussions, including discussions of areas for research. The CDC Disability and Health Team initiated a funding stream for research into the secondary conditions of individuals with disabilities, and it also supported statewide disability and health programs and projects. As a result of these CDC-supported initiatives and the strategic plans of NCMRR, NIDRR, and other funding sources, a science base for secondary conditions is developing.

On another front, the American Association of Health and Disability was established. The mission of this professional and advocacy organization is the prevention of additional health complications and secondary conditions in people with disabilities and the encouragement of health promotion and wellness programs that will assist people with disabilities to attain and maintain a positive health status. This national organization promotes interactions and information sharing among consumers, professionals, and agencies regarding secondary conditions and wellness for individuals with disabilities.

KEY DIMENSIONS OF SECONDARY CONDITIONS

No single seminal article has defined and enumerated secondary conditions. Various definitions and lists of conditions have appeared in articles and book chapters, on websites, and in promotional material (Pope and Tarlov, 1991; Lollar, 1994; Brandt and Pope, 1997; Coyle et al., 2000; U.S. Department of Health and Human Services, 2000; Simeonsson et al., 2002; Traci et al., 2002; Turk and Weber, 2005). Notwithstanding certain differences, these discussions generally specify some common key dimensions, in particular, that a secondary condition

- has a causal relationship to the primary condition,
- may be preventable,
- may vary in its expression and the timing of its expression,
- may be modified, and
- may increase the severity of the primary condition.

The most important and defining of these elements is that a secondary condition is related to a primary condition that is a risk factor for its development. In general, the secondary condition would not exist in the individual but for the presence of the primary condition, although additional factors (such as a lack of appropriate medical care) may contribute to the development of the secondary condition. Examples of common secondary conditions (some of which may also develop in their own right as primary conditions) include

- pain,
- osteoporosis,
- renal insufficiency,
- chronic lower limb edema,
- pressure ulcers,
- obesity,
- depression, and
- insulin-resistant diabetes mellitus (in individuals with spinal cord injuries).

As defined by the IOM, a secondary condition involves a physical or mental health problem. Some view the term more broadly to include social problems, such as isolation or relationship problems. This interpretation simply reproduces the general concepts of societal or environmental limitations and dilutes the concept of disability. Secondary conditions defined as health and medical conditions focus the attention on a distinct group of conditions.

Secondary conditions are likely preventable, although the degree of preventive success depends, in part, on many factors, including the underlying mechanisms linking the primary and secondary conditions. Social, personal, and knowledge barriers may impede prevention. Broad social barriers include negative attitudes toward disability; community environments that limit physical access to medical and other services and opportunities; and a lack of funding and other policy support for research, medical services, and additional elements of a successful prevention program. Moreover, individuals with disabilities may have personal characteristics or traits that affect their responsiveness to interventions. Resiliency is one such characteristic that has been recognized as an important variable in successful outcomes.

Certainly, the state of medical science and engineering technology affects the understanding, prevention, and management of secondary conditions. In some cases, research has led to a recognition that a health problem that was once thought to be an independent (or comorbid) condition is actually linked to a disability, for example, diabetes and spinal cord injury, as described by William Bauman in his paper in Appendix M of this workshop report. Such advances in medical knowledge must be disseminated to providers and consumers if it is to be effectively applied to prevent or manage secondary conditions.

In addition, as science or technology progresses, previously expected outcomes may change. Evidence of this comes from the advances in treatment techniques for spasticity that reduce or prevent certain secondary conditions. For example, spasticity and hypertonicity have often been at the base of significant contractures and deformities that limit function, increase the risk for pressure ulcers, and cause pain. Twenty years ago, options for management consisted of only a few medications. Orthopedic surgery was often the only long-standing management option. Over the past 10 years, additional oral medications, botulinum toxin injections, and intrathecal baclofen have changed the incidence and types of anticipated contractures and deformities. Children with cerebral palsy now have access to these interventions, and as they grow and mature, their contractures are often less severe. Surgical interventions are sometimes avoided or delayed.

Secondary conditions vary in the nature and the expression of their manifestations in association with a primary disabling condition. Having a particular disability does not necessarily lead to all secondary conditions associated with that primary disability. For example, not all children with cerebral palsy will have contractures, and some contractures will be more severe than others. Similarly, not all people with spinal cord injuries who have a neurogenic bladder (which results from disruption of the nerve supply to the bladder) will have renal insufficiency. The time of onset of a secondary condition may also vary from person to person. As an example, pain for people with cerebral palsy may become notable in the late teens, early 20s, or late 30s; and onset may be dependent on the individual's level of function and activity.

Secondary conditions may also be modified by a variety of factors. Anticipatory care may allow early recognition and intervention. However, developmental, personal, and contextual factors may modify problem recognition or treatment strategies. An example is neurogenic bladder and incontinence in individuals with cerebral palsy. Periodic incontinence in a 5-year-old may be ignored or not recognized as a symptom of a secondary condition, whereas such incontinence is not ignored in a 20-year-old who is looking for increased socialization. However, after 20 years of incontinence and possibly recurrent infections, the individual may experience associated chronic reflux and renal insufficiency. In addition, the interventions fashioned for a 5-year-old are quite different from those fashioned for a 20-year-old. Potentially, earlier recognition of incontinence in an older child or adolescent with cerebral palsy would prompt a timely and full evaluation, the recognition of a neurogenic component, and an intervention to prevent renal abnormalities.

Some secondary conditions, for example, deconditioning, are associated with different types of primary conditions that involve motor limitations. With ongoing investigation into lifelong disabilities and health conditions, more common groupings and risk factors may become more obvious.

The addition of secondary health conditions to a primary condition may increase the level of disability and decrease the quality of life for an individual. Secondary health conditions may require more medical attention, further complicate daily routines, and increase the need for support services. The secondary condition may become the primary medical condition or the individual's dominant medical problem. Once a secondary condition comes into existence, personal, social and environmental factors may modify the condition or its impact.

TAXONOMIES OF DISABILITY

A variety of taxonomies of disability covering primary, secondary, and other conditions have been used in clinical activities, in scholarly publications and education programs, and in policy proceedings regarding disabilities and their relationship to health and function. The traditional clinical taxonomies used to describe disability employ terms such as *primary disabling condition* or *primary condition, associated conditions, comorbidities, aging,* and *health.* This terminology is used within the narrow context of disability; however, the context can certainly be broadened to include chronic medical conditions as such, for example, diabetes and hypertension. Within a more traditional medical taxonomy of disability, secondary conditions can be distinguished not only from primary conditions but from also comorbidities and other concepts.

Primary conditions are the fundamental sources of disabilities (defined as limitations in the ability to perform certain socially expected roles and tasks). The clinical focus for a disabling condition may change over time. For example, in individuals with spinal cord injuries, neurogenic bladder and the consequent renal insufficiency may become the most disabling conditions to an individual. For someone with motor and cognitive impairments as a result of a traumatic brain injury, the cognitive impairment may come to be seen as a more important source of limitation over time.

Associated conditions are aspects of the pathology of the primary condition; they are expected—if not universal—features or characteristics of the condition itself. In individuals with cerebral palsy, for example, spasticity is an associated condition, that is, an aspect or part of upper motor neuron impairment; spasticity is not a secondary condition. Other associated conditions generally related to cerebral palsy are seizures and mental retardation; they are aspects of the condition, although not all those with cerebral palsy experience them. Among individuals with spinal cord injuries, associated conditions include neurogenic bladder and bowel and insensate skin. Associated conditions in individuals with traumatic brain injuries with significant motor impairments are typically cognitive or behavioral impairments and spasticity. Again, these are not secondary conditions; they can usually be expected on the basis of the existing pathology.

Comorbidities are health conditions unrelated to the primary condition, in essence, unassociated conditions. There may be pre-existing familial or genetic reasons for these conditions, but there is usually no known causal association with the primary disabling conditions. An example is cancer in an individual with cerebral palsy.

Research may uncover a previously unsuspected link between an apparent comorbidity and a primary disabling condition. The link between insulin-resistant diabetes and spinal cord injury has been identified only during the past 15 years. Understanding the relationships among medical conditions has much to do with the state of the science.

Complications of surgical, pharmaceutical, and other treatments also need to be recognized. In some cases, such treatment complications may be more serious and disabling than the primary or secondary condition being treated.

Aging happens regardless of the presence or the absence of disability. Aging is a birth-to-death developmental process and an anticipated decline in organ system function that may be modified but not prevented by genetics or environmental factors. For example, it is scientifically supported that exercise for people at any age can improve motor performance. People with disabilities, however, have a smaller reserve capacity for performance and function that may negatively affect their aging processes (Figure J-1). Exercise, the use of adaptive equipment, and other environmental factors may still enhance performance. Some problems associated with accelerated aging (e.g., early-onset deconditioning) may be viewed as secondary conditions.

In Figure J-1, the small rectangle represents the usual curve of skill attainment to a typical peak performance quotient, followed by a gradual loss of performance over time, if it is assumed that no exercise or focused performance training activity is carried out. The triangle represents a physically trained individual, who will show a higher maximum performance quotient related to exercise and activity and who will maintain a higher level of performance over time, if it is assumed that continued activity and exercise are performed. The large rectangle represents adult-onset disabil-

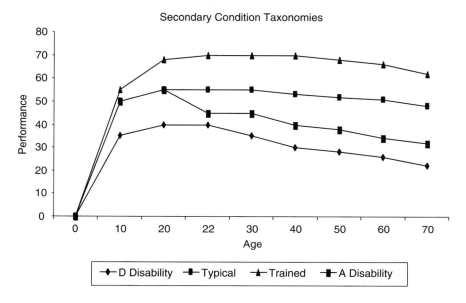

FIGURE J-1   Conceptual model of aging with different characteristics.
D Disability = developmental disability; A Disability = adult-onset disability.

ity. A person with adult-onset disability shows a typical initial attainment of skills followed by a significant drop in function after an acute event, the return of some but not the previous level of performance, and a faster age-related decline in performance over time. Finally, the diamond represents the pattern for someone with a developmental disability who is unable to achieve the typical performance quotient and who shows a faster decline in function. Note the lower performance capacity of the disability-related function and, therefore, the likely more limited reserve capacity for changes in health or the addition of medical conditions.

Health is a continuum, not the absence of impairment or disease. For individuals with disabilities, health status is dependent on the management of the chronic disease process, the maintenance or restoration of function, and the prevention of secondary conditions to the extent possible. In recent decades, the emphasis has increasingly been on health and wellness for people with disabling conditions.

Beyond the traditional clinical perspective on disabilities and other conditions, two models of disability merit attention. Both the *International Classification of Functioning, Disability and Health* (ICF) model and the enabling-disabling process—or the IOM model—have been described elsewhere (World Health Organization, 2001; Pope and Tarlov, 1991; Brandt and Pope, 1997). Each model defines the changing nature of disability and function relative to modifying factors. Both encompass health as well as medical conditions. Both models attempt to illustrate the entwined nature of function with health, the environment, personal characteristics, and quality of life. Both models also try to represent the continuum of disability. They have proposed useful conceptual distinctions. The IOM model, for example, distinguishes pathology (e.g., nerve damage) from impairment (e.g., muscle atrophy), functional limitation (e.g., the inability to grasp an object), and disability (e.g., the inability to work certain jobs). The ICF model makes a distinction between activities and participation that others have criticized as in need of further clarification or modification (see, e.g., Gale Whiteneck's paper in Appendix B of this workshop report).

Although neither the ICF nor the IOM graphic model includes secondary conditions as an explicit element, both are consistent with an understanding of primary conditions as a risk factor for secondary conditions. Both are likewise consistent with an understanding that environmental factors and personal choices or traits can affect the development of secondary conditions and the extent to which primary or secondary conditions become disabling. The 1997 version of the IOM model emphasizes quality of life for people with limitations or disabilities as another variable that may be affected by environmental factors and personal characteristics.

CONCLUSION

A secondary condition is a mental or physical health condition that is related to the primary disabling condition or primary health condition. Secondary conditions can be variable in expression, and the timing of their onset is variable. They are likely preventable, although the state of medical science may provide few prevention options for some conditions. Secondary conditions can be modified by many factors. With progression, secondary conditions can increase the severity of the disability or decrease the quality of life.

This understanding of secondary conditions further validates the experiences of people with lifelong disabilities. That is, people with disabilities go through the typical health and aging processes, in addition to idiosyncratic changes related to their particular disabilities.

Although it is an often misunderstood term, secondary condition has been embraced as an important aspect of lifelong disability. The definition has become clearer over time, and there is more agreement regarding the need to limit the term to health conditions. Broadening of the definition beyond health conditions serves to dilute both the concept of secondary conditions and the key elements of disability. Issues of participation, quality of life, and environment are important factors in the classification of function and disability. Despite disagreements regarding the definition, the national discussion has brought forth consideration of lifelong issues for people with disabilities.

REFERENCES

Brandt EN Jr., Pope AM, eds. 1997. *Enabling America: Assessing the Role of Rehabilitation Science and Engineering.* Washington, DC: National Academy Press.

Coyle CP, Santiago MC, Shank JW, Ma GX, Boyd R. 2000. Secondary conditions and women with physical disabilities: a descriptive study. *Archives of Physical Medicine & Rehabilitation* 81:1380–1387.

Heidegger M. 1964. *Basic Writings*, 2nd ed. San Francisco, CA: Harper.

Lollar DJ, ed. 1994. *Preventing Secondary Conditions Associated with Spina Bifida or Cerebral Palsy: Proceedings and Recommendations of a Symposium.* U.S. Department of Health and Human Services, Washington, DC: The Spina Bifida Association of America.

Pope AM, Tarlov AR, eds. 1991. *Disability in America: Toward a National Agenda for Prevention.* Washington, DC: National Academy Press.

Simeonsson RJ, McMillen JS, Huntington GS. 2002. Secondary conditions in children with disabilities: spina bifida as a case example. *Mental Retardation and Developmental Disabilities Research Reviews* 8:198–205.

Traci, MA, Seekins T, Szalda-Petree A, Ravesloot C. 2002. Assessing secondary conditions among adults with developmental disabilities: a preliminary study. *Mental Retardation* 40:119–131.

Turk MA, Weber RJ. 2005. Congenital and childhood-onset disabilities: age-related changes and secondary conditions in mobility impairments. In *Physical Medicine & Rehabilitation: Principles and Practice*, 4th ed. DeLisa JA, ed. Philadelphia, PA: Lippincott Williams & Wilkins.

U.S. Department of Health and Human Services. 2000. *Healthy People 2010* (Conference Edition, in two volumes). Washington, DC: U.S. Department of Health and Human Services.

World Health Organization (WHO). 2001. *International Classification of Functioning, Disability and Health.* Geneva, Switzerland: World Health Organization.

K

A User's Perspective on Midlife (Ages 18 to 65) Aging with Disability

June Isaacson Kailes *

P eople with significant disabilities and chronic conditions are aging and living much longer than they did in previous generations. Since we are not dead yet, the question is not, will we live; the question is, how well will we live? We need health care that helps us add life to years, not just years to life. Today's disability-specific health care treats many who live with a long-term disability as if we cease to exist after childhood or after acute or rehabilitation interventions.

We confront a "black hole" when seeking disability competent services. Our options in our quest for experienced professionals and comprehensive services are few. Our choices, if we are lucky, are to see pediatrics-focused health care professionals with teddy bears on their business cards or geriatrics-focused health care providers who sometimes incorporate a multidisciplinary team approach.

I write this paper from the perspective of someone who is a living, aging-with-disability "laboratory." My life-long disability is cerebral palsy. I am also a breast cancer survivor. My work in health, wellness, and aging with disability bridges the consumer and the provider worlds. Several decades of concentration on health as an advocate, writer, educator, consult-

*June Isaacson Kailes, Associate Director, Center for Disability Issues and the Health Professions, Western University of Health Sciences, Pomona, California. The analyses and views presented in this workshop paper are those of the author and not necessarily those of the Institute of Medicine Committee on Disability in America: A New Look.

194

ant, researcher, and health care professional allow me to speak not only from my own experience but from the experiences of many people who are aging with disability.

I, like many of my peers, had an early introduction to the so-called golden years and the aging experience, what our disability subculture sometimes refers to as "crip (short for crippled) years." When I talk with older people without disabilities about their aging experiences, I often identify with what they describe and think to myself, "I'm already there!"

There is progress in identifying secondary and associated conditions specific to aging and living with a disability. However, this work has not translated into effective interventions. For many of us, maneuvering through the complex health care system is a dense minefield full of

- physical, communication, program, and medical equipment barriers;
- "no-logic" bureaucracies;
- professionals with few, if any, specific competencies in treating disabling conditions;
- fragmented and dysfunctional services; and
- a lack of focus on living well with long-term disability and conditions.

It is a system lacking any semblance of disability-related literacy, competency, and clinical expertise. Successful navigation of the system takes enormous energy, razor-sharp advocacy, and considerable health literacy. These are necessary survival skill sets that few people have and that only a few more are able or willing to acquire.

The comments in this paper cover recommendations regarding planning "with" and not "for" people with disabilities, defining disability, the law, tracking progress, health policy and benefits, and research priorities.

PLAN WITH US AND NOT FOR US

Planning for and not with people with disabilities reflects an old paradigm: "a lot about us without us." People with disabilities need to be involved not in token ways (not just advisory) but in major significant and powerful ways. It is important to include in the research and practice processes qualified people with disabilities who understand and who can think through issues from a cross-disability perspective. Qualified people with disabilities should be included as investigators, contributors, collaborators, and managers. People with disabilities also need to be included, not excluded, from randomized clinical trials that test the effectiveness of interventions such as new medications and surgical procedures.

It is time to embrace the approach "nothing about us without us!" Being diligent in seeking qualified people with disabilities and taking advantage of the wealth, depth, and breadth of information available from the disability community yields positive payoffs.

DEFINE DISABILITY BROADLY

The 2000 U.S. census found that people with disabilities represent 19.3 percent of the 257.2 million people age 5 years old and older in the civilian noninstitutionalized population, or nearly one in five people. By adopting a broad definition of disability, no one is left behind when the broad spectrum of people with disabilities and activity limitations is included.

Preparing to accommodate people with disabilities often translates into being better equipped to serve all people. Given the approaching wave of the baby boom generation, people who live with disabilities today are truly "the canaries in the health care mine."

As people age, disability rates rise significantly. Most people, if they live long enough, will age into disability. As time alters our bodies, activity and functional limitations become natural occurrences.

Medical, technology, legal, and social advances keep more people with disabilities, chronic conditions, and activity limitations alive, healthy, productive, and functioning independently in their communities. Do not think of disability as a condition that affects the "special" or the "unfortunate few." Disability is just one variation on the diversity of being human, and it is a common characteristic and occurrence within the human experience.

The concept that people either have a disability or do not have a disability perpetuates misperceptions about the nature of disabilities and activity limitations. Disability should not be viewed as something you have or you don't have. Activity limitations exist along a continuum of gradation and duration (partial to total or temporary to permanent) that affect almost everyone at some point in their lives. Traditional narrow definitions of disability are not appropriate.

Governmental departments and policies have 60-plus different definitions of disability. That problem must be resolved. We need to think about disability more broadly, as people with disabilities and other activity limitations make up a sizable portion of the general population. Disability should be defined functionally in a unified and comprehensive way.

IMPLEMENT THE LAW

I, along with many others, have spent 15 years working to implement the Americans with Disabilities Act (ADA). The positive payoffs of this law in our environment are apparent and significantly contribute to helping people with disabilities be productive. The level of implementation of ADA in health care, however, lags far behind its level of implementation in many other public accommodation sectors.

The health care system overlooks its obligation to ensure compliance with ADA. Inadequate compliance is a major contributor to many of the documented health disparities that people with disabilities experience. Compliance involves not only attention to physical access but also attention to accessible medical equipment, communication, and programs.

- *Medical equipment* that needs to be usable by people with disabilities and activity limitations includes weight scales, examination tables (whose height should be adjustable), examination chairs, and other diagnostic and radiological equipment that facilitates access to routine care, preventive care, diagnostic tests, and necessary treatments. When a physician is unable to perform an appropriate examination or get an accurate weight because a patient cannot use a traditional scale or cannot get onto or is not assisted with getting onto an examination table, then the patient may receive a lower quality of health care. The patient might receive an inaccurate diagnosis because the physician may not have sufficient information. A patient with a disability or activity limitations might miss the benefit from the early detection and treatment of a developing condition as a result of the lack of availability of accessible medical equipment.

- *Accessible communications* provide explanations, directions, and other content by means that are understandable and usable by people with reduced or no ability to speak, see, or hear or who have cognitive limitations in learning and understanding.

- *Physical access* means removing physical barriers so that people can get to, enter, and use parking (curb cuts, ramps), examination, treatment, dressing, rest rooms, and other facilities. Depending on the facility and its location, creating access may mean the installation or construction of ramps, automatic door openers, curb cuts, widened doorways and exam and treatment rooms, and accessible and safe pathways from parking and public transit stops.

- *Program access* refers to services, programs, or activities that, when viewed as a whole, are accessible to and usable by people with disabilities. In addition to altering facilities, equipment, and communication methods, programs may assign personnel to assist individuals with disabilities and provide services at alternative sites if primary sites cannot be readily used so that those programs are accessible.

One step in strengthening accessibility for people with disabilities is stronger ADA-related enforcement and training efforts in all areas of health care. In addition, clearer and stronger tax incentives could encourage health care providers to improve access. Although much is known about how to improve access, an area that needs attention and resources is the development and enforcement of standards for accessible medical equipment.

ESTABLISH A BASELINE

We must clearly document the progress that has been made since the Institute of Medicine (IOM)'s publication of *Disability in America* in 1991 (Pope and Tarlov, 1991) and *Enabling America* in 1997 (Brandt and Pope, 1997).

- What has been accomplished in what areas?
- What are the significant findings?
- What has made a difference in peoples' lives?

To be effective, it is critical that we use evaluation and progress tracking tools. We need a report card that tracks progress.

REFORM HEALTH CARE POLICIES AND BENEFITS

Many of the following policy comments reflect an underlying message: "pay now or pay more later." An initial denial of services because of antiquated and shortsighted policies and inaccessible medical facilities and equipment subsequently results in the use of more expensive services downstream.

Health care policies that affect the access to health care of people with disabling conditions and activity limitations originate from an era when many people with disabilities did not age; they just died. Some of these policies focus primarily on preventing fraud and abuse. Policies and benefits specific to the definition of medically necessary, access to technology, care coordination, and evaluations need to be updated to reflect the current needs of people aging with activity limitations.

Medical Necessity

Definitions and interpretations of "medical necessity" play a critical role in determining what services people receive. Existing practices of denying needed services leads to short-term savings and long-term costs.

Policies must change to incorporate into this definition the prevention of decline and deterioration, in addition to the significant improvement of health status. For example, coverage should allow people with disabilities or activity limitations to obtain, maintain, and repair the right technology and to receive periodic evaluations by physical, occupational, and exercise therapists and those who provide other ancillary services that help prevent or mitigate functional loss.

Technology

Coverage of and access to the right technology translate into living better and longer. The question remains, given today's health care, how do you get it?

The pivotal role that assistive technologies and durable medical equipment (DME) play in preventing or reducing secondary conditions and injuries must be recognized. This includes, but is not limited to, hearing aids, grab bars and other safety devices, railings, canes, magnifiers, buttonhooks, speech synthesizers, augmentative communication devices, powered mobility devices, magnification equipment, sophisticated prosthetic limbs, environmental control units, powered and lightweight wheelchairs, and voice-output blood glucose meters.

These kinds of devices play a critical role in helping people with activity limitations of all ages maintain or improve their overall health and mental health, participation, independence, productivity, and integration in the home, in the classroom, in the workplace, and in the community. This technology helps prevent costly medical problems due to mental or physical deterioration (like depression, pressure sores, and injuries) as well as help reduce personal assistance costs.

Continuing to view wheeled mobility equipment as a "convenience item" is absurd. As I recently explained to Blue Cross (to make the case for reimbursement for yearly scooter batteries and several other small items that would continue to extend the life of my 15 year old, chronically airline-abused scooter), "I am not using this scooter to make a fashion statement!"

Shortsighted policies that allow payment only for stripped-down, noncustomized, and sometimes inexpensive devices like heavy manual wheelchairs cause preventable problems downstream, like upper-extremity injuries and pressure ulcers whose treatment requires high-cost interventions. The denial of coverage for wheelchair cushions can mean a payment of $50,000 to surgically repair a pressure sore later. The denial of coverage for low-cost grab bars may mean the expensive treatment of broken bones and other injuries later. Public and private payers must recognize improvements in function and prevention of primary and secondary injuries when they determine whether assistive devices, technologies, and related services are "medically necessary."

Increased federal funding must be committed to build the evidence base on the efficacy and cost-effectiveness of coverage of these devices and services.

Centers for Medicare and Medicaid Services must change Medicare's antiquated "in-the-home" wheelchair coverage policy, which restricts coverage of mobility devices only to those devices that are reasonable and necessary for use inside a person's home. By denying a basic mobility tool, this restriction is more costly in the long run and limits the independence, health, and community integration of people with disabilities who rely on wheelchairs to function outside of their homes.

Many people like me can get around their homes by "wall walking" and "furniture surfing" or by using a standard-issue manual wheelchair, cane, or walker. Outside the home, however, these methods are unsafe and confining. Many of us could easily have been in the group of people whose benefits deny them access to liberating technology.

The antiquated policy restrictions and interpretations cited above continue to unnecessarily

- confine, imprison, devalue, and oppress people with disabilities of all ages by compromising our health, independence, self-sufficiency and social connections;
- increase health and safety risks (and the development of conditions such as those associated with isolation); and
- increase the cost of treating often predictable and preventable downstream conditions that are already expensive to treat (and which are, ironically, covered by public and private insurance with little question).

Care Coordination

Make available high-quality, clinically competent care coordination for people who need assistance navigating the health care system. For example, people with multiple and complex health issues, including individuals who are living with several conditions, such as emphysema, diabetes, heart conditions, obesity, arthritis, and high blood pressure, are often overwhelmed and lost in a fragmented system.

Elements of care coordination of particular importance to many people with disabilities include fostering of a person-centered approach that honors the goal of achieving maximum self-determination while supporting independent living values, such as dignity, independence, individuality, privacy, and choice.

Comprehensive Health Evaluations

Disincentives that limit health care professionals' ability to offer comprehensive evaluations should be eliminated. Comprehensive health evaluations are available only for the elite chief executive officers. These are evaluations that many people would benefit from and welcome. However, the consequences and downstream costs of not periodically offering them to higher-risk people living and aging with disabilities are much more significant.

These evaluations are important, because individual needs, readiness, and timing for the incorporation of technology and adaptive strategies techniques change. The information learned in an express and compressed rehabilitation stay or outpatient visit often needs to be reinforced, refreshed, revisited, and enhanced. The need is the same for people who have life-long disabilities as well as people who acquire disabilities later in life.

Public and private insurance should cover comprehensive, periodic, coordinated, timely screenings, evaluations, and services tailored to the individual's age, sex, disability, chronic conditions, lifestyle, and personal history. What is described here is the ideal model. Even small steps toward the implementation of this model would indicate progress. In the ideal world, such evaluations should include a single-visit, one-stop evaluation that focuses on routine screening, improving functional capacity, and preventing decline and deterioration. Evaluations should center on the whole person and should consist of

- assessments by a multidisciplinary team of health care professionals who effectively solve problems together (as needed, a nurse, physician, physical therapist, occupational therapist, orthotist, social worker, mental health professional, care coordinator, fitness specialist, dentist, optometrist, and others);
- technology-specific tune-ups, which involve health education; preventive strategies regarding repetitive stress; and muscle underuse, overuse, and misuse injuries; as well as any safety product recalls;
- nutritional and fitness assessments;
- an optional on-site workplace assessment that covers areas such as seating and ergonomics;
- assessments and plans for preventing known health complications secondary to a disability and for preserving functional abilities with a focus on anticipating how such abilities may change with age;
- an easy-to-understand report that is given to the patient along with an individual health and wellness plan that is reviewed annually, revised as needed, and developed in partnership with the individual and the health care team; and
- fully funded follow-up services for the individual's health and wellness plan.

One specific example of the kind of up-to-date evaluation and information that such an approach would offer involves rehabilitation education for those using a wheelchair. A person would be informed that transferring from the wheelchair to a car by swinging one's body while holding onto the doorframe is a technique that will eventually cause significant shoulder pain. The person would review newer and less physically costly techniques in person, and these techniques would be augmented with reinforcing written and audiovisual materials.

BUILD THE SCIENCE BASE

If science does not focus on the intersection among the body, the environment, and health care policy, the enduring contributions will fall short. I can tell story after story illustrating aging with disability-specific problems, but anecdotal data do not carry much weight. Without respected data, we are just advocates with opinions.

A national large-scale epidemiological study of people with disabilities (similar to aging studies) is needed. Such a study should receive multi-disciplinary, multicollaborative, and multiagency funding. In addition, research needs to

- validate or disprove the merits and cost-effectiveness of periodic comprehensive evaluations;
- be reality based and focus on what can be accomplished to improve care given limited health care resources;
- focus on methods and models that will help reorient and transform the approach in health care that too often equates disability, chronic conditions, and activity limitations with an inability to work;
- focus on the prevention and mitigation of secondary and associated conditions; the research (reviewed by others) documents the prevalence of common secondary conditions like pain, depression, obesity, and fatigue across disability groups;
- focus on functional limitations; given the complexity and diversity of disability and the low prevalence of many conditions, research should focus on functional limitations across disabilities and not discrete diagnostic groups (for example, people with cerebral palsy have some characteristics in common, but variations in abilities and limitations manifested in vastly different ways are more common); there are common functional limitations that need attention across groups with different types of disabilities;
- incorporate cost-effectiveness and health economics components; this sometimes gives advocates the additional data that they need to make the case for improving health care policies and interventions;
- reduce the time between the use of common practices and the implementation of best practices;
- be coordinated across relevant federal agencies;
- guard against the "silo" effect by infusing disability content throughout other, nondisability-focused health research, for example, the array of institutes and centers at the National Institutes of Health; and

---

BOX K-1
Directions for Research on Health Living with a Disability

- Do individuals who acquire disabilities at different ages in the life cycle differ in the types, frequencies, and numbers of chronic health conditions that they experience after the onset of their primary disability? What are the differences, and which groups are at the greatest risk?
- What is the effect of exercise on preventing increasing levels of disability among individuals with specific types of disabilities?
- Does participation in certain kinds of sports for people with physical disabilities accelerate musculoskeletal difficulties?
- What steps should be incorporated in the early years of a disability to prevent or reduce future musculoskeletal problems? Is "use it or lose it" a sound strategy, or would voluntary curtailment of the intensity and scope of certain activities at an early age translate into fewer musculoskeletal difficulties in later years? What trade-offs need to be considered early in life, e.g., the rigors of walking with crutches and the upper-extremity muscle deterioration that it may cause as opposed to using a wheelchair, particularly if one's career depends on upper-extremity muscles?
- What are the long-term effects of disability-related physical and drug therapies and surgeries?
- Will osteoporosis become a major problem for people with physical disabilities? Should screening for osteoporosis occur earlier for people with mobility disabilities than for people without disabilities? What interventions are effective? When should they start?
- What strategies regarding aging well with a disability could be adopted from sports medicine, because the analogy is that many people with physical disabilities use their bodies more like athletes than other people? Could people benefit from this knowledge with regard to exercise, diet, assistive devices, medication and energy conservation?
- What is the impact of exercise and activity on the functional independence and overall health status of individuals with physical disabilities?

- give greater focus to ways of promoting healthy living with a disability that have direct, immediate, and practical applications. Box K-1 includes some questions about aging with a disability—which I have collected from my peers—that could be integrated into this research.

Research focused on DME, assistive technologies, and related services should emphasize several topics. These include

- determining if there is an evidence base regarding the efficacy and cost-effectiveness of coverage;
- determining how devices improve functional ability and reduce costs by decreasing pain and wear and tear on joints;

- studying if there are long-term savings and costs related to paying for customized technology;
- exploring whether strategies for the prevention of secondary conditions should accompany the delivery of various types of DME (e.g., whether, when wheeled mobility is prescribed, overweight and obesity prevention services and guidance on how to protect overused muscles and joints should be part of the service package);
- determining if coverage for repairs to a device, as well for training regarding the use and maintenance of a device, extends the life of the device and reduces its replacement cost;
- reducing the weight, size, and costs of devices and improving their ease of operation;
- documenting whether there are any differences between the use of customized assistive technology and noncustomized assistive technology in long-term physical and financial costs; and
- documenting or disproving the existence and scope of the "woodwork effect."

Resistance to modernizing policies is often based on fear of the so-called woodwork effect. That is, if more generous benefits are available, unimaginable numbers of beneficiaries will emerge "from the woodwork" to seek the service. Is there any validity to the use of the woodwork effect by policy makers and insurance carriers as an excuse not to improve policy? Is this an excuse that actually costs more in the long run?

THE CHARGE TO IOM

For me and my peers, this updating of *Disability in America* by IOM is serious business. It is about "getting it right" in areas that are essential to our health and independence. It is about giving many of us the tools and services that we need to keep going, to be productive, and to prevent the world from unnecessarily closing in on us and becoming confining. It is about translating the words and the mantras like "quality living in the community" into reality. Life is short, so be productive and focus on converting the words to reality so that they do not remain empty promises.

REFERENCES

Brandt EN Jr., Pope AM, eds. 1997. *Enabling America: Assessing theRole of Rehabilitation Science and Engineering.* Washington, DC: National Academy Press.
Pope AM, Tarlov AR, eds. 1991. *Disability in America: Toward a National Agenda for Prevention.* Washington, DC: National Academy Press.

L

Impact of Exercise on Targeted Secondary Conditions

*James H. Rimmer and Swati S. Shenoy**

Regular exercise has been recognized as one of the most important health behaviors for reducing the risk of chronic diseases and improving overall health.[19] There is strong evidence that exercise leads to improved physiologic fitness; extends longevity; and protects against the development of coronary heart disease, hypertension, type 2 diabetes, obesity, osteoporosis, colon cancer, breast cancer, lung cancer, and clinical depression.[13] As a result of this supportive literature base, regular exercise is considered one of the most essential health behaviors for reducing the risk of various health conditions and is listed as one of the primary target goals in the U.S. Department of Health and Human Services' *Healthy People 2010*, a document that identifies preventable threats to the nation's health and sets goals for reducing these threats.[18]

Less is known about the potential benefits of exercise in reducing secondary conditions in people with disabilities. The epidemiologic work that has confirmed the benefits of exercise in the general population has typically excluded individuals with physical, cognitive, and sensory disabilities. This has left an enormous gap in the literature in terms of understanding if

*James H. Rimmer, Ph.D., Professor of Disability and Human Development, Department of Disability and Human Development, College of Applied Health Sciences, University of Illinois at Chicago. Swati S. Shenoy, P.T., M.S., Department of Disability and Human Development, College of Applied Health Sciences, University of Illinois at Chicago. The analyses and views presented in this workshop paper are those of the authors and not necessarily those of the Institute of Medicine Committee on Disability in America: A New Look.

similar "doses" of exercise can have the same health benefits for people with disabilities.

In recent years there has been a modest but growing increase in the number of exercise-related studies that have targeted people with disabilities. Although the majority of these studies are not randomized controlled trials (RCTs) and had limited sample sizes, they are part of a growing effort among researchers to understand the effects of exercise in improving health among people with disabilities.[1,2,5,6,7,8,9] However, there is a limited amount of data on the effects of exercise in reducing or mitigating specific secondary conditions that are related to a primary disabling condition.[10,15]

LITERATURE SEARCH

This paper reviews 10 RCTs that tested an exercise intervention to ameliorate the following secondary conditions: deconditioning, fatigue, and pain. Two primary disabling conditions were targeted: multiple sclerosis and spinal cord injury. A glossary at the end of this paper describes the assessment instruments used in the studies reviewed. To identify relevant studies, we conducted a literature search for the period from 1990 to 2005. The databases searched were PubMed/MEDLINE and Cumulative Index to Nursing and Allied Health Literature (CINAHL). The keywords used to identify peer reviewed articles were "exercise," "physical activity," "secondary conditions," "disability," "multiple sclerosis," and "spinal cord injury." The studies selected had to fulfill the following criteria: (1) the enrolled subjects had to have a spinal cord injury or multiple sclerosis; (2) the intervention targeted deconditioning, fatigue, or pain; (3) the trial involved a prospective randomization methodology; (4) the treatment involved some type of exercise regimen; and (5) the study was published in English. A total of 10 articles satisfied the inclusion criteria.

DECONDITIONING

Deconditioning is associated with low levels of physical fitness (e.g., low levels of aerobic power and muscle strength and endurance, higher fat to lean muscle ratio, and poor flexibility) and often occurs as a result of high levels of sedentary behavior. It leads to a loss of cardiorespiratory endurance and musculoskeletal function, subsequently reducing a person's ability to perform various physical tasks, including activities of daily living, such as dressing and bathing, and instrumental activities of daily living, such as transfers, rolling up ramps, walking, and wheeling.

Six RCTs examined the effects of exercise on deconditioning in individuals with spinal cord injuries (one study) or multiple sclerosis (five studies). A brief review of each study is described below, followed by a summary of the overall findings.

Hicks and colleagues[9] conducted an RCT of supervised progressive exercise training in 34 subjects with spinal cord injuries (time postinjury, >1 year; age range, 19 to 65 years; lesion level, C4 or below; intervention group, 21 subjects; control group, 13 subjects) to examine the effects of a long-term exercise training protocol on strength and cardiovascular endurance. Subjects in the exercise intervention group trained 90 to 120 minutes per day, 2 days per week. The training protocol included a warm-up consisting of wheeling around an indoor track or low-intensity arm ergometry and gentle upper-extremity stretching. The aerobic portion involved arm ergometry for 15 ± 30 minutes at an intensity level of approximately 70 percent maximum heart rate (a rating of 3 to 4 on the 11-point Borg rating scale). Initially, the subjects performed two arm ergometry bouts of 5 ± 10 minutes, which were gradually increased to two bouts of 15 ± 20 minutes as the training progressed. These two bouts were interspersed with resistance training exercise. The resistance training component consisted of exercises with a wall pulley, free weights, and an Equalizer weight machine. The subjects performed their resistance exercises in a circuit system, which consisted of two sets of each exercise (50 percent of 1-RM, which is the maximum amount of weight that can be lifted one time by a particular study subject) and which then progressed to three sets (70 to 80 percent of 1-RM) after the fourth week. The resistance loads were reassessed approximately every 6 weeks to ensure a constant training intensity. A wide variety of exercises targeted the upper torso (i.e., forearm-wrist, biceps, back, chest, abdominals, shoulder, triceps, and legs). Subjects in the control group were offered a bimonthly education session (together with the exercise group) on topics that included exercise physiology for individuals with spinal cord injuries, the occurrence of osteoporosis after a spinal cord injury, and relaxation techniques. Control subjects were also given the opportunity to join the exercise program once the 9-month study ended. The evaluations for 1-RM strength and arm ergometry were obtained at 3, 6, and 9 months, respectively. The results indicated that a 9-month training program of structured exercise two times per week produced significant increases in submaximal power output (81 percent; $p < 0.05$) and significant increases in upper body muscle strength (19 to 34 percent; $p < 0.05$). The exercise group was able to perform significantly more work at a given heart rate compared with the amount of work performed at baseline. The implications of these findings were that subjects could perform certain physical tasks much easier after this 9-month training program, which would hypothetically lead to greater independence. However, this association was never tested.

Petajan and colleagues[15] conducted a 15-week RCT involving aerobic exercise with 46 individuals with multiple sclerosis. Subjects were randomly assigned to an exercise group (n = 21) or a nonexercise (control) group (n = 25). Six subjects were excluded for reasons unrelated to the study, and two subjects were dropped because of an exacerbation. Outcome measures included maximal aerobic capacity; isometric strength; body composition; blood lipids; performance in daily activities; mood, fatigue, and disease status as measured by the Profile of Mood States (POMS), Fatigue Severity Scale (FSS), and Sickness Impact Profile (SIP); the Kurtzke Expanded Disability Status Scale (EDSS); and neurological examination. The subjects trained 3 days per week for 40 minutes per session using a combination of arm/leg cycling on a stationary bicycle. Exercise sessions consisted of a warm-up (5 minutes) and cool down (5 minutes); 30 minutes of cycling at 60 percent of VO_{2max}; and 5 to 10 minutes of stretching that focused on the posterior muscles of the lower leg, thigh, and back. Compared with values at baseline, the exercise group demonstrated significant increases in VO_{2max} (22 percent), physical work capacity (48 percent), upper- and lower-extremity strength, skin fold thickness and triglyceride levels. The results of EDSS were unchanged except for improved bowel and bladder function. The exercise group showed improved SIP scores (physical dimension) in ambulation, mobility, body care, and movement. The investigators noted that the gains in fitness were associated with enhanced social integration and improvements in physical and psychological functions.

Mostert and Kesselring[11] conducted a 4-week aerobic exercise training program with 37 subjects who had one of the following types of multiple sclerosis: relapsing-remitting, chronic-progressive, or relapsing-progressive. All subjects were in an inpatient rehabilitation program. Subjects with multiple sclerosis were randomly assigned to an exercise training group (MS-ET) or a nonexercise training or nonintervention (MS-NI) group. The subjects in the latter group received physical therapy but did not engage in any other physical activity. Another control group consisted of 26 subjects without multiple sclerosis matched with the MS-ET and the MS-NI groups by age, gender, and activity level. Eleven of the 37 subjects with multiple sclerosis were excluded or dropped out of the study, leaving a total of 13 subjects in each group (the MS-ET and MS-NI groups). Subjects performed a graded exercise test to measure peak aerobic capacity (VO_{2peak}). The training component consisted of five 30-minute sessions of stationary cycling per week for 3 to 4 weeks. The results indicated that there were no changes in peak aerobic capacity (VO_{2peak}), although the maximum work rate did improve (+11 percent) in the training group. The investigators noted that the low training volume (3 to 4 weeks) might not have been high enough to improve fitness. Other improvements included increased health perception (vitality, +46 percent; social interaction, +36 percent) and activity level (+17 percent). No changes in these measures were observed in the MS-NI group or the control group without multiple sclerosis. Overall, the researchers considered the rate of compliance with the training program to be low (65 percent).

Romberg and colleagues[16] conducted an RCT with subjects with multiple sclerosis to evaluate the effects of a progressive 6-month exercise training program consisting of 3 weeks of inpatient rehabilitation and 23 weeks of home exercise on walking and other aspects of physical function. The subjects (n = 114; age range, 30 to 55 years) had mild to moderate multiple sclerosis on the basis of their EDSS scores, which were between 1.0 and 5.5. The subjects were randomly assigned to either the exercise group (n = 56) or the control group (n = 58). The outcome measures included walking speed (7.62- and 500-meter-walk tests), maximal isometric torque of knee extensor and flexor muscles (dynamometer), upper-extremity endurance (weightlifting test), peak oxygen uptake, and static balance. The groups were evaluated at baseline and 6 months. Data for only 95 subjects were included in the analyses because of withdrawals or exclusion because of illness. The intervention consisted of inpatient rehabilitation (weeks 1 to 3), followed by a progressive home-based exercise program (weeks 4 to 26). Ten supervised strength training and aerobic exercise sessions were conducted during the inpatient rehabilitation. Trained physiotherapists instructed the patients individually on the home exercise program. Aerobic training during weeks 1 to 3 consisted of aquatic training, and during weeks 4 to 26 the subjects were encouraged to continue with aquatic training or with their earlier mode of aerobic exercise (the specific modes were not reported). The results indicated that 91 (96 percent) of the 95 subjects who enrolled in the study were able to complete it. However, this was after a screening process that identified 276 eligible subjects, 162 of whom were not eligible for the study for several reasons, including the fact that they were out of the age range of the study, their EDSS score was out of the range for the study, they had some other disease or medical condition, they could not be contacted, or they did not want to participate. Walking speed improved significantly on both the 7.62-meter-walk (p = 0.04) and the 500-meter-walk (p = 0.01) tests. In the 7.62-meter-walk test, the exercise group had a 12 percent decrease in time, whereas the controls had a 6 percent decrease. On the 500-meter-walk test, the exercise group decreased their time by 6 percent and there was no change for the controls. There were no reported changes in lower-extremity strength, VO_{2peak}, static balance, or manual dexterity. Even though the researchers concluded that exercise had a significant effect on increasing functional performance and was considered safe by individuals with mild to moderate multiple sclerosis, the measures typically improved in exercise trials (i.e., VO_{2peak} and lower extremity strength) were not demonstrated.

DeBolt and McCubbin[5] conducted an RCT to examine the effects of an 8-week home-based resistance exercise program on balance, power, and mobility in adults with multiple sclerosis. The subject pool consisted of 29 women with multiple sclerosis (mean age, 50.3 ± 8.5 years) and 8 men with multiple sclerosis (mean age, 51.1 ± 7.1 years). The subjects were stratified by disability level, as determined by EDSS, and age and were randomized into an intervention group ($n = 19$) or a control group ($n = 17$). The intervention consisted of 5 to 10 minutes of warm-up activities (walking) and stretches, 25 to 30 minutes of strengthening exercises, and 5 to 10 minutes of whole-body stretching. The exercises included chair raises, forward lunges, step-ups, heel-toe raises, and leg curls. Weighted vests were used to increase the intensity of the training regimen. The progression of intensity was based on the strength training periodization model: the initial vest resistance was set at 0.5 percent of body weight and increased by percentages of body weight (0.05 to 1.5 percent) every 2 weeks. During weeks 1 and 3 the participants were instructed to perform two sets of 8 to 12 repetitions of each exercise, and during weeks 2 and 4 they were instructed to perform three sets of 8 to 12 repetitions of each exercise (hypertrophy phase). During weeks 5 to 8, the participants decreased the number of exercises to two sets of 8 to 10 repetitions (strength and power phase). The control group members were given the opportunity to learn the home-based resistance exercises at the end of posttesting and were also given a home exercise video. Bimonthly home visits and weekly phone contacts were conducted for both groups. The results indicated a significant improvement in leg extensor power in the exercise group ($p < 0.004$). However, measures of balance and mobility did not show any changes.

Patti and colleagues[14] conducted an RCT to evaluate the effects of a 12-week comprehensive outpatient rehabilitation program on the quality of life in individuals with multiple sclerosis. Individuals with multiple sclerosis ($n = 111$) were recruited from a sample of 407 eligible subjects on the basis of the following inclusion criteria: laboratory-confirmed multiple sclerosis, an EDSS score between 4.0 and 8.0, and age between 18 and 65 years. The eligible subjects were randomly assigned to the treatment group ($n = 58$) or a control group on a treatment waiting list ($n = 53$). The intervention consisted of a comprehensive outpatient rehabilitation program (6 weeks), followed by a 6-week self-initiated home exercise program. The control group on the waiting list was offered the comprehensive outpatient rehabilitation program at the end of 12 weeks. The outcome measures were the EDSS, the SF-36 health-related quality of life survey, the Beck Depression Inventory (BDI), the Tempelaar Social Experience Checklist (SET), and the Fatigue Impact Scale (FIS). The results indicated that the EDSS score remained unaffected in both groups. For the treatment group, all health-related quality-of-life components on the various components of the SF-36 improved significantly, including physical functioning, bodily pain, general health, and social functioning ($p < 0.001$) and vitality and emotional and mental health ($p < 0.05$). Additionally, there was a significant reduction in fatigability and a significant improvement in social functioning and depression, as measured by FIS, SET and BDI, after the 12-week intervention ($p < 0.001$).

In summary, the six RCTs reported on in this section targeted improvements in physical fitness (i.e., aerobic power, muscle strength, and endurance) or physical function (measures of mobility), with the intent ot reduce the effects of deconditioning. The total aggregate sample that participated in the intervention arm was 21 subjects with spinal cord injuries and 156 subjects with multiple sclerosis. The sample sizes in the intervention arm ranged from 13 to 58. All of the studies reported positive findings on one or more outcome measures associated with deconditioning, but there were wide variations between studies. This may be related to the substantial heterogeneity in age, gender, and level of disability. The studies of individuals with multiple sclerosis indicated that individual patterns of disease progression may or may not have matched well between the control and the experimental groups. Similarly, all of the studies included subjects with various types and severities of multiple sclerosis. With small sample sizes, this becomes an even greater issue because alterations in health or function could skew the findings for either the control group or the experimental group. Only two studies reported a power analysis,[5,16] and one of those studies indicated that the power was less than 80 percent.[26] One study performed an intention-to-treat analysis,[16] but the other studies reported their findings only for subjects who remained in the study. It is possible that subjects who agreed to participate in an exercise trial may have had higher levels of baseline function or health, which may limit the findings to a subgroup of the targeted population. Several participants dropped out of each of the studies because of compromised health status, a lack of interest, or other factors.

FATIGUE

Fatigue is a common secondary condition that affects individuals with multiple sclerosis. It can be expressed as general or systemic fatigue; muscle fatigue without exercise; and cognitive fatigue, which is indicated by reduced attention, memory, and information processing. Only four RCTs that targeted fatigue reduction in individuals with multiple sclerosis were identified.

Surakka and colleagues[17] conducted an RCT consisting of a 3-week supervised exercise program followed by 23 weeks of home exercise to examine the effects of aerobic and strength training on motor fatigue of knee flexor and extensor muscles in individuals with multiple sclerosis. The subject pool consisted of 95 subjects with mild to moderate disability who were randomly assigned to an exercise group (n = 47) or a control group (n = 48). The outcome measures were the Fatigue Index, subjective fatigue measured by the Fatigue Severity Scale (FSS) and EDSS. The intervention phase consisted of five supervised resistance exercise sessions and five aerobic exercise sessions. The resistance exercise was conducted in a circuit training format, beginning with a 10-minute warm-up, followed by 10 exercises with 10 to 15 repetitions in two sets. The exercises were performed with pressurized air resistance machines, with weight stack machines, or against gravity. The exercise load was 50 to 60 percent of 1-RM. The load was increased or decreased on the basis of the evaluation at the end of the third session. The aerobic program consisted of a variety of gymnastic exercises in shoulder-deep water with the temperature maintained at 28°C (82.4°F). The session started with a 5- to 7-minute warm-up, followed by 20 to 25 minutes of aerobic exercise, and ended with a 5- to 8-minute cool down. The exercise intensity was maintained at 65 to 70 percent of the age-predicted maximum heart rate (MHR). If the subject was unable to participate in the aquatic program, a 30- to 35-minute stationary cycling program was used.

The home exercise program lasted 23 weeks, with four exercise sessions per week during weeks 1 to 17 and five exercise sessions per week during weeks 18 to 23. The subjects were provided with two different elastic therabands for the upper and the lower extremities that were used for training. The participants in the control group were asked to continue with their normal daily routine. The results showed decreases in the AFI in the exercise group (p < 0.007) and a reduction in motor fatigue in knee flexion (p < 0.001) but not in extension in female subjects only after 6 months of exercise training.

Oken and colleagues[12] conducted a 6-month parallel-group (two or more different groups of patients) RCT to determine the effects of yoga and aerobic exercise on fatigue in 69 individuals with multiple sclerosis (12 subjects did not complete the study, leaving a total of 57 subjects). The subjects were randomly assigned to one of three groups: (1) Iyengar yoga (n = 22) (a form of hatha yoga that focuses on physical alignment of the body in various poses) with home practice, (2) aerobic exercise (n = 15) on a recumbent or dual-action stationary cycle with a home program, and (3) a control group on a waiting list (n = 20). The Iyengar yoga intervention was performed 1 day a week for 90 minutes. The subjects were trained in 19 poses (not all poses were completed each week), which were performed in a chair, against the wall, or while the subject was sitting on the floor. Each pose was held for approximately 10 to 30 seconds, with rest periods between poses of 30 seconds to 1 minute. The aerobic exercise sessions were held 1 day a week, along with home exercise, and consisted of bicycling on a recumbent or dual-action (arms and legs) stationary cycle. All exercises started and ended with a 5-minute stretching routine that involved the cycling muscles. The heart rate (HR) was not recorded, and the subjects were instructed to exercise at a very light to moderate intensity (modified Borg Rating of Perceived Exertion of 2 to 3). Outcomes measures for fatigue at baseline and at the end of 6 months were measured with the Multidimensional Fatigue Inventory (MFI); POMS, which includes measures of fatigue and vigor; and SF-36. The results indicated that both intervention groups showed a significant improvement on the general fatigue component of the MFI ($p < 0.01$) and the energy and fatigue component of the SF-36 energy and vitality dimension ($p < 0.001$).

Petajan and colleagues[15] conducted a 15-week RCT of aerobic training with 54 individuals with multiple sclerosis who were randomly assigned to an exercise group or a control group (see the study design discussed above in the section on deconditioning). For the exercise group, POMS depression and anger scores were significantly reduced at weeks 5 and 10, and fatigue was reduced at week 10. The exercise group improved significantly on all components of the physical dimension of SIP and showed significant improvements for social interaction, emotional behavior, home management, total SIP score, and recreation and pastimes. No changes on the FSS were observed for the exercise or the no-exercise control group. Exercise also had a positive impact on factors related to quality of life.

Mostert and Kesselring[11] conducted a 4-week aerobic exercise training program with 26 subjects (13 experimental and 13 control) involved in an inpatient rehabilitation program (see the study design discussed above in the section on deconditioning). The results indicated that, compared with the level of fatigue at baseline, the participants in the training group demonstrated a tendency toward less fatigue, although the researchers noted that the difference was not significant.

PAIN

Pain is one of the most common secondary conditions reported by people with disabilities.[3] In particular, musculoskeletal pain in the neck and shoulder region are commonly observed in individuals with spinal cord injuries and is exacerbated by wheelchair transfers and propulsion.[1,2,3,4] Only four exercise-related RCTs that targeted pain reduction in individuals with spinal cord injuries were identified.

Hicks and colleagues[9] targeted reduction in pain as one of their primary outcomes (see the study design discussed above in the section on deconditioning). The results indicated that a 9-month training regimen consisting of cardiorespiratory endurance and resistance exercise decreased the level of self-reported pain in individuals with spinal cord injuries. The researchers suggested that exercise be used as a prophylactic measure for improving pain tolerance in this population.

Ginis and colleagues[8] conducted an RCT of aerobic and resistance training with 34 individuals with traumatic spinal cord injuries (23 men and 11 women; mean age, 38.6 ± 11.7 years; average duration postinjury, 10.4 years; 14 had complete spinal cord injuries and 13 had incomplete spinal cord injuries). The participants were matched for years postinjury and relative mortality risk and were then randomly assigned to either an exercise group ($n = 21$) or a control group ($n = 13$), a ratio of 2:1. The treatment group trained two times per week in small groups of three to five participants. Each session included a 5-minute stretching routine, 15 to 30 minutes of arm ergometry exercise, and 45 to 60 minutes of resistance exercise. Initially, the exercise intensity for the aerobic component was 70 percent of MHR, but this was progressively increased on the observation of a decrease in perceived exertion or HR. The results indicated that there were significant improvements ($p < 0.05$) in perceived quality of life and better physical self-concept and a significant decrease ($p < 0.05$) in pain compared with the findings for the controls.

Patti and colleagues[14] (as discussed above) evaluated the effects of a comprehensive outpatient rehabilitation program on the quality of life in individuals with multiple sclerosis. All health-related quality-of-life components—physical functioning, role limitations due to physical health problems (role physical), bodily pain, general health, and social functioning—significantly improved in the treatment group ($p < 0.001$).

Curtis and colleagues[4] analyzed the effectiveness of a 6-month exercise protocol on shoulder pain in wheelchair users ($n = 42$). The subject pool consisted of a cluster sample recruited from the community. The average age was 35 ± 8 years, and the average duration of wheelchair use was 14 ± 9 years. The subjects were randomly assigned to a treatment group ($n = 21$) or a control group ($n = 21$). The subjects in the treatment group received 60 minutes of educational training that instructed them in five daily shoulder exercises. These exercises consisted of two static stretching exercises to increase the flexibility of the anterior shoulder muscles and three resistive strengthening exercises for the posterior shoulder muscles. The subjects performed all exercises independently while they were seated in their wheelchairs, and lightweight elastic exercise bands were used for resistance. The subjects with tetraplegia used wrist straps to accommodate a weak or absent grasp response. An instructional session was included to provide an overview of functional shoulder anatomy, the purpose of the exercises, and a demonstration of each exercise. The treatment group was instructed to perform stretching exercises twice daily, five times each, with a 20- to 30-second hold of each position for a prolonged stretch and to perform the strengthening exercises once daily with three sets of 15 repetitions. Bi-weekly phone calls were made to monitor performance and problems. The Wheelchair Users Shoulder Pain Index (WUSPI) was used to evaluate pain at baseline and at bimonthly intervals. The results showed that 75 percent of the subjects reported a history of shoulder pain since the initiation of wheelchair use. The average initial performance-corrected WUSPI (PC-WUSPI) score for the 42 subjects was 17.7 ± 21.3 with a range of 0 to 103.2. (A low score on the PC-WUSPI indicates lower levels of pain intensity.) More than 83 percent of the subjects (35 of 42) completed the 6-month study. The subjects in the treatment group decreased their PC-WUSPI scores by an average of 39.9 percent, whereas the decreases for the control group were only 2.5 percent. The study demonstrated that a small number of flexibility and resistive exercises had a positive effect on the reduction of shoulder pain in a population of wheelchair users.

SUMMARY OF STUDIES REVIEWED

The studies that we have reviewed used various methodologies, assessment tools, and exercise doses to address various health issues associated with people with multiple sclerosis and spinal cord injuries: deconditioning, fatigue, and pain. The studies reported under deconditioning used quality of life as their primary endpoint, which included both physiological and psychological measures. In the future, a more focused research agenda should use specific doses and modalities of exercise to address specific secondary conditions. Moreover, studies should be more homogeneous in terms of the age, health status, and functional levels of the study subjects and should use a consistent methodology and training dose to enhance the generalizability of the findings to certain subgroups of disabilities.

All of the studies reviewed in this paper had several different outcomes (e.g., physical and emotional well-being, quality of life, reduced fatigue, and increased fitness), used a variety of interventions and doses of exercise (length of study, frequency, duration, intensity, and modality), and had widely different inclusion and exclusion criteria within each disability group. A few studies included individuals in a wide age range and with a wide range of functional levels. This may have attenuated the potential effects of the intervention on a certain subgroup within the larger sample (e.g., younger versus older subjects). Although the use of heterogeneous populations makes it easier to recruit subjects (e.g., by including individuals with paraplegia and tetraplegia in the same study) and obtain higher levels of statistical power, generalizability is limited because of variations in the levels of health and function within disability groups.

It has become widely accepted that exercise promotes good health and reduces the risk of chronic conditions. However, it is less clear what doses of exercise are effective for reducing or mitigating the effects of various secondary conditions in people within different disability types and, within a certain disability, between individuals with different functional levels.

The lack of data pertaining to the frequency, intensity, duration, and modality components of an exercise prescription for individuals with various disabilities has limited the utility of exercise as a viable treatment for secondary conditions. While exercise is presumed to be beneficial for all individuals (with or without a disability), data on dose-response are critical for understanding and providing appropriate, targeted interventions that have a clinically meaningful effect in reducing the risk of, minimizing, or eliminating certain secondary conditions.

Researchers must also explore the possibility that certain individuals with the same disability may require a greater dose or a lower dose of exercise, depending on their genetic history, functional level, and the severity of the secondary condition being targeted (e.g., pain, fatigue, depression, and deconditioning). Some individuals may not respond favorably to a certain dose of exercise or physical activity, whereas others may drop out because of an injury or exacerbation. In one of the RCTs reviewed in this paper,[9] 10 of 21 subjects (47.6 percent) who were randomized to the exercise arm dropped out of the study because of illness, transportation difficulties, or time conflicts. This is a major concern in research with disabled populations and should be addressed in future clinical trials.

SPECIFIC RESEARCH RECOMMENDATIONS

1. Prospective observational studies should be conducted to determine the frequency, intensity, and duration of physical activity associated with reducing the symptoms of targeted secondary conditions (e.g., deconditioning, fatigue, and pain). Epidemiological studies will offer greater opportunities to obtain an understanding of the effects of various forms of structured exercise and general physical activity on the incidence, risk, or reduction of secondary conditions in individuals with disabilities.

2. The heterogeneity between and within disability groups and the low incidence of many disabilities make it extremely difficult to obtain adequate sample sizes when subjects are recruited from one setting. Multicenter trials are necessary to achieve adequate statistical power and to be able to generalize the findings of those trials to certain subgroups within the targeted disability (e.g., older versus younger individuals, individuals with higher levels of functioning versus those with lower levels of functioning, male versus female subjects, individuals with paraplegia versus those with tetraplegia, and individuals with progressive multiple sclerosis versus those with relapsing-remitting multiple sclerosis). A structured protocol that tar-

gets a homogeneous subset of the population identified (e.g., young adults with paraplegia) and that employs the same testing instruments, procedures, and training regimen must be established.

3. RCTs are needed to examine exercises of various types and doses (by frequency, intensity, and duration). There is still a lack of information on what types of programs or interventions are the most effective for ameliorating specific secondary conditions. Evidence-based practice guidelines must be established from well-designed studies.

4. Group versus individual exercise, such as tai chi or yoga, may have an additional social benefit, which may improve outcomes but which may also confound the benefit of the specific dose of exercise. Future studies should control for the social aspect of exercise to obtain accurate data on the exercise regimen itself versus the social benefits associated with exercising in a group.

5. Numerous self-report assessment tools have been developed to measure changes in deconditioning, fatigue, and pain. It is difficult to make comparisons between studies when the instruments are not the same or are not explained in detail to make critical comparisons between them. The use of a consistent set of instruments that measure the reductions in specific secondary conditions should be explored so that data from various studies can be compared.

6. Although the studies reviewed here were mostly supportive of the role of exercise in reducing deconditioning, fatigue, and pain, none explained the physiological, musculoskeletal, or neurological mechanisms associated with these changes. With more sophisticated imaging and laboratory techniques, it may now be possible to identify the more subtle biological changes associated with exercise training.

7. Innovative strategies for the recruitment of individuals who generally do not volunteer for research studies must be explored. Because most experimental research is conducted with volunteers, it is difficult to generalize the study's findings to the entire subgroup. People who volunteer for exercise-related research may generally be younger or may have a higher functional level. This is a common problem in experimental research, but it may be an even greater problem for people with disabilities because sample selection is limited to a small subset of the population and barriers such as transportation limit opportunities for participation in clinical research.

8. Several studies emphasized the unique aspects of improving social integration and quality of life. It would be helpful to understand how these self-report measures are associated with more objective measures, such as quantitative assessment of an increase in community participation (i.e., an increased number of out-of-home social activities, a greater amount of time engaging in social events, increased rates of employment, and more social

contacts). The idea that exercise can improve psychological functioning and quality of life is an intriguing one, and should be measured with more objective monitoring techniques.

9. Specific secondary conditions, such as deconditioning, fatigue, and pain, must be more clearly defined. There are various types of deconditioning (e.g., low muscle strength, poor cardiorespiratory endurance, and lack of flexibility or balance), fatigue (e.g., physical and mental), and pain (e.g., neurogenic and musculoskeletal). Researchers targeting the reduction of these secondary conditions must be certain that the sample groups are similar on the basis of the defined characteristics of the secondary conditions.

10. There needs to be stronger collaboration between researchers whose work focuses on a specific disability group or secondary condition. Government funding agencies that support model systems involved in tracking the health status of a specific disability group (e.g., spinal cord injury, traumatic brain injury), should consider funding similar networks that conduct intervention research aimed at reducing specific secondary conditions.

CONCLUSION

Very few RCTs have targeted the reduction of secondary conditions in people with disabilities. There is a strong need for a new frontier of research that identifies the effective doses of structured exercise regimens and general physical activity needed to reduce various physical, psychological, social, and environmental secondary conditions in individuals with disabilities.

Understanding how exercise can affect various secondary conditions is a line of research that must be given a higher priority among funding agencies, in the same regard that other prophylactic measures, such as the use of medication and assistive technology, are scientifically supported with public and private funding. Evidence-based exercise guidelines associated with the reduction of various secondary conditions will require more empirical evidence before private and public health insurers will pay for these programs or services.

REFERENCES

1. Bizzarini E, Saccavini M, Lipanje F, Magrin P, Malisan C, Zampa A. (2005). Exercise prescription in subjects with spinal cord injuries. Arch Phys Med Rehabil, 86(6):1170–1175.
2. Bougenot MP, Tordi N, Betik AC, Martin X, Le Foll D, Parratte B, Lonsdorfer J, Rouillon JD. (2003). Effects of a wheelchair ergometer training programme on spinal cord-injured persons. Spinal Cord, 41(8):451–456.

3. Coyle CP, Santiago MC, Shank JW, Ma GX, Boyd R. (2000). Secondary conditions and women with physical disabilities: a descriptive study. Arch Phys Med Rehabil, 81:1380–1387.

4. Curtis, KA, Drysdale GA, et al. (1999). Shoulder pain in wheelchair users with tetraplegia and paraplegia. Arch Phys Med Rehabil, 80(4):453–457.

5. DeBolt LS, McCubbin JA. (2004). The effects of home-based resistance exercise on balance, power, and mobility in adults with multiple sclerosis. Arch Phys Med Rehabil, 85(2):290–297.

6. Ditor DS, Latimer AE, Ginis KA, Arbour KP, McCartney N, Hicks AL. (2003). Maintenance of exercise participation in individuals with spinal cord injury: effects on quality of life, stress and pain. Spinal Cord, 41(8):446–450.

7. Ginis KA, Latimer AE, Hicks AL, Craven BC. (2005). Development and evaluation of an activity measure for people with spinal cord injury. Med Sci Sports Exerc, 37(7): 1099–1111.

8. Ginis KA, Latimer AE, McKechnie K, Ditor DS, McCartney N, Hicks L. (2003). Using exercise to enhance subjective wellbeing among people with spinal cord injury: the mediating influences of stress and pain. Rehabil Psych, 48(3):157–164.

9. Hicks AL, Martin KA, Ditor DS, Latimer AE, Craven C, Bugaresti J, McCartney N. (2003). Long-term exercise training in persons with spinal cord injury: effects on strength, arm ergometry performance and psychological well-being. Spinal Cord, 41(1): 34–43

10. Institute of Medicine. (1991).Prevention of secondary conditions. In: Pope AM, Tarlov AR, (eds.), Disability in America: Toward a National Agenda for Prevention. (pp. 214–241). Washington, DC: National Academy Press.

11. Mostert S, Kesselring J. (2002). Effects of a short-term exercise training program on aerobic fitness, fatigue, health perception and activity level of subjects with multiple sclerosis. Mult Scler, 8(2):161–168.

12. Oken BS, Kishiyama S, Zajdel D, Bourdette D, Carlsen J, Haas M, Hugos C, Kraemer DF, Lawrence J, Mass M. (2004). Randomized controlled trial of yoga and exercise in multiple sclerosis. Neurology, 62(11):2058–2064.

13. Paffenbarger RS, Morris JN, Haskell WL, Thompson PD, Lee I-M. (2004). An introduction to the Journal of Physical Activity and Health. J Phys Activity Health, 1:1–3.

14. Patti F, Ciancio MR, Reggio E, Lopes R, Palermo F, Cacopardo M, Reggio A. (2002). The impact of outpatient rehabilitation on quality of life in multiple sclerosis. J Neurol, 249(8):1027–1033.

15. Petajan JH, Gappmaier E, White AT, Spencer MK, Mino L, Hicks RW. (1996). Impact of aerobic training on fitness and quality of life in multiple sclerosis. Ann Neurol, 39(4):432–441.

16. Romberg A, Virtanen A, Ruutiainen J, Aunola S, Karppi SL, Vaara M, Surakka J, Pohjolainen T, Seppanen A. (2004). Effects of a 6-month exercise program on patients with multiple sclerosis: a randomized study. Neurology, 63(11):2034–2038.

17. Surakka J, Romberg A, Ruutiainen J, Aunola S, Virtanen A, Karppi SL, Maentaka K. (2004). Effects of aerobic and strength exercise on motor fatigue in men and women with multiple sclerosis: a randomized controlled trial. Clin Rehabil, 18(7):737–746.

18. U.S. Department of Health and Human Services. (2000). Healthy People 2010. Washington, DC: U.S. Department of Health and Human Services.

19. U.S. Department of Health and Human Services. (1996). Physical Activity and Health: A Report of the Surgeon General. Atlanta, GA: U.S. Department of Health and Human Services, Centers for Disease Control and Prevention, National Center for Chronic Disease Prevention and Health Promotion.

GLOSSARY OF ASSESSMENT INSTRUMENTS
USED IN THE STUDIES REVIEWED

AFI: Ambulatory Fatigue Index

AFI is a 500-meter walking test. Subjects are asked to walk at their maximum speed.

BDI: Beck Depression Inventory

BDI is a self-administered 21-item self-report scale that measures the supposed manifestations of depression and takes approximately 10 minutes to complete.

EDSS: The Kurtzke Expanded Disability Status Scale

EDSS is a method of quantifying disability in individuals with multiple sclerosis. EDSS quantifies disability in eight functional systems and allows neurologists to assign a functional system score in each of the eight areas. The functional systems are pyramidal, cerebellar, brainstem, sensory, bowel, bladder, visual, and cerebral. EDSS steps 1.0 to 4.5 refer to people with multiple sclerosis who are fully ambulatory. EDSS steps 5.0 to 9.5 are defined by impairment related to ambulation.

FI: Fatigue Index

FI is the ratio between the integral of muscle strength decay over time and maximal voluntary contraction using a knee muscle dynamometer. The fatigue index was defined as the ratio of the force F at time t (F_t) to the maximum force during stimulation (F_{max}): $FI = F_t/F_{max}$.

FIS: Fatigue Impact Scale

FIS evaluates the impact of fatigue on physical function (10 items), cognitive function (10 items), and psychosocial function (20 items).

FSS: Fatigue Severity Scale

FSS is designed to measure the impact of fatigue on function using nine statements for which subjects rate their level of agreement.

MFI: Multidimensional Fatigue Inventory

The MFI self-assessment questionnaire measures five dimensions of fatigue: general fatigue, physical fatigue, reduced activity, reduced motivation, and mental fatigue.

MOS SF-36 Health Survey: the Medical Outcomes Study 36-Item Short-Form Health Survey

Same instrument as the SF-36. Initially, the SF-36 was developed to survey health status in the Medical Outcomes Study. It is a measure of health status designed for use in clinical practice, research, health policy evaluations, and general population surveys. It includes eight scales that assess the following general health concepts: physical functioning, role limitations due to physical health problems (role physical), bodily pain, general health perceptions, vitality, social functioning, role limitations due to emotional problems (role emotional), and mental health.

MSIS-29: 29-item Multiple Sclerosis Impact Scale

MSIS-29 can be used to measure therapeutic outcomes in persons with multiple sclerosis. It consists of 29 items: (1) 3 items dealing with limited abilities and (2) 26 items related to the symptoms or the consequences of the illness.

MSWS-12: 12-item Multiple Sclerosis Walking Scale

MSWS-12 is a questionnaire that asks the patient to self-rate the degree of limitation in walking due to multiple sclerosis experienced in the prior 2 weeks for each of 12 activities.

POMS: Profile of Mood States

The POMS provides a method to assess transient, fluctuating mood states. The key areas measured are tension-anxiety, anger-hostility, fatigue-inertia, depression-dejection, vigor-activity, and confusion-bewilderment.

SIP: Sickness Impact Profile

SIP describes relative functional limitations across 12 specific areas: ambulation, body care and movement, mobility, emotional behavior, social interaction, alertness behavior, communication, work, sleep and rest, eating, home management, and recreation and pastimes.

M

Secondary Conditions with Spinal Cord Injury

*William A. Bauman**

The secondary consequences of spinal cord injury may be medical, neurological, musculoskeletal, or urological. This paper discusses the medical consequences of spinal cord injury and describes a few of the pulmonary, cardiac, body compositional, metabolic, gastrointestinal, and dermatological issues confronting individuals with such injuries. In another paper presented at the IOM workshop, Margaret Turk (Appendix J) listed the secondary medical disabilities that are associated with spinal cord injuries and suggested that they have been accepted into mainstream medical knowledge, which is quite different than what was accepted just a few years ago.

PULMONARY AND CARDIOVASCULAR DISEASES

In the 1940s and 1950s most individuals with spinal cord injuries died of urinary complications soon after their injury, but today their longevity approaches that of the general population. Because individuals with spinal cord injuries are living longer, researchers have the opportunity to appreci-

---

*William A. Bauman, M.D., Director, Rehabilitation Research and Development Center of Excellence for the Medical Consequences of Spinal Cord Injury, James J. Peters VA Medical Center, and Professor of Medicine and Rehabilitation Medicine, Mount Sinai School of Medicine, New York City. The analyses and views presented in this workshop paper are those of the author and not necessarily those of the Institute of Medicine Committee on Disability in America: A New Look.

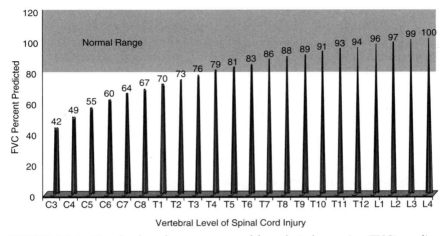

FIGURE M-1 Fitted values for percentage of forced vital capacity (FVC) predicted by level of complete motor lesions. C = cervical; T = thoracic; L = lumbar.
SOURCE: Compiled from data presented by Linn et al. (2001).

ate their secondary disabilities. In individuals with chronic spinal cord injuries, as in the able-bodied population, the common causes of morbidity and mortality are pulmonary and cardiovascular diseases. For example, Gale Whiteneck has found that, similar to the able-bodied population, cardiovascular disease is a leading cause of death in those with spinal cord injuries (Whiteneck et al., 1992). He and his colleagues have reported that among individuals who survive more than 30 years after their injury, 46 percent of all deaths are the result of a fatal cardiovascular event; among those older than 60 years, cardiovascular disease is responsible for 35 percent of all deaths. Heart and lung diseases may not be an immediate cause of death, but they potentially cause further functional impairment and require additional expenditures of resources in those with greater disabilities.

Individuals with spinal cord injuries are classically described as having restrictive ventilatory dysfunction, although in those with higher cord lesions, there is also evidence of airflow obstruction. The higher the spinal cord lesion that an individual has, the greater compromise of the muscles of respiration and the more difficult it is to breathe and cough effectively. If cough is reduced or absent, the clearance of secretions is impaired, which, in turn, can lead to atelectasis and, possibly, pneumonia. Those individuals who have lesions that are at thoracic level 4 or higher have been reported to have an ability to forcibly exhale that falls below the normal range, as evidenced by a forced vital capacity below 80 percent of the levels predicted for able-bodied subjects matched for age, gender, race, and height (Figure M-1).

At present, the clearance of pulmonary secretions for such individuals is accomplished by pharmacological interventions, by the use of pulmonary rehabilitation modalities, or with mechanical devices, including those that produce insufflation-exsufflation and those that electrically stimulate the muscles used for respiration. However, these interventions are often inadequate. As such, therapeutic strategies need to be developed to help those with higher spinal cord lesions to cough more effectively. If such interventions are efficacious, they would be expected to reduce the pulmonary causes of morbidity and mortality.

Individuals with cervical spinal cord injuries have heightened cholinergic airway tone and exhibit nonspecific airway hyperreactivity similar to that found in asthmatic subjects. These individuals also report worsening breathlessness after exposure to cold air, hot air, and secondary smoke. Inhaled bronchodilators are efficacious in improving airflow in those with higher cord lesions, although it has not been determined whether the regular use of these medications is associated with reduced morbidity or mortality. It is also not known whether exposure to common air pollutants, such as sulfur dioxide, causes bronchoconstriction in those with tetraplegia, although these pollutants might be expected to cause airway hyperreactivity. Members of my research unit will address this question in collaboration with Henry Gong, Chief of Environmental Health Service, Rancho Los Amigos National Rehabilitation Center.

METABOLIC SYNDROME

Those with spinal cord injuries have an increased tendency to develop what is now commonly referred to as the "metabolic syndrome." These individuals become insulin resistant, have associated carbohydrate and lipid abnormalities, and tend to be relatively overweight. Furthermore, those with paraplegia have an increased prevalence of hypertension, a condition not found in individuals with higher cord lesions.

Lipid Abnormalities

The primary lipid abnormality in those with spinal cord injuries is a low serum high-density lipoprotein (HDL) cholesterol ("good" cholesterol) level. The proportion of individuals with spinal cord injuries with normal serum low-density lipoprotein (LDL) cholesterol concentration, a modifiable risk factor for coronary artery disease, is similar to that in the able-bodied population. However, normal LDL levels may lull the health care provider into a sense of complacency that may be ill founded. This possibility is discussed below in greater detail.

The protective effect of serum HDL cholesterol is predominantly by

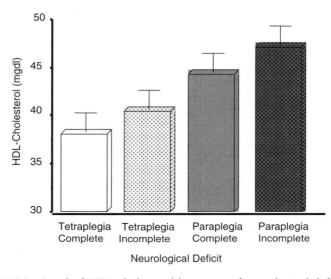

FIGURE M-2   Level of HDL cholesterol by extent of neurological deficit.
SOURCE: Compiled from data presented by Bauman et al. (1998a).

reverse cholesterol transport, which removes cholesterol from the periphery (vessel wall and macrophages) and transports it to the liver. Other beneficial mechanisms of action of serum HDL cholesterol include antioxidant, anti-inflammatory, direct vascular, antiplatelet, and anticoagulant effects. When the serum HDL cholesterol falls below 40 milligrams per deciliter (mg/dL), the morbidity risk ratio rises above unity.

Higher, more complete spinal cord lesions result in greater neurological impairment, which are associated with lower serum HDL cholesterol levels; those who have the least impairment have the highest serum HDL cholesterol levels (Figure M-2). At present, there is no specific recommendation for a therapeutic goal for the serum HDL cholesterol level. However, the Framingham study has shown that for every 1-milligram-per-deciliter (mg/dL) fall in the serum HDL cholesterol concentration, there is about a 2 to 3 percent increase in the risk of having a cardiac event (Castelli et al., 1986).

Interventions used to raise the serum HDL cholesterol level, as in the able-bodied population, include diet, activity, and drug therapy. A three-center collaborative study (sponsored by the National Institute of Disability and Rehabilitation Research of the U.S. Department of Education) is under way to investigate the effect of Niaspan, a long-acting niacin preparation, on increasing HDL cholesterol levels and reducing the rate of vascular disease among individuals with spinal cord injuries. Smoking cessation is also associated with a rise in serum HDL cholesterol levels.

The conventional risk factors have been shown to account for only about half the total risk of a cardiac event. Thus, it may be worthwhile to touch on other emerging risk factors for coronary artery disease: LDL particle number, the lipoprotein(a) concentration, and the plasma homocysteine level. Evidence indicates that individuals with the metabolic syndrome have smaller, denser, and more atherogenic LDL particles. For the same absolute level of serum LDL cholesterol, if the amount of LDL particles in the circulation is increased, the risk of vascular disease is increased. If the caring physician were to base a therapeutic decision solely on the absolute concentration of serum LDL cholesterol, no treatment may be initiated. However, the risk of coronary artery disease may be elevated if the number of LDL particles is considered, as has recently been shown in several epidemiological studies.

Higher levels of lipoprotein(a) are atherogenic. It had been thought that the level of activity affected the serum lipoprotein(a) concentration. Contrary to expectation, the distribution of lipoprotein(a) levels in individuals with spinal cord injuries was similar to that in an age- and a gender-matched able-bodied population (Bauman et al., 1998b).

Elevated plasma homocysteine levels are vasotoxic. The concentrations of plasma homocysteine have been reported to be higher in those with spinal cord injuries than in a reference able-bodied population (Bauman et al., 2001).

Insulin Resistance

What are the determinants of insulin resistance? Body composition and an individual's level of activity largely influence insulin sensitivity. Increased adiposity and decreased muscle mass are associated with insulin resistance, as are decreased levels of activity and fitness.

Changes in body composition in individuals with spinal cord injuries occur immediately after the acute injury in a dramatic fashion and continue insidiously for years. There is an obvious and immediate loss of muscle tissue after an acute spinal cord injury, but for decades after the injury there is also a progressive, incremental loss of lean body tissue and a relative gain of adiposity. The mechanisms for this include paralysis and immobilization, as well as a possible reduction in anabolic forces (serum testosterone and growth hormone/insulin-like growth factor levels) and an elevation of catabolic hormone (angiotensin 1 and cortisol) levels. A study performed in conjunction with the Rancho Los Amigos National Rehabilitation Center showed that the percentage of total lean tissue in the body declined more rapidly in individuals with spinal cord injuries of all ages than in a matched able-bodied population (Figure M-3).

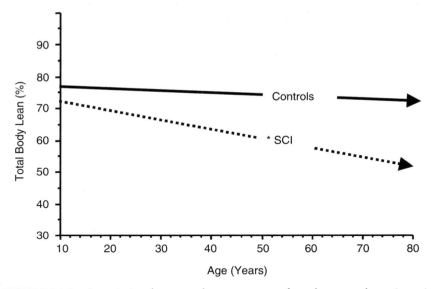

FIGURE M-3 Association between the percentage of total percent lean tissue in the body and age for able-bodied controls (solid arrow; slope = –0.102; r^2 = 0.02) compared with that for individuals with spinal cord injuries (SCI) (dashed arrow; slope = –0.275; r^2 = 0.10) (*, $p < 0.0001$).
SOURCE: Compiled from data presented by Spungen et al. (2003).

In the able-bodied population, the body mass index (BMI) is a surrogate measure of adiposity. A person with a spinal cord injury who has a BMI of 25.0 kilograms per meter squared (kg/m^2) has 10 to 15 percent more total body fat than an able-bodied individual with the same BMI (Figure M-4). Therefore, this commonly relied upon surrogate measure of adiposity in the able-bodied population grossly underestimates the true level of adiposity in those with spinal cord injuries.

Individuals with the highest and the most complete spinal cord injuries are at the lowest end of the activity spectrum. They have lost the greatest amount of muscle and are relatively fatter than individuals with lower cord lesions. Is there a greater risk of developing insulin resistance and problems with carbohydrate handling in those with the greatest neurological impairment? Those with high and complete spinal cord injuries have a 73 percent chance of having an abnormality in the ability to handle oral carbohydrates, either impaired glucose tolerance or diabetes mellitus, whereas other groups with spinal cord injuries (incomplete tetraplegia, complete paraple-

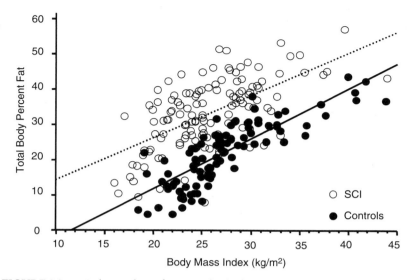

FIGURE M-4   Relationship of percent body fat to BMI for individuals with spinal cord injuries (SCI) compared with that for controls.
SOURCE: Spungen et al. (2003). Used with permission.

gia, and incomplete paraplegia) have significantly lower percentages (Figure M-5). Individuals with higher cord lesions (tetraplegia) have a higher prevalence of hyperinsulinemia than those with lower cord lesions (53 and 37 percent, respectively).

Individuals with spinal cord injuries have a cluster of risk factors for heart disease. What can be done to favorably modify the risk? The use of oral hypoglycemic agents in the general population has been shown to delay the progression from normal glucose tolerance or impaired glucose tolerance to diabetes. Serum HDL cholesterol may be raised by increasing the level of activity. The maintenance of a steady exercise routine is inherently difficult in able-bodied persons, and it is certainly no less difficult in those with spinal cord injuries. It should be noted that evidence suggests that small increases in fitness are associated with favorable metabolic changes, such as increases in serum HDL cholesterol levels. Thus, even modest improvements in the level of activity should be considered and pursued. When indicated, diet or pharmacological interventions, or both, should also be used to increase the serum HDL cholesterol concentration. Smoking cessation should be encouraged as another way to favorably affect the lipid profile.

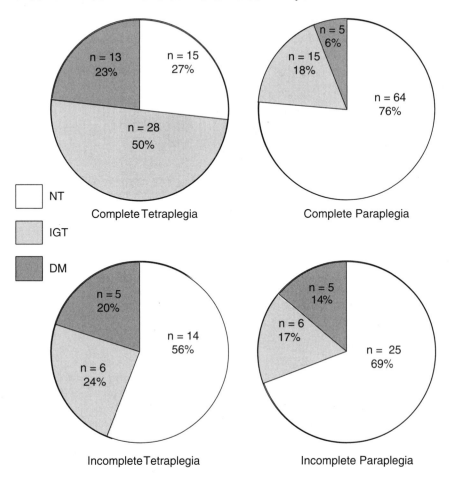

FIGURE M-5   Oral glucose tolerance by level of neurological deficit. NT = normal glucose tolerance; IGT = impaired glucose tolerance; DM = diabetes mellitus. SOURCE: Compiled from data presented by Bauman et al. (1999).

BOWEL EVACUATION

Individuals with spinal cord injuries often have difficulty with bowel evacuation. Bowel care can be extremely time-consuming and often inadequate, leaving the individual with the potential for accidents. Attendant care may be required as well, causing a loss of independence and privacy. Reduced bowel motility in those with spinal cord injuries is postulated to be due to defective or relatively reduced parasympathetic tone to the gut.

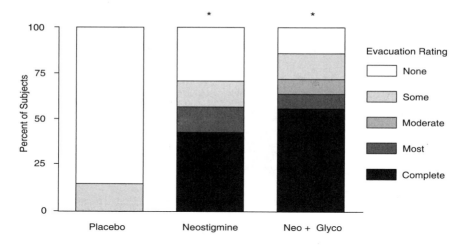

FIGURE M-6   Bowel evacuation after the administration of neostigmine or neo-stigmine and glycopyrrolate compared with that after administration of a placebo (*, $p < 0.01$ for both drugs compared with placebo).
SOURCE: Compiled from data presented by Korsten et al. (2005).

Increased gut motility and bowel evacuation after administration of a cho-linergic agent have been reported in individuals with spinal cord injuries. Because cholinergic agents are associated with adverse effects on the heart (bradycardia) and lung (bronchoconstriction), glycopyrrolate, a partial cho-linergic antagonist or blocker, has successfully been administered in con-junction with neostigmine, a cholinergic medication. Glycopyrrolate suc-cessfully blocks the adverse cardiopulmonary effects but preserves the effect of neostigmine on the bowel to produce evacuation (Figure M-6).

OSTEOPOROSIS

Osteoporosis in the appendicular skeleton is a source of morbidity in individuals with spinal cord injuries. Bone loss occurs very rapidly at the time of injury, and although this loss slows, it continues for years after the injury. In a study with identical twins, when an interpair difference score was determined—that is, when the bone mineral density (or bone mineral content) of the twin without a spinal cord injury was subtracted from that of the twin with a spinal cord injury—an estimate of the bone loss in the twin with a spinal cord injury can be generated. It was found that with longer duration of injury, more bone is lost in the lower extremities and pelvis (regions of the skeleton below the level of the lesion).

Bone loses its architectural structure by a loss of trabeculae and intervening struts as early as 1 or 2 years after acute immobilization. Once the normal architecture or connectivity is lost, the quality of bone is severely compromised, and this qualitative loss appears to be irreversible. Thus, bone loss must be prevented at the time of injury. To date, this has not yet been successfully accomplished in a clinically useful manner. The possibility exists that the prevention of bone loss may be feasible by the administration of an antiresorptive agent (e.g., a bisphosphonate) in conjunction with an osteoblastic agent or mechanical stimuli immediately after paralysis.

VITAMIN D DEFICIENCY

Individuals with spinal cord injuries have been shown to be vitamin D deficient. In one study, about one-third of military veterans with spinal cord injuries were vitamin D deficient, as were those at university hospitals and other community medical centers (unpublished findings). In the presence of vitamin D deficiency, parathyroid hormone (PTH) levels are elevated. An increase in the PTH level is often associated with increased bone turnover and bone loss. The Food and Nutrition Board of the Institute of Medicine recommends the consumption of 200 units of vitamin D per day until age 50 years and 400 units per day in those aged 50 years and older. In one study, 800 units of vitamin D per day were provided for 12 months to 40 individuals with spinal cord injuries (Figure M-7). At the baseline, 33

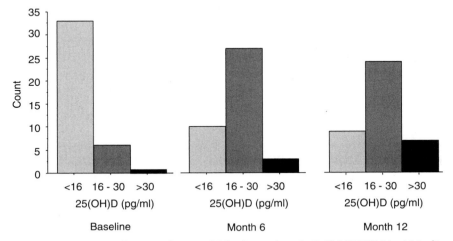

FIGURE M-7   Distribution of serum 25-hydroxyvitamin D [25(OH)D] in 40 individuals with spinal cord injuries who received supplementary vitamin D (800 units per day for 12 months).
SOURCE: Bauman et al. (2005). Used with permission.

subjects (83 percent) had vitamin D levels that were below the absolute lower limit of normal. After 12 months of vitamin D replacement therapy, 9 subjects (23 percent) had levels that remained below the normal range, and after 12 months 23 subjects (58 percent) had levels between 16 to 30 picograms per milliliter (pg/mL). Individuals with vitamin D levels between 16 and 30 pg/mL may be referred to as relatively vitamin D deficient because the plateau is not yet reached for maximum vitamin D-facilitated calcium absorption or for maximum PTH suppression. The significance of preventing osteoporosis would be to improve employment and personal activities, as well as afford psychological benefits.

PRESSURE ULCERS

Pressure ulcers occur in all immobilized individuals and are common in those with spinal cord injuries. They are a tremendous source of morbidity and carry with them a high cost of care. The cost of care rendered for pressure ulcers in hospitals, nursing homes, and home care nationwide has been estimated to be about $8 billion to $10 billion each year. In January 2005, the Cooperative Studies Program of the U.S. Department of Veterans Affairs funded a study to address pressure ulcer care in veterans with spinal cord injuries. The primary objective is to determine if inpatients with spinal cord injuries who have a full-thickness pressure ulcer of the pelvic region and who receive optimized clinical care and an oral anabolic agent for 24 weeks or less have a greater percentage of full healing than those who receive placebo and the same clinical care. The expectation is to learn the percentage of full-thickness ulcers that healed completely; the healing rate; and the effects of nutrition, inflammatory, and endocrine factors on pressure ulcer healing.

CONCLUSION

In summary, most individuals with spinal cord injuries have learned to adapt to being paralyzed. The secondary complications may have a greater impact on quality of life than the loss of ambulation. The knowledge gained from studying the secondary consequences of spinal cord injuries can be transferred, in large measure, to other disabilities or immobilizing conditions. The cost of investigating the problems associated with the medical consequences of spinal cord injuries is slight compared with the cost of care after neglecting them.

REFERENCES

Bauman WA, Spungen AN. Carbohydrate and lipid metabolism in chronic spinal cord injury. *Journal of Spinal Cord Medicine* 2001; 24:266–277.

Bauman WA, Adkins RH, Spungen AM, Kemp BJ, Waters RL. The effect of residual neurological deficit on serum lipoproteins in individuals with spinal cord injury. *Spinal Cord* 1998a; 36:13–17.

Bauman WA, Adkins RH, Spungen AM, Herbert R, Schecter C, Smith D, Waters RL. Individuals with extreme inactivity do not have abnormal serum Lp(a) levels. *Horm Metab Res* 1998b; 30:601–603.

Bauman WA, Adkins RH, Spungen AM, Waters RL. The effect of residual neurological deficit on oral glucose tolerance in persons with chronic spinal cord injury. *Spinal Cord* 1999; 37(11):765–771.

Bauman WA, Adkins RH, Spungen AM, Waters RL, Kemp BJ, Herbert V. Levels of plasma homocysteine in a population of persons with spinal cord injury. *J Spinal Cord Med* 2001; 24:81–86.

Bauman WA, Morrison NG, Spungen AM. Vitamin D replacement therapy in persons with spinal cord injury. *Journal of Spinal Cord Medicine* 2005; 28:203–207.

Castelli WP, Garrison RJ, Wilson PWF, Abbott RD, Kalousdian S, Kannel WB. Incidence of coronary heart disease and lipoprotein cholesterol levels: the Framingham Study. *Journal of the American Medical Association* 1986; 256:2835–2838.

Gordon DJ, Probstfield JL, Garrison RJ, Neaton JD, Castelli WP, Knoke JD, Jacobs DR Jr, Bangdiwala S, Tyroler HA. High-density lipoprotein cholesterol and cardiovascular disease. Four prospective American studies. *Circulation* 1989; 79(1):8–15.

Korsten MA, Rosman AS, Ng A, Cavusoglu E, Spungen AM, Radulovic M, Wecht J, Bauman WA. Infusion of neostigmine-glycopyrrolate for bowel evacuation in persons with spinal cord injury. *American Journal of Gastroenterology* 2005; 100(7):1560–1565.

Linn WS, Spungen AM, Gong H Jr, Adkins RH, Bauman WA, Waters RL. Forced vital capacity in two large outpatient populations with chronic spinal cord injury. *Spinal Cord* 2001; 39(5):263–268.

Spungen AM, Adkins RH, Stewart CA, Wang J, Pierson RN Jr., Waters RL, Bauman WA. Factors influencing body composition in persons with spinal cord injury: a cross-sectional study. *Journal of Applied Physiology* 2003; 95:2398–2407.

Whiteneck GG, Charlifue SW, Frankel HL, Fraser MH, Gardner BP, Gerhart KA, Krishnan KR, Menter RR, Nuseibeh I, Short DJ, et al. Mortality, morbidity, and psychosocial outcomes of persons spinal cord injured more than 20 years ago. *Paraplegia* 1992; 30(9):617–630.

N

Depression as a Secondary Condition in People with Disabilities

Bryan Kemp, Ph.D.[*]

D epression is one of the world's most common health problems in the general population, affecting more than 5 percent of all people (Schulberg et al., 1999). In the United States, about 15 percent of the general population will suffer from a major depressive disorder at some time in their life (U.S. Department of Health and Human Services, 1993), and to cost the economy $40 billion annually (Robinson et al., 2005). Major depression is especially disabling, but even moderate depression affects daily functioning. Depression has been estimated to be as disabling as congestive heart disease, severe arthritis, and early dementia (Wells et al., 1989).

Depression among people who already have a disability is an especially important and complicated issue. Depression is one of the most common, if not the most common, secondary conditions associated with disability. When it is left untreated, depression can cause inordinate personal suffering, increased disability, additional health problems, and stress in others. It is only recently that there has been any focus on secondary conditions in people who have a disability. The 1991 IOM report *Disability in America* devoted a chapter to the topic and included depression in the discussion

---

[*]Bryan Kemp, Ph.D., Director, Rehabilitation Research and Training Center on Aging with a Disability, Rancho Los Amigos National Rehabilitation Center, and Professor of Medicine and Psychology, Program in Geriatrics, University of California, Irvine. The analyses and views presented in this workshop paper are those of the author and not necessarily those of the Institute of Medicine Committee on Disability in America: A New Look.

234

(Pope and Tarlov, 1991). Previously, most preventive research and policy efforts focused on prevention of the primary impairment, such as a spinal cord injury, cerebral palsy, or brain trauma. It is now recognized that it is just as important, if not more important, to address the inordinately high rate of secondary conditions that people with disabilities have.

An entire chapter of the recently published report *Healthy People 2010* was related to disability and secondary conditions in people with disabilities (U.S. Department of Health and Human Services, 2001). Through this focused attention, the report sought to "promote the health of people with disabilities, prevent secondary conditions, and eliminate disparities between people with and without disabilities in the United States" (p. 3). Of the variety of secondary conditions that occur in people with primary impairments, depression was pointed out as being particularly important. Although there were relatively few data available at the time, that report highlighted the fact that people who have a disability reported having more days of pain, depression, and anxiety and fewer days of vitality during the previous month compared with the rates among people without a disability. That report also emphasized the need for more research, particularly applied research, on the problem of depression among people with disabilities.

A growing focus in the disability community today is the recently noted increase in life expectancy among people with impairments and chronic disabilities, including people with the most severe impairments. For example, life expectancy for a person with a spinal cord injury has increased more than 1,000 percent in the last 40 years (Sasma et al., 1993). Other groups with impairments such as cerebral palsy, polio, rheumatoid arthritis, and Down syndrome are showing similar increases in life expectancy. This aging of people with disabilities has resulted in what appears to be increased secondary conditions as people grow older. Recent research on these conditions (Kemp and Mosqueda, 2004) indicates that as people age with a disability they are at an even higher risk of secondary conditions than they were earlier in their lives. Changes such as a loss of function, increased pain, increased fatigue, and multiple medical problems present new challenges and new stresses to people with disabilities. These new challenges and stresses have a strong likelihood of resulting in difficulties adjusting and a possible increase in the likelihood of depression.

This paper describes what is known about the nature of depression in people with disabilities, its prevalence in groups of people with physical impairments, its possible causes and consequences, the assessment and treatment of depression in people with disabilities, and future research and practice needs. It is clear that better understanding, recognition, and treatment of depression for people with disabilities is an important avenue for improving a range of outcomes that are important to the people with disabilities. For example, it is hard to imagine that people who have a disability and who are also depressed stand much of a chance of having a good quality of life. It is also likely that people who have a disability and who are depressed are likely to suffer even more health problems. The primary care physicians who encounter people with disabilities are relatively untrained and unsophisticated in dealing with the multiple medical, social, and psychological issues that a person with a disability may have. Improving the understanding of depression and its treatment can help primary care physicians and others better address these needs in people with disabilities.

SECONDARY CONDITIONS AND COMORBIDITIES

Disability in America defines a secondary condition as a new pathology, impairment, functional limitation, or disability that is causally linked to a primary disabling condition (Pope and Tarlov, 1991). In other words, according to the report, the secondary condition would not occur or would be less likely to occur without the existence of the primary condition. Secondary conditions can have either a direct or an indirect causal relationship to the primary impairment. A common direct relationship is one between a pressure sore and a spinal cord injury. Without the spinal cord injury, it is likely that the person would not have developed a pressure sore. Depression is likely an example of a condition with an indirect causal relationship to the primary impairment, because high levels of stress (from the physical environment, interpersonal relations, and health problems) result in an increased risk of hypertension, fatigue, increased disability, and, possibly, depression. Because there is rarely a one-to-one correspondence between a primary impairment and a secondary condition (everyone with the primary impairment does not get the secondary condition), it would perhaps be better to say that the primary impairment increased the risk of a secondary condition through either a direct or an indirect mechanism. Thus, it can be seen that people with disabilities are more vulnerable to certain other conditions. Furthermore, as people with disabilities age, the effects of aging may interact with the disability to further increase vulnerability. Many people with disabilities report that their secondary health conditions are more troublesome—and often are more disabling—than their primary condition.

A comorbidity is a condition that is not related to an individual's primary impairment. For example, some forms of cancer may occur in people with a disability without being directly or indirectly caused by the primary disability. People who have a disability may still get the flu, although they may not get it at a higher rate than anybody else. From a practical point of view, the presence of a primary impairment, an increased risk of secondary conditions, increased vulnerability because of aging with a disability, and the ordinary risks of sustaining any comorbid conditions make people with disabilities unique in terms of their health and health care needs. Hence, the prevention of secondary health problems among people with disabilities would do a lot to improve the quality of their lives and, furthermore, would decrease the risks of hospitalization and further disability.

DEPRESSION AS A SECONDARY CONDITION

Depression clearly fits within the definition of a secondary condition. This is especially evident if one focuses on the higher rate of depression among people with disabilities compared with that among the general population. It is unlikely that there is a direct causal relationship between having a disability and developing a depressive disorder because not everyone who has a disability becomes depressed, and as evidence indicates, there is practically no relationship between the severity of the disability and the occurrence of depression (see below).

Depression does appear, however, to be indirectly related to having a disability. The indirect link between depression and disability could be mediated by a variety of mechanisms, but the increased stresses that frequently accompany having a disability are likely. This issue will be further explored below; however, it is clear that having a disability exposes a person to higher rates of economic, environmental, interpersonal, health, and vocational problems than the rates found in the nondisabled population. These increased stresses and the challenges of coping with them appear to contribute to the higher rates of depression among people with disabilities.

Ultimately, depression is a biopsychosocial disorder both in its causes and in its consequences. There are physical aspects to the disorder in terms of central nervous system and autonomic nervous system changes, there are psychological changes in terms of thinking and emotion, and there are social aspects to depression in terms of support from others and the consequences on others. Therefore, having a depressive disorder when one also has a disability may lead to additional problems that will in turn cause more complications. Understanding the mechanisms involved in the development of depression secondary to a disability is essential for both the prevention and the treatment of depression as well as the possibility of reducing other health problems. For example, it is quite common for a person who has a spinal cord injury and who is depressed to not look after himself or herself very well. Consequently, the rates of pressure sores tend to be higher among people who have a depressive disorder. Pressure sores represent one of the most expensive and devastating secondary health problems for people with spinal cord injuries. Yet, it is not possible to fully reduce the rate of pressure sores in this population without also understanding the mechanisms by which pressure sores occur through the avenue of a depressive disorder.

DEFINING AND MEASURING DEPRESSION AMONG PEOPLE WITH DISABILITIES

Three major issues complicate research on and clinical interventions for depression among people with disabilities. The first issue is defining depression, the second issue involves the measurement of depression as it applies to people with disabilities, and the third issue concerns the environmental barriers to obtaining proper clinical interventions for people who have a disability and who are depressed.

The *Diagnostic and Statistical Manual of Mental Disorders* (DSM-IV) (American Psychiatric Association, 1995) states that depression is not a single entity but rather a spectrum of disorders that are classified on the basis of the number, severity, type, and progressiveness of the symptoms and their durations and effects on an individual's function. The central feature of all depressive disorders is an altered mood state that is not normal for that person. This altered mood state may include sadness and melancholia; but it may also include, and frequently does include, irritability or apathy. Other symptoms of depression that need to be present to meet a full diagnosis include those from the categories of cognition, behavior, and physiology. These other symptoms may include changes in appetite or sleep, fatigue or excess subjective pain, decreased energy, or changes in digestion. They may also include thoughts of hopelessness and helplessness or, possibly, even thoughts of suicide. Frequently, the cognitive impairment is also such that the person is incapable of thinking rationally; and reports of memory problems or attention deficits are also frequent. Behavioral symptoms may include not looking after one's self, not interacting with others in a meaningful or appropriate manner, not following instructions for medical care, and not engaging in meaningful or pleasurable activities. Unfortunately, some of the confusion in the literature and the lack of ability to compare findings result from investigators using the term "depression" to apply to any of the range of disorders across the spectrum.

The diagnosis of depression is ultimately determined after an extensive evaluation. Anything short of that represents some approximation of depression. Instruments that have been developed to assess and measure depression can come close to obtaining true rates of depression if they have been properly designed and validated for the population in question. The population of people with disabilities is unique in terms of the use of instruments to measure depression. The problem is that scales that include a large proportion of physiological symptoms (e.g., pain, fatigue, and digestive problems) may be assessing the effects of a disability or true health problems rather than depression.

Several screening instruments have been developed to help identify people who may be depressed. They include but are not limited to the Beck Depression Inventory (Beck et al., 1961), the Zung Self-Rating Depression Scale (Zung, 1965), and the Centers for Epidemiological Studies Depression Scale (Radloff, 1977). All of these scales are used both for nondisabled people and for people with disabilities. At least two screening instruments are especially helpful in identifying depression in groups of people with disabilities. They are the Older Adult Health and Mood Questionnaire, developed by Kemp and Adams (1995), and the Geriatric Depression Scale, developed by Yesavage and colleagues (1983). Although these two tools were developed from work with a geriatric population, the primary thing that they were trying to compensate for was not age but the presence of the chronic disabling conditions that frequently accompany age. These scales have been used in studies that have included adults with disabilities who were not necessarily part of the geriatric population and have produced many important findings.

It is important to accurately screen for and assess depression in people who have a disability because even relatively minor or moderate levels of depression have been found to have a major impact on health, activities of daily living, and interpersonal relationships among people with disabilities (Hybels et al., 2001). This fact highlights the importance of recognizing and treating all forms of depression, but it also highlights the need to be able to differentiate the different degrees of depression for research purposes. To the extent that studies report either full diagnostic workups or report the results from instruments validated against full workups, they will reflect better data.

The third issue, environmental barriers to proper treatment for people with disabilities who are depressed, relates to how people with disabilities are viewed by clinicians and how they obtain access to services. The major obstacle to the proper treatment of depression, especially major depression, is getting it identified. The high rate of depression among people with disabilities (and other "minority" groups) implies that it is not being properly identified and treated.

PREVALENCE OF DEPRESSION
AMONG PEOPLE WITH DISABILITIES

Estimates of the prevalence of depression among people with disabilities vary greatly, depending on the nature of the measurement method, when the measurement was taken relative to the time of onset of the disability, the kind of impairment, and the definition of depression being used.

The overall rate of depression among individuals with disabilities reported in *Healthy People 2010* was about 28 percent (U.S. Department of Health and Human Services, 2001). This finding was based primarily on one question asked in the National Health Interview Survey: "During the past 30 days, how often did you feel so sad that nothing could cheer you up?" That question was then followed up with another question if the person answered positively: "All together, how much did these feelings interfere with your life or activities: a lot, some, a little, or not at all?" The rate of agreement with this statement was 7 percent among people without disabilities.

Other studies have also found rates higher than those cited above. For example, Fuhrer and colleagues (1993) reported a rate of depression of about 40 percent among people with spinal cord injuries. Hughes and colleagues (2001) reported that the rate was even higher among women with spinal cord injuries, and the Consortium for Spinal Cord Injury (1998) established the rate of depression in people with spinal cord injuries to be about 25 percent. Dickens and colleagues (2003) reported that the rate of depression, as measured by standardized methods, was 39 percent among people with rheumatoid arthritis.

Over the last 10 years, the Rehabilitation Research and Training Center on Aging with a Disability and Aging with Spinal Cord Injury has conducted studies of depression among people with various impairments to help establish rates of depression. Krause and colleagues (2001) reported on the rate of depression among more than 1,300 people with spinal cord injuries. The overall prevalence was 42 percent. In a sample of people with cerebral palsy, the rate of depression was also found to be 40 percent. Rates of up to 50 percent and higher have been found among people who have had a stroke (Robinson, 2003). These rates include the rates of both moderate and major depression. In each of these cases, approximately half of the cases of depression were severe and major. Figure N-1 displays the rates of moderate and major depression in groups of people with various types of disabling conditions.

Depression among people with disability is as common as disabling arthritis, heart disease, and diabetes combined in the general population. According to the National Center for Health Statistics (1989), the rates of conditions causing activity limitations across all ages in the United States were as follows: arthritis, 12 percent; heart disease, 11 percent; asthma, 4 percent; orthopedic impairments, 21 percent; and diabetes, 3 percent. In 1990, the Centers for Disease Control and Prevention initiated the first national colloquium dedicated to the prevention of secondary conditions after a spinal cord injury (Graitcer and Maynard, 1990). This colloquium met at Craig Hospital in Denver, Colorado. The topic of depression was considered to be so important that it was made the number one psychological issue to be addressed as a secondary condition in people with spinal

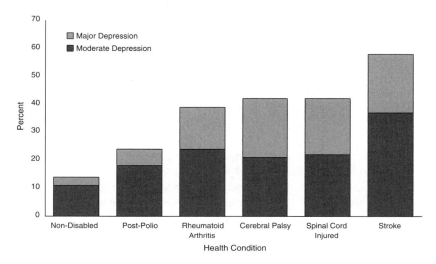

FIGURE N-1   Depression prevalence among people with different types of disabling conditions.
SOURCES: Robinson (2003), Kemp and Krause (1999), Krause et al. (2001), Dickens and Creed (2001), and Rehabilitation Research and Training Center on Aging with a Disability (2003).

cord injuries. Several types of research needs were outlined, including more epidemiological research and research on prevention and care.

In summary, the overall rate of depressive disorders, including both moderate and severe depression, among people with physical disabilities appears to be somewhere between 25 and 50 percent, with approximately half of these cases being major depression. Therefore, one person in four or one person in three who has a primary physical impairment likely also has a depressive disorder. This rate is approximately four times higher than that in the nondisabled population. This figure points to the necessity for regular, routine screening for depression among people with disabilities who consult health providers. However, it fails to recognize the fact that many people who are depressed and who have disabilities do not have a primary health care provider and lack adequate screening for this problem.

CAUSES OF DEPRESSION AMONG PEOPLE WITH DISABILITIES

Understanding the causes of depression in people with disabilities is an important and complex issue for both clinical and research purposes. Clinically, if practitioners believe that depression is caused by the disability, they may be less inclined to provide optimal care because they may believe that if nothing can be done to cure the disability, then nothing can be done to cure the depression. Therefore, depression may wrongly become viewed as "normal" for people with disability. Research is needed to help identify the true causes of depression so that ways to prevent it and to treat it can better be identified.

Depression does not appear to be a direct result of having a disability. In many studies it has been shown that there is little or no relationship between the severity of impairment or the degree of disability and the rate of depression as measured. For example, McColl and Rosenthal (1994) studied 70 people with spinal cord injuries of various ages and with various durations of disability. They found no relationship between the level of spinal cord injury, scores on the Functional Independence Measure, age, or the duration of the injury and depression. Similarly, in the study by Fuhrer and colleagues (1992), the rates of depression among people with paraplegia were the same as the rates among people with tetraplegia. In the study by Robinson (2003), depression was found to be unrelated to the size or the location of the stroke. In a large-scale study of more than 1,300 people with spinal cord injuries, Krause and colleagues (2001) found no relationship between the level of the spinal cord injury and the rate of depression that was measured. The higher rate of depression in people with disabilities is likely the result of the disability per se. It is therefore more likely that depression relates to disability in an indirect manner.

One model that may help explain such a relationship is a general stress and coping model. This kind of model, described by Lazarus and Folkman (1984) and Haley and colleagues (1987), describes stress and coping as a dynamic interplay involving five primary variables. They argue that the interplay between these five variables helps to determine the outcome from potentially stressful life situations, such as having a disability. These five variables are (1) the number and nature of negative life events that a person faces; (2) the person's view or appraisal of those events in terms of the perceived degree of threat to his or her future and current well-being; (3) the support that the person receives from other people, both instrumentally and emotionally; (4) the coping methods that the person uses to help deal with these stressors; and (5) the person's underlying personality. By understanding each of these variables and the interplay among them, research has been able to account for differences in outcomes, such as depression, given the same objective life events, such as a disability.

It has been argued that among people who do not adjust well to stressful life events and who become depressed, problems or deficits in one or more of these areas is likely. For example, those who become depressed are more likely to have a higher number of negative life events over a given period of time than people who are not depressed. Dickens and Creed (2001) studied people with rheumatoid arthritis longitudinally and found that depression occurred following a deterioration in functional ability. Moreover, deterioration in the activities that the person regarded as especially important (e.g., family and recreation) had the highest correlation with the onset of depression. A 10 percent reduction in valued activities was followed by a 700 percent increase in the rate of depression in the following year. Similarly, people who become depressed are likely to interpret these events in more negative terms than people who do not become depressed (Elliott et al., 1991; Cairns and Baker, 1993). Also, people who become depressed are less likely to have resources in terms of income or support from others to help deal with the stressful life events.

It is likely that differences in these kinds of variables are the source of the differences between rates of depression in nondisabled and disabled individuals. It is clear from the results presented earlier that the level of disability and the severity of impairment are related to the likelihood of depression.

In the study by McColl and Rosenthal (1994), depression was negatively related to social support but not to the level of injury. The statistical correlation (r) between depression and social support was –0.55, indicating a moderate to strong negative relationship. Additionally, people who have a disability have more health problems than people who do not have a disability, and the number of health problems has been found to correlate positively with depression (Kemp et al., 1997; Tate et al., 1994).

Depression is also related to the coping method in people with disabilities. Tate and colleagues (1993) found that people with polio who were depressed had poorer coping methods than people with polio who were not depressed. The same was found for people with multiple sclerosis (Lynch et al., 2001) and spinal cord injuries (Shulz and Decker, 1985). They found that coping methods that are more negative, such as escape-avoidance coping, typically correlates about 0.40 with negative outcomes such as depression in people with spinal cord injuries. People who are less likely to be depressed also appear to have more positive attitudes toward their disabilities (Kemp et al., 1997). Thus, mounting evidence suggests that aspects of stress and coping are predictive of depression. Moreover, because people with disabilities live with the disability long term and experience multiple stressors, they may develop more negative appraisals about what to expect in the future. Certainly, difficulties with obtaining adequate health care, maintaining employment, and economic survival and the ongoing pain and discouragement could lead to more negative appraisals. An important piece of research would be to test this kind of model with people who are depressed and those who are not depressed but who have equivalent disabilities. Figure N-2 presents this general stress and coping model.

The other advantage of a model like this is that it could help direct prevention and intervention efforts toward reducing depression. That is,

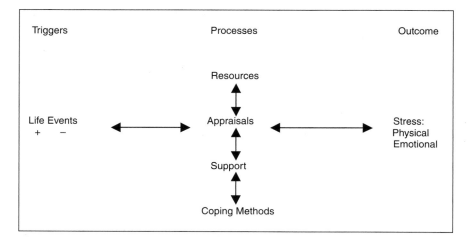

FIGURE N-2 A general model of psychological stress and coping.
SOURCES: Adapted from Lazarus and Folkman (1984) and Haley et al. (1987).

each of those five variables is something that can, for the most part, be modified and that can be improved to treat depression. For example, if the number of negative life events in a person with a disability is high and comprises such things as health problems, economic problems, and housing problems, then efforts should be directed toward improving those areas of the person's life. If the difficulty was with the use of inappropriate coping methods, then efforts could be used in counseling to explore other coping methods and try to reduce stress.

CONSEQUENCES OF DEPRESSION FOR
PEOPLE WITH DISABILITY

Depression has multiple consequences for a person with a disability, including effects on longevity, function, community activities, and quality of life. Morris and colleagues (1993) studied over a 10-year period the rates of survival of depressed and nondepressed people who had had a stroke. After 10 years the probability of survival for the nondepressed group was approximately 65 percent, whereas the probability of survival was approximately 30 percent for the depressed group. The difference between the groups increased exponentially each year. The mechanisms involved in the differential survival rates were thought to be more indirect than direct. That is, it was probably not a result of differential suicide rates but, rather, differences in compliance with medications, adherence to health programs, engagement in exercise, cessation of smoking, and regular follow-up examinations.

Wells and colleagues (1989) concluded that depression and chronic medical conditions had unique and additive effects on patient dysfunctioning. Dickens and Creed (2001) showed that depression added significantly to the health and social problems of people with rheumatoid arthritis, even when they controlled for the degree of disease. Krause and colleagues (2001) found that people with spinal cord injuries who were depressed used more alcohol and had more hospitalizations than people who were not depressed.

In studies at the Rehabilitation Research and Training Center on Aging with Disability, colleagues and I have monitored people longitudinally over 5-year spans. In one of those studies, we examined changes in activities of daily living among people with disability by status on a depression scale. The results showed that over a 5-year period, activities of daily living decreased nearly twice as much for people who were depressed compared to people who were not depressed. In another study, Kemp and colleagues (2004) assessed community activities and life satisfaction in people with spinal cord injuries who were depressed. Those individuals participated in one-third the number of community activities compared with the number for the nondepressed individuals, and their life satisfaction scores were 40 percent below those for people who were not depressed. In and of itself, the level of spinal cord injury had no effect on these findings.

TREATING DEPRESSION

Although the literature contains scores of articles about depression and disability, relatively few of them concern the treatment of depression. In a recent article, Elliott and Kennedy (2004) reviewed an extensive range of studies in the spinal cord injury literature with the purpose of finding and evaluating the quality of intervention studies directly concerned with the treatment of depression. They found many correlates and concomitants of depressive symptoms among people with spinal cord injuries, but they could find only nine treatment studies that met the criteria for inclusion in their review. Three of the studies were psychological interventions, five studies described antidepressant therapy, and one study reported on the effects of electrical stimulation. Only one of these studies used a randomized assignment to treatment and control groups, but that study excluded people with major depression. Most studies of psychological interventions focused on support groups, counseling, and peer groups. Furthermore, many of the studies focused on inpatients who were undergoing rehabilitation at the same time. Relatively few studies have focused on people living with a disability long term in the community.

King and Kennedy (1999) performed a study that shows both a way to treat depression in people with disabilities and a way to help prevent it. They used a group approach called the Coping Effectiveness Training (CET) program, which was grounded in the stress and coping model of Lazarus and Folkman (1984). A total of 38 inpatients with spinal cord injuries were divided into treatment and control groups. The treatment group had lower rates of depression at the end of the study. Moreover, the social interaction and reappraisals of the disability were the most important factors in alleviating depression. Such programs as this one could be used to help prevent depression in people with disabilities.

Recently, Kemp and colleagues (2004) studied the effects of treating major depression in people with spinal cord injuries using a combination of psychotherapy and antidepressant medication. They used a quasiexperimental design in which the comparison group declined treatment but was monitored over a similar period of time as those who elected to receive treatment. That study evaluated three outcomes. The first involved changes on a 22-item scale for the measurement of depression. The second was an 11-item life satisfaction scale in which each item was rated on a 4-point scale, with 1 being "mostly dissatisfied" and 4 being "mostly satisfied." A 16-item community activities checklist that measured the number of times during the last 7 days that a person had engaged in a variety of community activities was also included. Over a 6-month course of treatment, there was a 57 percent reduction in the rate of depressive symptoms among the treated individuals, whereas there was no reduction in symptoms among those who declined treatment. Moreover, approximately half the participants in the treated group were either not depressed or had lower degrees of depression by the end of the treatment. Finally, those who received treatment showed an increase in community activities that corresponded to decreases in depressive symptoms and also showed a 40 percent increase in life satisfaction compared with that at the beginning of the treatment. More studies testing treatment interventions are needed to help deal with this important problem. The results of that study are presented in Figure N-3.

One area of research that is needed should determine whether people with disabilities who are also depressed are recognized, properly assessed, and properly treated by their primary physicians. There is relatively little information on this phenomenon, but it is an area of great concern. Considering the fact that Krause and colleagues (2001) found a 40 percent rate of depression and found that very few people were treated implies that this problem goes relatively unrecognized or untreated in the community. In that study, more than 525 people met the criteria for moderate or major depression, yet none of them was being treated. As the country moves toward a managed care model of the provision of health care, with the short appointment times that are part of that model, it will be even more

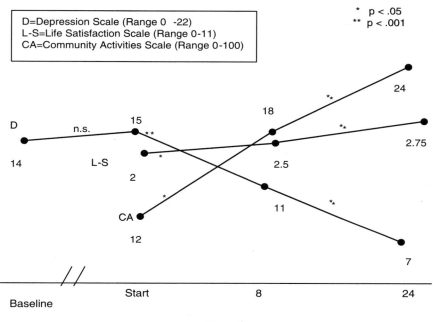

FIGURE N-3   Effects of treatment on depression. n.s. = not significant.
SOURCE: Kemp et al. (2004).

important to be able to screen individuals quickly and accurately and to refer them for further assessment and treatment.

NEEDED RESEARCH

Research on depression and disability is needed, particularly in the following areas: (1) determination of whether primary care physicians are accurately identifying people with disabilities who are depressed; (2) determination of whether people who have a disability and are depressed are being adequately treated; (3) testing of the interventions that best help people who are depressed and who have a disability; (4) testing of a stress and coping model in a sample of people with disabilities; (5) assessment of the effects of consumer education and various interventions to help prevent depression, such as the teaching of methods to help people cope with stress; (6) determination of the length of treatment interventions that are optimal for people with disabilities; (7) identification of whether peer counseling is a good adjunct component to standard care for people with disabilities; (8) identification of strategies to help prevent the occurrence of depression in the population of people at risk who have a disability; (9) further study of the effects of depression on other health problems in people with disabilities; and (10) the development and cross-validation of more instruments for the identification of depression in people with disabilities.

CONCLUSIONS

Depression is a common and serious secondary condition among people with disabilities. The rates of moderate and major depression combined are between 25 and 50 percent across impairment groups. Both moderate and major depression can have serious consequences on health status, functional abilities, longevity, interpersonal relations, and quality of life. It appears likely that the disability and its underlying impairment are not direct causes of depression in people with disabilities. Instead, other factors, such as those involved in a stress and coping model, are likely more important. Issues such as the number and nature of negative life events, social support, coping methods, and one's outlook and viewpoint about stresses and coping appear to be more important than the disability itself. There are several important issues in studying depression among people with disabilities, including the proper definition of depression, the development and use of instruments that take into account their unique health problems, and finally, the proper treatment of depression by reducing some of the environmental and professional training issues that stand in the way. The evidence to date suggests that when proper treatment is provided, depression can be improved and other outcomes are also improved, such as quality of life and community participation. Research is needed in this area to investigate other avenues of treatment and to help validate the approaches that help the best.

REFERENCES

American Psychiatric Association. (1995). *Diagnostic and Statistical Manual of Mental Disorders*, 4th ed. Washington, DC: American Psychiatric Association.

Beck, A.T., Ward, C.H., Mendelson, M., Moch, J., and Erbaugh, J. (1961). An inventory for measuring depression. *Archives of General Psychiatry*, 4, 53–63.

Cairns, D. and Baker, J. (1993). Adjustment to spinal cord injury: a review of coping styles contributing to the process. *Journal of Rehabilitation*, 59, 30–33.

Consortium for Spinal Cord Injury. (1998). *Depression Following Spinal Cord Injury: A Clinical Practice Guideline for Primary Care Physicians*. Washington, DC: Paralyzed Veterans of America.

Dickens, C. and Creed, F. (2001). The burden of depression in patients with rheumatoid arthritis. *Rheumatology*, 40, 1327–1330.

Dickens, C., Jackson, J., Tomenson, B., Hay, E., and Creed, F. (2003). Association of depression and rheumatoid arthritis. *Psychosomatics*, 44(3), 209–215.

Elliott, T.R. and Kennedy, P. (2004). Treatment of depression following spinal cord injury: an evidenced-based review. *Rehabilitation Psychology*, 49(2), 134–139.

Elliott, T.R., Godshall, F., Herrick, S., Witty, T., and Spruell, M. (1991). Problem-solving appraisal and psychological adjustment following spinal cord injury. *Cognitive Therapy Research*, 15, 387–398.

Fuhrer, M.J., Rintala, D.H., Hart, K.A., Clearman, R., and Young, M.E. (1992). Relationship of life satisfaction to impairment, disability, and handicap among persons with spinal cord injury living in the community. *Archives of Physical Medicine and Rehabilitation*, 73, 552–557.

Fuhrer, M.J., Rintala, D.H., Hart, K.A., Clearman, R., and Young, M.E. (1993). Depressive symptomotology in persons with spinal cord injury who reside in the community. *Archives of Physical Medicine and Rehabilitation*, 74, 255–260.

Graitcer, P.D. and Maynard, F.M. (1990). Psychosocial secondary disabilities. In P.O. Graitcer and F.M. Maynard (eds.). *First Colloquium on Preventing Secondary Disabilities among People with Spinal Cord Injuries*. Atlanta, GA: U.S. Department of Health and Human Services. Pp. 71–77.

Haley, W.E., Levine, E.G., Brown, S.L., and Bartolucci, A.A. (1987). Stress, appraisal, coping and social support as predictors of adaptational outcome among dementia caregivers. *Psychology of Aging*, 2, 323–330.

Hughes, R.B., Swedlund, N., Petersen, N., and Nosek, M.A. (2001). Depression and women with SCI. *Topics in Spinal Cord Injury Rehabilitation*, 7: 16–24.

Hybels, C.F., Blazer, D.G., and Pieper, C.F. (2001). Toward a threshold for subthreshold depression: an analysis of correlates of depression by severity of symptoms using data from an elderly community sample. *Gerontologist*, 41(3), 357–365.

Kemp, B. and Adams, B. (1995). The Older Adult Health and Mood Questionnaire: a new measure of geriatric depressive disorder. *Journal of Geriatric Psychiatry and Neurology*, 8, 162–167.

Kemp, B. and Mosqueda, L. (eds.). (2004). *Aging with a Disability: What the Clinician Needs to Know*. Baltimore, MD: The Johns Hopkins University Press.

Kemp, B., Adams, B., and Campbell, M. (1997). Depression and life satisfaction in aging polio survivors versus age matched controls. *Archives of Physical Medicine and Rehabilitation*, 78, 187–192.

Kemp, B.J. and Krause, J.S. (1999). Depression and life satisfaction among people ageing with a disability: a comparison of post-polio and spinal cord injury. *Disability and Rehabilitation*, 21(5/6), 241–249.

Kemp, B.J., Kahan, J.K., Krause, J.S., Adkins, R.H., and Nava, G. (2004). Treatment of major depression in individuals with spinal cord injury. *Journal of Spinal Cord Medicine*, 27, 22–28.

King, C. and Kennedy, P. (1999). Coping effectiveness training for people with spinal cord injury: preliminary results of a controlled trial. *British Journal of Clinical Psychology*, 38(Pt.1), 5–14.

Krause, J.S., Kemp, B., and Coker, J. (2001). Depression after spinal cord injury: relation to gender, ethnicity, aging, and socioeconomic indicators. *Archives of Physical Medicine and Rehabilitation*, 81, 1099–1109.

Lazarus, R.S. and Folkman, S. (1984). *Stress, Appraisal and Coping*. New York: Springer Publishing Co.

Lynch, S.G., Kroeneke, D.C., and Denney, D.R. (2001). The relationship between disability and depression in multiple sclerosis: the role of uncertainty, coping and hope. *Multiple Sclerosis*, 7, 411–416.

McColl, M.A. and Rosenthal, C. (1994). A model of resource needs of aging spinal cord injured men. *Paraplegia*, 32, 261–270.

Morris, P.L.P., Robinson, R.G., Andrzejewski, M.S., Samuels, J., and Price, T.R. (1993). Association of depression with 10-year post-stroke mortality. *American Journal of Psychiatry*, 150, 124–129.

National Center for Health Statistics. (1989). Questionnaires from the National Health Interview Survey, 1980–84. Vital and Health Statistics, Series 1, No. 24, DHHS Publication (PHS) 90-1302. Washington, DC: U.S. Government Printing Office.

Pope, A.M. and Tarlov, A.R. (eds.). (1991). *Disability in America: Toward a National Agenda for Prevention*. Committee on a National Agenda for the Prevention of Disabilities, Division of Health Promotion and Disease Prevention, Institute of Medicine. Washington, DC: National Academy Press.

Radloff, L.S. (1977). The CES-D scale: a self-report depression scale for research in the general population. *Applied Psychological Measures*, 1, 385–401.

Rehabilitation Research and Training Center on Aging with a Disability, Rancho Los Amigos National Rehabilitation Center. (2003). Rates of Depression among Adults with Cerebral Palsy. Unpublished data.

Robinson, R.G. (2003). Post-stroke depression: prevalence, diagnosis, treatment and disease progression. *Biology Psychiatry*, 54(3), 376–387.

Robinson, W.D., Geske, J.A., Prest, L.A., and Barnacle, R. (2005). Depression treatment in primary care. *Journal of the American Board of Family Practice*, 18(2), 79–86.

Sasma, G.P., Patrick, C.H., and Feussner, J.R. (1993). Long-term survival of veterans with traumatic spinal cord injury. *Archives of Neurology*, 50, 909–913.

Schulberg, H.C., Katon, W.J., Simon, G.E., and Rush, A.J. (1999). Best clinical practice: guidelines for managing major depression in primary medical care. *Journal of Clinical Psychiatry*, 60(7), 19–26.

Shulz, R. and Decker, S. (1985). Long-term adjustment to physical disability: the role of social support, perceived control and self-blame. *Journal of Personality and Social Psychology*, 48, 1162–1172.

Tate, D., Kirsch, N., Maynard, F., Peterson, C., Forshheimer, M., Roller, A., and Hansen, N. (1994). Coping with the late effects. Differences between depressed and non-depressed polio survivors. *American Journal of Physical Medicine and Rehabilitation*, 73, 27–35.

Tate, D.G., Forschheimer, M., Kirsch, N., Maynard, F., and Roller, A. (1993). Prevalence and associated features of depression and psychological distress in polio survivors. *Archives of Physical Medicine and Rehabilitation*, 74, 1056–1060.

U.S. Department of Health and Human Services, Agency for Health Care Policy and Research. (1993). *Depression in Primary Care: Volume 1, Diagnosis and Detection*. Clinical Practice Guideline Number 5. AHCPR Publication 93-0550. Rockville, MD: U.S. Department of Health and Human Services, Agency for Health Care Policy and Research.

U.S. Department of Health and Human Services. (2001). *Healthy People 2010*: Disability and Secondary Conditions. Vision for the Decade. Proceedings and recommendations of a symposium, Atlanta, Georgia. December 4–5, 2000. Washington, DC: U.S. Department of Health and Human Services.

Wells, K.B., Stewart, A., Hays, R.D., Burnam, A., Rogers, W., Daniels, M., Berry, S., Greenfield, S., and Ware, Jr., J.E. (1989). The functioning and well-being of depressed patients: Results from the medical outcomes study. *Journal of the American Medical Association*, 262(7)6, 914–919.

Yesavage, J.A, Brink, T.L, Rose, T.L., Lum, O., Huang, V., Adey, M.B., and Leirer, V.O. (1983). Development and validation of a geriatric depression screening scale: a preliminary report. *Journal of Psychiatric Research*, 17, 37–49.

Zung, W.W.K. (1965). A self-rating depression scale. *Archives of General Psychiatry*, 12, 63–70.

O

Promoting Health and Preventing Secondary Conditions Among Adults with Developmental Disabilities

*Tom Seekins, Meg Traci, Donna Bainbridge, Kathy Humphries, Nancy Cunningham, Rod Brod, and James Sherman**

D isability is one of the nation's most significant public health issues (Pope and Tarlov, 1991). For example, Berkowitz and Green (1989) estimate that the annual medical costs for disabilities are as high as $79.3 billion. A major contributor to activity limitations due to impairments is secondary conditions, preventable health problems that occur after the acquisition of a primary impairment (Brandt and Pope, 1997; Marge, 1988; Seekins et al., 1991).

Among the population with disabilities, an estimated 2 million to 4 million people have intellectual or developmental disabilities. This group accounted for 35 percent of all disability years in 1986 (Pope and Tarlov, 1991). Furthermore, mental retardation ranks first among all chronic conditions causing activity limitations among people of all ages (LaPlante, 1989). Arguably, secondary conditions play a significant role in limiting the participation of individuals with intellectual or developmental disabilities in community life (Pope, 1992).

*Tom Seekins, Ph.D., Meg Traci, Ph.D., Donna Bainbridge, Ed.D., Kathy Humphries, Ph.D., Nancy Cunningham, Rod Brod, Ph.D., The Rural Institute, University of Montana, Missoula. James Sherman, Ph.D., Department of Applied Behavioral Science, University of Kansas, Lawrence. This research has been supported by grants from the National Center on Birth Defects and Developmental Disabilities of the Centers for Disease Control and Prevention. The analyses and views presented in this workshop paper are those of the authors and not necessarily those of the Institute of Medicine Committee on Disability in America: A New Look.

Although many adults with intellectual or developmental disabilities live with members of their own family, since the late 1960s community-based services have emerged as the dominant public model for supporting individuals with intellectual or developmental disabilities. Chief among the options now available in each state is a network of group homes and supported living arrangements. Prouty and colleagues (2005) estimated that 420,202 adults with developmental disabilities live in 148,520 of these arrangements nationwide.

In the process of deinstitutionalization and the building of a system of community supports, policy makers emphasized residential and employment options. Health, on the other hand, tended to be equated with medical care; and the responsibility for managing the overall health of this population was assigned to medical providers. As a result, little systematic work that integrates efforts to encourage healthy lifestyles has been found. Frey and colleagues (2001) conducted a literature review to identify intervention programs targeting the top 20 secondary conditions found in a series of studies of this population. Of the more than 2,000 studies that they reviewed, only 25 met the minimum criteria of prevention and empirical evaluation.

Researchers, policy makers, and service providers have developed a wide range of empirically derived programs for the general population; but these efforts typically exclude or ignore the needs of people with disabilities. The Surgeon General of the United States thus called for a significant and systematic effort to address the health and wellness needs of people with intellectual or developmental disabilities (U.S. Surgeon General, 2002). This paper outlines one model for conducting research in this area and briefly summarizes the relevant findings from one series of studies. This approach involves contextually appropriate research based on a surveillance model for a targeted population.

CONCEPTUAL FRAMEWORK OF SECONDARY CONDITIONS

Secondary conditions have been defined as any condition to which a person with a primary diagnosis is more susceptible and may include medical, physical, emotional, family, or community problems (Lollar, 2001). From the perspective of tertiary prevention, it is important to diagnose and treat secondary conditions to limit their impact on an individual. Alternatively, the impact of secondary conditions might be managed. Figure O-1 outlines a conceptual model for understanding secondary conditions. In this model, physiological, environmental, and behavioral risk and protective factors are seen as influencing limitations due to secondary conditions. For example, a change in living arrangements to a less restrictive arrangement may increase limitations due to isolation. Alternatively, the change

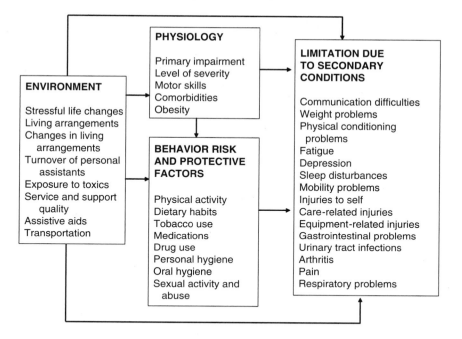

FIGURE O-1   Relationship between environmental, physiological, and behavioral risk and protective factors and limitations due to secondary conditions. Changes in risk and protective factors can influence the experience of limitations in participation. The finding of correlations between variables helps identify possible targets for intervention.

may increase the likelihood that an individual may use tobacco and indirectly influence the experience of limitations due to secondary conditions.

In practice, such a model must be applied to a population living within a context. One way to do this is through a surveillance system that incorporates services directed at identified health problems (Graitcer, 1987). Figure O-2 depicts the major components of such a model for adults with intellectual or developmental disabilities living in supported arrangements. Starting at the far right, annual assessments of the health of the targeted population of adults with intellectual or developmental disabilities living in supported living arrangements are conducted, for example, by a designated health coordinator, program staff, and consumers themselves. Data from such assessments are compiled and provided to state program planners. These planners use the data to identify and prioritize targets for intervention. They also mobilize resources to deliver information, training, and support to local service staff. New interventions and treatments are then

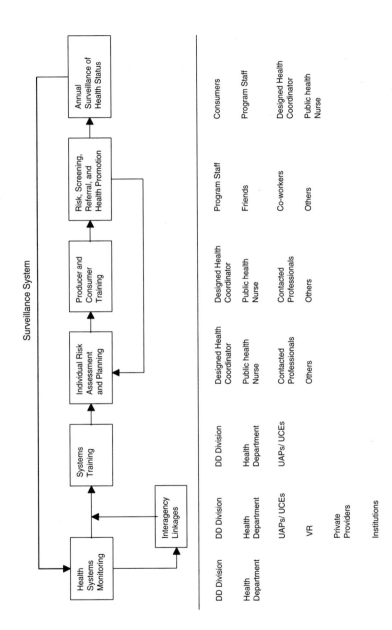

FIGURE O-2 Surveillance systems for secondary conditions in the population of adults with intellectual and developmental disabilities living in supported arrangements.

integrated into the local service system. The surveillance loop is closed when annual assessments are again conducted. Progress can be assessed and new priorities can be established.

ASSESSING SECONDARY CONDITIONS AND RISK FACTORS

Surprisingly little research has been done to assess secondary conditions among adults with intellectual or developmental disabilities (Hayden and Kim, 2002; Horowitz et al. 2000; Robertson et al., 2000). In a series of studies supported by the Centers for Disease Control and Prevention and the Montana Developmental Disability Council, we conducted several assessments of limitations due to secondary conditions, the associated risk and protective factors, and the rates of use of medical services.

Assessing Secondary Conditions

As a first key step in developing a systematic, evidence-based approach to preventing and managing secondary conditions among adults with intellectual or developmental disabilities living in supported arrangements, we developed and validated a secondary conditions surveillance instrument in a series of studies (Traci et al., 2002). The Health and Secondary Conditions Instrument for Adults with Developmental Disabilities (HSCIADD), was designed to measure limitation in participation due to 45 secondary conditions of concern to this population, risk for secondary conditions associated with 3 categories of risk variables (11 lifestyle variables, 4 physiological risk variables, and 21 environmental risk and protective variables), and medical service utilization measures. Limitation due to each secondary condition was reported on a 4-point Likert scale ranging from zero (no limitation) to three (significant/chronic limitation of activities; limits activity 11 or more hours per week).

Four measures were calculated for each secondary condition, including: (1) the percentage of respondents endorsing an item, (2) the prevalence per 1,000 population, (3) the average severity rating of that item, and (4) a problem index. The percentage endorsing an item was calculated by dividing the number of respondents who rated a secondary condition as 1, 2, or 3 by the total number of respondents to the item. Prevalence rate was calculated by dividing the number of persons endorsing an item by the total number of respondents, then multiplying by 1,000. An average severity rating for each secondary condition was calculated by dividing the sum of severity ratings by the number endorsing the item. A problem index was calculated by multiplying the percentage endorsing a secondary condition by the condition's average severity rating. This fourth measure combines

TABLE O-1   Top Ranked Secondary Conditions

Secondary Conditions	Percent Endorsing	Prevalence per 1,000	Average Severity	Problem Index
Communication difficulties	53	526	1.80	95
Physical conditioning problems	47	466	1.49	78
Weight problems	41	411	1.62	66
Persistence problems	42	417	1.56	66
Personal hygiene problems	41	407	1.56	64
Oral health problems	39	390	1.64	64
Problems with mobility	28	281	1.91	54
Memory problems	31	309	1.59	49
Vision problems	31	312	1.53	47
Joint and muscle pain	28	277	1.65	46
Depression	29	293	1.54	45
Fatigue	30	299	1.47	44
Balance problems	26	256	1.63	42
Sleeping problems	23	234	1.52	35

SOURCE: Traci et al. (2002).

both frequency of occurrence and severity. Thus, the problem index ranks the most severe secondary conditions experienced by the most respondents. Table O-1 presents the top 14 secondary conditions reported in one sample as rank ordered by use of a Problem Index, a calculation used to identify the most significant problem experienced by the most people.

It is noteworthy that a rating of average severity reported by those who experience a problem produces a different order among all items. In this sample, cancer and diabetes (not shown here) were the most limiting secondary conditions but were experienced by far fewer respondents. Thus, they did not rise to the top of this analysis. From a public health perspective, decisions about which secondary conditions should be targeted are influenced by the number of individuals experiencing a condition, the severity of the limitation, the availability of potential interventions, and the cost-benefit of those interventions.

Individual items may reflect underlying groupings. In another study (Bainbridge et al., 2005), we conducted a factor analysis of data from 320 respondents collected in five waves over 12 months. Table O-2 shows the eight multi-item factors and their individual item components. In addition, five single items did not group with any others: gastrointestinal problems, allergies, osteoporosis, hypotension, and pressure sores.

TABLE O-2   Secondary Condition Factors and Items Represented

Factor	Item Components
Hygiene	Oral health and personal hygiene
Social interaction and access	Access, mobility, vision, communication
Psychological	Conditioning, cardiovascular, weight, respiratory, nutrition
Orientation	Balance, injury, memory
Pain	Joint and muscle pain, contractures, arthritis
Elimination and digestive	Bladder, bowel, urinary problems
Equipment	Failure, injuries to self and others

SOURCE: Bainbridge et al. (2005).

Assessing Risk Factors

This process of surveillance also allows researchers to examine possible linkages between risk and protective factors and the degree of limitation due to secondary conditions. As with secondary conditions, surprisingly little research has been done to assess health risk factors in this population. Havercamp and colleagues (2004) reported that adults with developmental disabilities in North Carolina were more likely to lead sedentary lifestyles and seven times as likely to report inadequate emotional support than adults without disabilities. Robertson and colleagues (2000) found that those living in less restrictive residential settings had poorer diets, were more likely to smoke, and experienced greater rates of obesity.

Behavioral Risk Factors

Seekins and colleagues (2005) collected a range of data on the risk and protective factors experienced by consumers of the Montana service system as part of developing a targeted surveillance system for that population. Consistent with other published findings, they found low levels of physical activity, poor nutrition, mediocre oral hygiene, and high levels of medication use. Several expected correlations appeared, including an increase in problems of physical conditioning with an increase in age, an increase in weight problems as junk food intake increases but a decrease in junk food intake as the intake of fruits and vegetables increases, and decreases in the number of medications as the number of days per week with raising heart rate increases. These are correlations, however, and suggest only possible targets for intervention.

Environmental Risk Factors

The new paradigm of disability places increased emphasis on the contributions of environmental variables to disability (Seelman and Sweeney, 1995; Steinfeld and Danford, 1999). For this population, the organization of the treatment environment plays a critical role in the health and wellness of adults with intellectual or developmental disabilities. These support environments generally involve the provision of personal assistance to the individual with a disability. Personal assistance is specifically identified as a critical contextual component by International Classification of Impairments, Disabilities and Health–2 (WHO, 1997, p, 235, Code No. e10300) and is provided by people generically referred to as personal assistants. For the many adults with intellectual or developmental disabilities living in group homes or supported living environments, someone else is primarily responsible for organizing the environment and ensuring that healthy behavior patterns are followed. As such, personal assistants play a significant role in the prevention and management of the secondary conditions experienced by adults with intellectual or developmental disabilities (Pope, 1992). Motivating direct care providers to consider health as a worthwhile investment is an important and yet largely unaddressed component of health management among adults with intellectual or developmental disabilities.

Unfortunately, data from a number of sources show that consumers experience a high rate of change in personal assistance providers (Felce et al., 1993; Larson and Lakin 1992; Mitchell and Braddock, 1993, 1994; Razza, 1993; Sharrard, 1992). Analyses of pilot data from a sample of 266 adults with intellectual or developmental disabilities found that 66 percent experienced a change in personal assistants over a 24-month period (Traci et al., 1999; Seekins et al., 1999). These individuals had significantly more secondary conditions overall and more injury-related secondary conditions than individuals without a personal assistant change. A 1-year longitudinal study found that limitations due to secondary conditions increased with a change in personal assistants but that higher levels of secondary conditions increased the likelihood that personal assistants would leave (Bainbridge et al., 2005). Stable personal assistance can contribute to the prevention and management of secondary conditions, whereas unstable personal assistance may contribute to the onset and severity of secondary conditions by disrupting the treatment environment at multiple levels (Seekins et al., 1999; Traci et al., 1999). As such, these preliminary data point to stability and the continuity of the personal assistance environment as a key risk and protective factor.

Another critical feature of the treatment environment involves the individual plan. The individual plan, required by law, directs services for consumers and is the blueprint of environmental organization. The individual plan directs the activities of personal assistants. One correlation between environmental arrangements and health outcomes that suggests an encouraging link is between having an individual plan that addresses a secondary condition and management of that condition. Traci and colleagues (2002) observed that limitations due to secondary conditions addressed by an individual plan were more likely to decline than secondary conditions not addressed by an individual plan.

DEVELOPING CONTEXTUALLY APPROPRIATE INTERVENTIONS

Researchers have established the effectiveness of a wide range of health practices that lead to beneficial outcomes for the general population. Few of these have been explored for use with populations of people with disabilities. A challenge to public health researchers involves the development and evaluation of interventions that can be used to manage or prevent secondary conditions in a support environment with high rates of change of support staff. In addition, the resources available to most public programs are meager. Moreover, staff of these programs must follow many complex regulations governing treatment and personal interactions with residents. As such, interventions must be simple and easy to use, as well as demonstrably cost-effective.

An Example of Oral Health

Bainbridge and colleagues (2004) examined the oral health microenvironments of individuals in supported living arrangements and conducted a pilot project to examine the effectiveness of a simple oral health behavior intervention. Microenvironments consisted of the immediate area—e.g., sink, medicine cabinet, mirror, and toothbrush holder—in which an individual typically keeps his or her oral health equipment and brushes his or her teeth. They found many simple opportunities to arrange the environment to promote hygiene, such as using toothbrush holders that keep individual toothbrushes separate.

They also conducted a pilot test of several strategies to promote brushing behavior. They recruited 12 adults with intellectual or developmental disabilities who received supported living services. Each participant could independently brush his or her own teeth and could understand simple instructions. A dentist examined each potential participant and determined that five individuals were ineligible because of missing teeth or untreated decay. One participant withdrew from the study, and two additional participants were recruited.

Importantly, the researchers piloted two measurement methods to assess the impact on dental health of toothbrushing. A dental hygienist who was unaware of the specific intervention used each measure to screen each

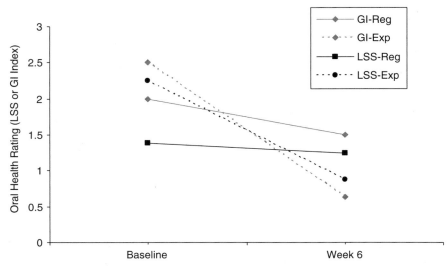

FIGURE O-3   Oral health ratings obtained by using two measures, the Gingivitis Index (GI) and the Lobene Stain Index (LSS), across regular (Reg) and novel (experimental [Exp]) toothbrushes during the baseline and at 6 weeks after the intervention. SOURCE: Bainbridge et al. (2004).

participant before the hygienist cleaned the participant's teeth. Screening was repeated at the start of the study to establish a comparable baseline and at the end of the pilot study. Participants were divided into three groups, with each group were assigned to use a different experimental brush—a double-headed manual brush, a sonic brush, or a mechanical rotary brush—on the one side of their mouth. As a control, participants used a regular, manual toothbrush on the other side of their mouth across the six weeks of the study. At baseline, the Gingivitis Index for the regular manual brush (control) condition was 2. At week 6, it was 1.5. At baseline, the Gingivitis Index for the experimental brush conditions was 2.5. At week 6, it was 0.63. At baseline, the Lobene Stain Index for the regular manual brush (control) condition was 1.38. At week 6, it was 1.25. At baseline, the Lobene Stain Index for the experimental brush conditions was 2.25. At week 6, it was 0.88. Figure O-3 presents selected data from this pilot test. (Both indexes have a range of 0 to 3 with lower numbers indicating better or more normal oral health.)

These results support the established findings that routine brushing reduces plaque, gingivitis, and debris. Furthermore, the investigators found that maintenance of a routine brushing schedule required minimal support time and cost.

Comprehensive Programs of Health Promotion

Although the development and validation of targeted interventions that demonstrate health improvement is a valuable endeavor, it is also important to explore methods for the systematic delivery of such interventions consistently and on a broad scale. Such models might focus on organizing the support environment and limiting reliance on staff. The program should fit seamlessly into the existing operations of service provider and be relatively easy to implement and manage. It should also be flexible and allow the framing of action steps related to any of the 467 objectives outlined in *Health People 2010* (U.S. Department of Health and Human Services, 2000). Finally, it should anticipate the emergence of new service models in which consumers live in settings providing increased independence and decreased levels of supervision.

Currently, we are developing The Wellness Club, a contextually appropriate intervention that is designed to serve as a mechanism that can be used to consistently address health and wellness issues within supported living arrangements. The Wellness Club is the system that we have designed for planning, implementing, and evaluating these action steps for Americans with developmental disabilities. It is a model system for organizing resources and supports to prevent and manage secondary conditions by building and maintaining healthy lifestyles. It embeds wellness education and the management of secondary conditions into a model of individual services based on principles and procedures of choice and applied behavior analysis. The Wellness Club consists of general wellness education and materials for providers and consumers, global assessments for individual planning, specific functional assessments for the design of an individual treatment plan, standard mechanisms for prompting and reinforcing healthy lifestyle behaviors, self-monitoring, and evaluation procedures. Such programs promote lifestyle changes through social engagement and making healthy living fun.

CONCLUSIONS

The new paradigm of disability places emphasis on the contribution of the environment to the outcomes of a disability. The national network of supported living arrangements provides an excellent example of the importance of environmental variables to health. More research should be conducted to obtain an understanding of the role of personal assistants in promoting and maintaining the health of the population with intellectual or developmental disabilities. In addition, we need to better understand how individualized plans can incorporate health and wellness goals.

A substantial body of research has demonstrated the health benefits of a wide range of lifestyle practices. The findings of this research provide one example an empirically derived health promotion strategy for adults with intellectual or developmental disabilities living in supported living arrangements. Importantly, such demonstrations must show how they may be easily incorporated into a system with many responsibilities and high rates of staff turnover.

Finally, a relatively small proportion of adults with intellectual or developmental disabilities live in supported living arrangements. Researchers should address the needs of this population who still live with their parents into late adulthood. Similarly, researchers and educators should explore models for introducing health promotion and lifestyle management into the education process for students with disabilities.

REFERENCES

Bainbridge, D.B., Traci, M.A., Seekins, T., Peterson, S., Huckebe, R., and Millar, S. (2004). *Oral Health Program for Adults with Intellectual and/or Developmental Disabilities: Results of a Pilot Study*. Missoula: Rural Institute on Disabilities, The University of Montana.

Bainbridge, D.B., Traci, M.A., Seekins, T., Brod, R., and Senninger, S. (2005). *The Effects of Direct Service Staff Stability-Instability on the Health of Adults with Intellectual and Developmental Disabilities in Supported Environments in Montana: A Final Report*. Missoula: Rural Institute on Disabilities, The University of Montana.

Berkowitz, M., and Green, C. (1989). Disability expenditures. *American Rehabilitation, 159*, 7–29.

Brandt, E.N., and Pope, A.M. (eds.) (1997). Disability and the environment. In *Enabling America: Assessing the Role of Rehabilitation Science and Engineering* (pp. 147–169). Washington, DC: National Academy Press.

Felce, D., Lowe, K., and Beswick, J. (1993). Staff turnover in ordinary housing services for people with severe or profound mental handicaps. *Journal of Intellectual Disabilities Research, 37*(2), 143–152.

Frey, L., Szalda-Petree, A., Traci, M.A., and Seekins, T. (2001). Prevention of secondary health conditions in adults with developmental disabilities: a review of the literature. *Disability and Rehabilitation, 23*(9), 361–369.

Graitcer, P. (1987). The development of state and local injury surveillance systems. *Journal of Safety Research, 18*, 191–198.

Havercamp, S.M., Scandlin, D., and Roth, M. (2004). Health disparities among adults with developmental disabilities, adults with other disabilities, and adults not reporting disability in North Carolina. *Public Health Reports, 119*, 418–426.

Hayden, M.G., and Kim, S.H. (2002). *Health Status, Health Care Utilization Patterns, and Health Care Outcomes of Persons with Intellectual Disabilities: A Review of the Literature* (p. 1391). Policy Research Brief. Minneapolis: Institute on Community Integration, University of Minnesota.

Horowitz, S.M., Kerker, B.D., Owens, P.L., and Zigler, E. (2000). The health status and needs of individuals with mental retardation. New Haven, CT: Department of Epidemiology and Public Health, Yale University School of Medicine and Department of Psychology. [Online.] http://www.specialolympics.org/NR/rdonlyres/e5lq5czkjv5vwulp5lx 5tmny4mcwhyj5vq6euizrooqcaekeuvmkg75fd6wnj62nhlsprlb7tg4gwqtu4xffauxzsge/ healthstatus_needs.pdf. Accessed January 4, 2005.

LaPlante, M.P. (1989). *Disability in Basic Life Activities across the Life Span. Disability Statistics Report 1.* San Francisco: Institute for Health and Aging, University of California.

Larson, S.A., and Lakin, K.C. (1992). Direct-care staff stability in a national sample of small group homes. *Mental Retardation, 30,* 12–22.

Lollar, D.J. (2001). Public health trends in disability: past, present, and future. In: Albrecht, G.L., Seelman, K.D., Bury, M. (eds.), *Handbook of Disability Studies* (pp. 754–771). Thousand Oaks, CA: Sage Publications, Inc.

Marge, M. (1988). Health promotion for persons with disabilities: moving beyond rehabilitation. *American Journal of Health Promotion, 2,* 29–44.

Mitchell, D., and Braddock, D. (1993). Compensation and turnover of direct-care staff in developmental disabilities residential facilities in the United States. I. Wages and benefits. *Mental Retardation, 31,* 429–437.

Mitchell, D., and Braddock, D. (1994). Compensation and turnover of direct-care staff in developmental disabilities residential facilities in the United States. II. Turnover. *Mental Retardation, 32,* 34–42.

Pope, A.M. (1992). Preventing secondary conditions. *Mental Retardation, 30,* 347–354.

Pope, A.M., and Tarlov, A.R. (eds.) (1991). *Disability in America: Toward a National Agenda for Prevention.* Washington, DC: National Academy Press.

Prouty, R.W., Smith, G., and Lakin, K.C. (2005) *Residential Services for Persons with Developmental Disabilities: Status and Trends Through 2004.* Minneapolis: Research and Training Center on Community Living, Institute on Community Integration.

Razza, N.J. (1993). Determinants of direct-care staff turnover in group homes for individuals with mental retardation. *Mental Retardation, 31,* 284–291.

Robertson, J, Emerson, E., Gregary, N., Hatton, C., Rutner, S., Kessissoglou, S., and Hallam, A. (2000). Lifestyle related risk factors for poor health in residential settings for people with intellectual disabilities. *Research in Developmental Disabilities, 21,* 469–486.

Seekins, T., Smith, N., McCleary, T., Clay, J., and Walsh, J. (1991). Secondary disability prevention: involving consumers in the development of policy and program options. *Journal of Disability Policy Studies, 1*(3), 21–35.

Seekins, T., Traci, M.A., and Szalda-Petree, A. (1999). Preventing and managing secondary conditions experienced by people with disabilities: roles for personal assistants providers. *Journal of Health and Human Services Administration, 22,* 259–269.

Seekins, T., Traci, M.A., Bainbridge, D. B., and Humphries, K. (2005). Toward secondary conditions risk appraisal for adults with intellectual or developmental disabilities. In W. Nehring (ed.), *Health Promotion with Persons with Intellectual or Developmental Disabilities.* Washington, DC: American Association on Mental Retardation.

Seelman, K., and Sweeney, S. (1995). The changing universe of disability. *American Rehabilitation,* Autumn-Winter, 2–13.

Sharrard, H. E. (1992). Feeling the strain: job stress and satisfaction of direct-care staff in the mental handicap service. *The British Journal of Mental Subnormality, 38,* 32–38.

Steinfeld, E., and Danford, G.S. (1999). *Enabling Environments: Measuring the Impact of Environment on Disability and Rehabilitation.* New York: Kluwer Academic/Plenum Publishers.

Traci, M.A., Szalda-Petree, A.C., and Seninger, S. (1999). Turnover of personal assistants and the incidence of injury among adults with developmental disabilities. Rural Disability and Rehabilitation Research Progress Report #3. Missoula, MT: Research and Training Center on Rural Rehabilitation Services, University of Montana.

Traci, M.A., Seekins, T., Szalda-Petree, A.C., and Ravesloot, C.H. (2002). Assessing secondary conditions among adults with developmental disabilities: a preliminary study. *Mental Retardation* 40, 119–131.

U.S. Department of Health and Human Services (2000). *Healthy People 2010: Understanding and Improving Health*, 2nd ed. Washington, DC: U.S. Government Printing Office.

U.S. Surgeon General (2002). *Closing the Gap: A National Blueprint to Improve the Health of Persons with Mental Retardation.* Washington, DC: U.S. Surgeon General.

WHO (World Health Organization). (1997). *ICIDH-2: International Classification of Impairments, Activities and Participation* [sic]. Geneva: WHO.

P

Biographical Sketches of Workshop Committee and Workshop Presenters[*]

Alan M. Jette, Ph.D., M.P.H., P.T. *(Committee Chair),* directs the Health and Disability Research Institute at Boston University. He also serves as professor of rehabilitation sciences at Boston University's Sargent College of Health & Rehabilitation Sciences and professor of social and behavioral sciences at Boston University's School of Public Health. He was a member of the Institute of Medicine committee to review the Social Security Administration's disability decision process research (1998 to 2002), which produced several workshops and reports. His research emphases include late-life exercise; evaluation of treatment outcomes; and the measurement, epidemiology, and prevention of late-life disability. He has published more than 125 articles on these topics in the rehabilitation, geriatrics, and public health literature.

Elena Andresen, Ph.D., is professor and chief of the Epidemiology Division, Department of Health Services Research, Management & Policy at the University of Florida Health Sciences Center and is also Research Health

---

[*]Following the workshop and with the initiation of the second phase of the disability study, additional members were appointed to the committee: Michael Chernew, Ph.D., professor of health management and policy, School of Public Health, University of Michigan; Margaret A. Turk, M.D., professor of physical medicine & rehabilitation, State University of New York Upstate Medical University at Syracuse; Gregg Vanderheiden, Ph.D., professor of industrial and biomedical engineering and director, Trace Research and Development Center, University of Wisconsin at Madison; and John Whyte, M.D., Ph.D., director, Moss Rehabilitation Research Institute, Philadelphia.

Scientist at the Rehabilitation Outcomes Center of Excellence at the North Florida/South Georgia Veterans Health System. She served on an Institute of Medicine committee tasked with developing an agenda for health outcomes research for elderly people and was a member of the Healthy People with Disabilities 2010 Work Group. With more than 60 publications, Dr. Andresen's training and interests include health services research and chronic disease epidemiology. She has developed and taught graduate-level courses in disability and health. Her funded research includes topics in disability epidemiology, aging, and surveillance measures of health for use in policy and planning. Dr. Andresen is a member of the Society for Epidemiologic Research, the International Society for Quality of Life Research, the Academy for Health Services Research and Policy, the American College of Epidemiology, and the American Public Health Association.

Dudley S. Childress, Ph.D., is professor of biomedical engineering and of physical medicine and rehabilitation in the McCormick School of Engineering and the Feinberg School of Medicine, Northwestern University. He is director of the Northwestern University Rehabilitation Engineering Program and the Northwestern University Prosthetics Research Laboratory and executive director of the Northwestern University Prosthetics and Orthotics Education Program. He is a member of the Institute of Medicine and served with the Committee on Assessing Rehabilitation Science and Engineering. Dr. Childress is the recipient of numerous honors and awards, including the Missouri Honor Award for Distinguished Service in Engineering and the Magnuson Award. He serves on the editorial board of the *Journal of Rehabilitation Research and Development* and has been a member of the Advisory Board, National Center for Medical Rehabilitation Research of the National Institutes of Health and the National Research Advisory Council of the U.S. Department of Veterans Affairs. His research and development activities are concentrated in the areas of biomechanics; human walking; artificial limbs; ambulation aids; and rehabilitation engineering, which includes the design and development of modern technological systems for amputees and other disabled people.

Vicki A. Freedman, Ph.D., is professor of health systems and policy at the University of Medicine and Dentistry of New Jersey's School of Public Health. Dr. Freedman is a demographer and chronic disease epidemiologist with expertise in disability measurement in older populations. She has published extensively on the topics of population aging, disability, and long-term care, including several widely publicized articles on trends in late-life functioning. Her current research emphasizes interventions for the promotion of late-life disability decline, the socioeconomic and the racial disparities and causes of late-life disability trends, and the role of assistive technology in ameliorating disability. She has served on more than a dozen national advisory panels for federal agencies, including the National Institute on Aging and the U.S. Department of Health and Human Services.

Patricia Hicks, M.D., is an assistant professor in the Division of General Academic Pediatrics in the Department of Pediatrics at the University of Texas Southwestern Medical School at Dallas and adjunct professor of law at Southern Methodist University. She is the director of the Residents' Continuity of Care Clinic in the residency training program, where she teaches residents and also cares for children with complex chronic health conditions and counsels and advises their families. Many of these children and families depend on medical devices. Her teaching responsibilities include clinical ethics and a course in law, literature, and medicine. As a member of the hospital's Information Systems Committee, she is involved with projects related to electronic medical records and database organization and design for research, reporting, and clinical decision support and monitoring. Dr. Hicks is also the mother of a son who relies on a varying array of life-sustaining medical devices that he uses at home and at school.

Lisa I. Iezzoni, M.D., M.Sc., is professor of medicine at Harvard Medical School and codirector of research in the Division of General Medicine and Primary Care, Department of Medicine, at Beth Israel Deaconess Medical Center in Boston. She is a member of the Institute of Medicine and has served on the Committee to Evaluate Measures of Health Benefits for Environmental, Health, and Safety Regulation; the Committee on Identifying Priority Areas for Quality Improvement; the Committee on Multiple Sclerosis; the Institutional Review Board Committee; and the Committee to Advise the National Library of Medicine on Information Center Services. Dr. Iezzoni and is on the board of directors of the National Quality Forum and serves on the editorial boards of major medical and health services research journals. A 1996 recipient of the Investigator Award in Health Policy Research from The Robert Wood Johnson Foundation, she is studying disability policy issues relating to mobility impairments. Dr. Iezzoni has published a textbook on risk adjustment for measuring health care outcomes and has conducted numerous studies for the Agency for Healthcare Research and Quality, the agency responsible for the Medicare program, and private foundations on a variety of topics. Her research interests include risk adjustment for measuring health care outcomes; developing and evaluating methods for assessing quality of care; and examining the personal and societal implications of disability, specifically, difficulty walking.

June Isaacson Kailes, M.S.W., L.C.S.W., is an adjunct professor and associate director at the Center for Disability Issues and the Health Professions,

Western University of Health Sciences. She is a disability rights advocate and is a national leader in the independent living movement. As a presidential appointee to the United States Access Board from 1995 to 2003, she served as its chair and vice chair. She also chaired the Committee on Telecommunication as well as served as the Board's liaison to the Telecommunication Access Advisory Committee and the Passenger Vessels Access Advisory Committee. Additionally, Ms. Kailes has held many offices on the boards of the National Council for Independent Living and the California Coalition of Independent Living Centers. With over 30 years of experience, she consults and trains managed care organizations, businesses, universities, state associations, government entities, centers for independent living, and other not-for-profit organizations.

Laura Mosqueda, M.D., is a board-certified geriatrician and family physician. She is the director of geriatrics at the University of California, Irvine (UCI), School of Medicine, where she is also a professor of family medicine and the Ronald W. Reagan Endowed Chair in Geriatrics. As the director of geriatrics, she oversees both clinical and academic programs that include clinical care for seniors and adults with disabilities, research projects and grants, education of health care professionals, and community outreach. In the clinical setting, Dr. Mosqueda implemented a multidisciplinary health assessment program for seniors and adults with disabilities, and was instrumental in the development of the UCI Senior Health Center (SHC), an outpatient setting that caters to the special needs of seniors and adults with disabilities. As the medical director of SHC, she has an outpatient clinical practice specifically for seniors and adults with disabilities. For more than 10 years, she was involved with the Rehabilitation Research and Training Center on Aging-Related Changes in Impairment for Persons Living with Physical Disabilities, a federally funded center headquartered at Rancho Los Amigos Medical Center in Downey, California. Additional research activities include a study on osteoporosis in adults with cerebral palsy and, more recently, a primary care initiative to improve access to care for adults with disabilities. Dr. Mosqueda coedited and contributed to a textbook entitled *Aging with a Disability: What the Clinician Needs to Know* (Johns Hopkins University Press, 2004). She is the founder of the Elder Abuse Forensic Center, which focuses on the abuse of elders and adults with disabilities. Areas of special interest include aging with a disability, dementia, abuse, and bioethics.

P. Hunter Peckham, Ph.D., is professor of biomedical engineering and orthopedics at Case Western Reserve University. He also serves as director for the Functional Electrical Stimulation Center at the Louis Stokes Veterans Affairs Medical Center and director of orthopaedic research for the Rehabilitation Engineering Center at MetroHealth Medical Center. He is a member of the National Academy of Engineering and serves on the Committee on Spinal Cord Injury: Strategies in a Search for a Cure. He is an expert in the areas of neural prostheses and the use of electrical stimulation of nerves to restore function in cases of central nervous system paralysis and holds multiple patents related to his work. Dr. Peckham is the recipient of numerous honors and awards for his innovative research, including the Paul B. Magnuson Award and the U.S. Food and Drug Administration Commissioner's Special Citation. In 2000, he was elected Engineer of the Year by *Design News*. In 1996–1997, he chaired the National Institutes of Health National Advisory Board to the National Center for Medical Rehabilitation Research.

James Marc Perrin, M.D., is director of the Division of General Pediatrics at the Massachusetts General Hospital (MGH) for Children and the MGH Center for Child and Adolescent Health Policy and a professor of pediatrics at Harvard Medical School. He has served on four Institute of Medicine committees, including the Committee on the Evaluation of Selected Federal Health Care Quality Activities, the Committee on Improving Quality in Long-Term Care, the Committee on the Quality of Long-Term Care Services in Home and Community-Based Settings, and the Workshop on Maternal and Child Health Under Health Care Reform. For the American Academy of Pediatrics, Dr. Perrin chaired the Committee on Children with Disabilities and a committee to develop a practice guideline for attention deficit hyperactivity disorder. He is past president of the Ambulatory Pediatric Association (APA) and founding editor of the APA journal *Ambulatory Pediatrics*. Dr. Perrin was a member of the Health Care Technology study section of the Agency for Healthcare Policy and Research, the National Advisory Council for the Agency for Healthcare Research and Quality, and the National Commission on Childhood Disability. He directs the MGH coordinating center for the Autism Treatment Network. His research has examined asthma, middle ear disease, children's hospitalization, and childhood chronic illness and disabilities.

WORKSHOP PRESENTERS

Jay Bhattacharya, M.D., Ph.D., is an assistant professor at the Center for Primary Care and Outcomes Research. Dr. Bhattacharya received both an M.D. degree and a Ph.D. degree in economics from Stanford University, the former in 1997 and the latter in 2000. Dr. Bhattacharya's research interests focus on the importance of insurance markets to the well-being of vulnerable populations. A primary focus of Dr. Bhattacharya's research is the population of individuals with limitations in activities of daily living. His

work has shown rising levels of disability among adult nonelderly populations in the United States over the past two decades. In related work, Dr.
Bhattacharya, along with his colleagues at RAND and Stanford University,
have developed a sophisticated demographic model to forecast Medicare
expenditures and the demand for long-term care. This Future Elderly Model
accounts for changing life expectancy, trends in disability in younger and
older populations, trends in chronic disease, and technological changes

William A. Bauman, M.D., is professor of medicine at the Mount Sinai
School of Medicine, New York, New York, with a secondary appointment
in rehabilitation medicine, and is a staff physician at the Veterans Affairs
(VA) Medical Center, Bronx, New York. He is board certified in internal
medicine, with a subspecialty in endocrinology and metabolism. In the
1980s, he received a career development award from the U.S. Department
of Veterans Affairs, under the mentorship of Rosalyn S. Yalow, Ph.D.,
Nobel Laureate in Physiology or Medicine. In 1989, he established and
remains director of the Spinal Cord Damage Research Center at the Mount
Sinai School of Medicine, with research activities at the VA Medical Center,
Bronx, New York. Under his guidance, clinician-investigators and scientists
have been studying the secondary disabilities of spinal cord injuries. The
varied and numerous contributions of this unit have been recognized at the
national and international levels. In 2001, the VA Rehabilitation Research
& Development Center of Excellence for the Medical Consequences of
Spinal Cord Injury was awarded to Dr. Bauman and his associates. He has
been active in the programs of the Spinal Cord Injury Model System of
National Institute on Disability and Rehabilitation Research, U.S. Depart-
ment of Education, at several medical centers, including the Mount Sinai
School of Medicine, the Kessler Institute of Rehabilitation, the Rancho Los
Amigos National Rehabilitation Hospital, and the University of Miami. Dr.
Bauman is chairman of a U.S. Department of Veterans Affairs cooperative
study entitled Anabolic Therapy on Pressure Ulcer Healing in Persons with
Spinal Cord Injury. He has served on the boards of directors for the American Paraplegia Society and the American Spinal Injury Association. He is
on the editorial boards of *Advances in Skin and Wound Care* and the
Journal of Rehabilitation Research & Development. In 2002, he has received the Excellence Award from the American Paraplegia Society. Dr.
Bauman has chaired the U.S. Department of Veterans Affairs Merit Review
study section on spinal cord injury.

Vicki A. Freedman, Ph.D. (see IOM committee biography).

Jack Guralnik, M.D., Ph.D., is acting chief of the intramural Laboratory of
Epidemiology, Demography and Biometry at the National Institute on Ag-

ing. He attended medical school in Philadelphia, and after receiving training in internal medicine at Georgetown University, he spent several years practicing medicine in community and public health clinics. He obtained an M.P.H. degree from the University of California, Berkeley, in 1982 and a Ph.D. in epidemiology in 1985. He is board certified in public health and general preventive medicine. He has been in the intramural epidemiology research program at the National Institute on Aging since 1985. His primary areas of interest in the epidemiology of aging include the study of physical functioning and disability, the prevalence and impact of multiple coexisting chronic conditions, factors associated with healthy aging, methods of assessment of health and functional status, and trends in the demographic and health status characteristics of the older population. He has published more than 325 journal articles and book chapters in these areas of aging research and has taught and lectured extensively in the United States and abroad.

June Isaacson Kailes, M.S.W., L.C.S.W. (see IOM committee biography).

Bryan J. Kemp, Ph.D., obtained a Ph.D. in clinical psychology and aging from the University of Southern California in 1971. He has worked in the fields of aging, rehabilitation, and mental health for more than 30 years and currently holds several related positions. At Rancho Los Amigos National Rehabilitation Center, he is director of Gerontology Outpatient Programs and director of the federally funded Rehabilitation Research and Training Center on Aging with a Disability. At the University of California at Irvine (UCI), Dr. Kemp is professor of medicine and psychology in the Program in Geriatrics. He is also the clinical psychologist on the Elder Abuse Forensic Center at UCI. He is the author of more than 150 articles, chapters, books, and invited lectures on aging-related issues, including the recently published text *Aging with a Disability: What the Clinician Needs to Know*. His areas of interest are aging with disability, geriatric depression, quality of life, and elder abuse.

Julie Keysor, Ph.D., P.T., is an assistant professor of physical therapy at the Sargent College of Health and Rehabilitation Sciences, Boston University. She received a doctorate in health behavior and health education from the University of North Carolina. She has master of science and bachelor of science degrees in physical therapy. Dr. Keysor's area of research is in preventing and minimizing disability among individuals with chronic functional limitations, with an emphasis on understanding the environmental determinants of disability as well as the personal motivational determinants of disability.

John Reiss, Ph.D., is chief of the Division of Policy and Program Affairs, Institute for Child Health Policy; and associate professor in the Department of Pediatrics, University of Florida, Gainesville. Dr. Reiss, who is a counseling psychologist by training, has focused much of his time and effort on facilitating collaborative action among public- and private-sector organizations at the federal, regional, and state levels and between families and professionals to improve the organization, financing, and delivery of health care for children and youth with special health care needs and to promote full partnership with families. From 1993 to 2003 he directed a series of Maternal and Child Health Bureau (MCHB)-funded projects that provided training and technical assistance to Title V Children with Special Health Care Needs (CSHCN) Program staff and other key stakeholders through yearly CSHCN Leadership Training Institutes; Tri-Regional Meetings; e-mail listservs; and web-based, video, and print materials. In 1998, Dr. Reiss began his work on the issue of health care transition. Currently, Dr. Reiss is the principal investigator for three health care transition projects: a 5-year National Institute on Disability and Rehabilitation Research (NIDRR)-funded research and training project on the transition of youth with special health needs from child-centered (pediatric) to adult-oriented health care; a 3-year contract from the Florida Title V CSHCN Program (Children's Medical Services) to develop a web-based health care transition training curriculum for program staff; and a contract from the Florida Developmental Disabilities Council to develop web-based health care transition training materials for families and youth. Through the NIDRR grant, Dr. Reiss also moderates a special-interest e-mail discussion group, which has more than 2,000 members internationally.

James H. Rimmer, Ph.D., is a professor in the Department of Disability and Human Development, College of Applied Health Sciences, University of Illinois at Chicago. For the past 25 years, Dr. Rimmer has been developing and directing health promotion programs for people with disabilities. He has published more than 70 peer-reviewed journal articles and book chapters on various topics in health promotion, physical activity, and disability. He is the director of two federally funded centers, the National Center on Physical Activity and Disability (www.ncpad.org) and the Rehabilitation Engineering Research Center on Recreational Technology and Exercise Physiology for Persons with Disabilities (www.rercrectech.org).

Tom Seekins, Ph.D., is the director of the Research and Training Center on Disability in Rural Communities at the University of Montana and the director of research for the Rural Institute on Disabilities. He received a Ph.D. from the University of Kansas in 1983. He has been involved in disability research and service for more than 25 years, emphasizing issues of consumer advocacy, rural health and disability, self-employment, independent living center services, rural transportation and housing, disability among American Indian tribes and reservations, and rural economic and community development. He has published extensively in the professional literature; presented reports of his work to numerous national, regional, state, and local organizations; and provided technical assistance to state and local programs. He has served as president of the American Association on Health and Disability and as president of the National Association of Rehabilitation Research and Training Centers. He is particularly interested in the intersection between disability and community development.

Rune J. Simeonsson, Ph.D., M.S.P.H., is professor of education, Research Professor of Psychology, and a fellow at the Frank Porter Graham Child Development Institute at the University of North Carolina at Chapel Hill. He also holds an appointment as adjunct professor in the Department of Psychiatry at Duke University. He is coordinator of the School Psychology Program and teaches graduate courses in psychological assessment and intervention, child development and disability and research design and analysis. His research interests reflect the intersection of child development, special education, and public health, focusing on issues in the assessment and classification of childhood disability and the promotion of child health and development. He is actively engaged in research and scholarship on human functioning and disability and currently serves as chair of a work group for the World Health Organization to develop a version of the International Classification of Functioning, Disability and Health for Children and Youth.

Ruth E.K. Stein, M.D., is professor of pediatrics at the Albert Einstein College of Medicine and former vice chairman in the Department of Pediatrics at the Albert Einstein College of Medicine and Children's Hospital at Montefiore. Her research on children's health and children with chronic conditions has been supported by a number of federal agencies and private foundations. For more than a decade she was director and principal investigator of the National Institute of Mental Health-supported Preventive Intervention Research Center for Child Health at Albert Einstein College of Medicine/Montefiore Medical Center. She has published extensively on children with chronic conditions, the measurement of outcomes for child health, and mental health issues in primary care. She was a charter member of the board of directors and executive committee of the Center for Child Health of the American Academy of Pediatrics. She is the editor of two books: *Caring for Children with Chronic Illness: Issues and Strategies* and *Health Care for Children: What's Right What's Wrong What's Next*. She is a member of the Board on Children, Youth, and Families of the National

Research Council and the Institute of Medicine and cochaired the Board's Committee on the Evaluation of Child Health (which recently published *Children's Health, The Nation's Wealth: Assessing and Improving Child Health*).

Margaret A. Turk, M.D., is professor of physical medicine and rehabilitation at the State University of New York Upstate Medical University at Syracuse, with a joint appointment in the Department of Pediatrics. She is also medical director of rehabilitation services at St. Camillus Health and Rehabilitation Center. Dr. Turk serves as the chair of the American Board of Physical Medicine and Rehabilitation. In addition to her clinical and administrative responsibilities, Dr. Turk is involved in rehabilitation research and has been funded by the Centers for Disease Control and Prevention over a 10-year period for projects related to secondary conditions of and health promotion for individuals with disabilities. Her publications and national and international presentations have been on pediatric rehabilitation, pediatric electrodiagnosis, tone management, adults with cerebral palsy, secondary conditions, health promotion in individuals with disabilities, and the health of women with disabilities. She participates with the New York State Department of Health Disability Prevention Program Working Group on Secondary Conditions, which she cochairs. She received the United Cerebral Palsy Research and Educational Foundation Isabelle and Leonard Goldenson Technology and Rehabilitation Award in 2004. She was recently appointed to the National Advisory Board on Medical Rehabilitation Research. She has served on the Medical Rehabilitation Research Subcommittee, National Institute of Child Health and Human Development, National Institutes of Health, and was chair of that subcommittee for 2 years. She participated in the Institute of Medicine report on rehabilitation science and engineering, *Enabling America*.

Gale Whiteneck, Ph.D., has been the director of research at Craig Hospital in Englewood, Colorado, since 1986. He is principal investigator for three federal projects, including the Rocky Mountain Regional Spinal Injury System, the Rocky Mountain Regional Brain Injury System, and a collaborative study of mortality after traumatic brain injury. Major investigations focus on spinal cord injury and traumatic brain injury program evaluation, functional assessment, handicap-participation measurement, environmental impact assessments, long-term outcomes, aging, and the cost of lifetime care. He is the author of three books, numerous articles, and the Craig Handicap Assessment and Reporting Technique and the Craig Hospital Inventory of Environmental Factors, which are used in the national spinal cord injury and traumatic brain injury databases and other disability research. Dr. Whiteneck has been invited to present award lectures to the

American Congress of Rehabilitation Medicine, The American Paralysis Society, the International Society of Paraplegia, and the American Spinal Injury Association. He served as a consultant to the World Health Organization for the revision of the *International Classification of Impairments, Disabilities and Handicaps* and the development of the *International Classification of Functioning, Disability and Health*.